Keep Out of Court

A Medico-Legal Casebook for Midwifery and Neonatal Nursing

AMELDA LANGSLOW LLB

Health Law Education

First published in 2014 by:

Health Law Education

2642 Daylesford Rd, Malmsbury (VIC) Australia, 3446

National Library of Australia Cataloguing-in-Publication entry : (paperback)

Author: Langslow, Amelda

Title: Keep Out of Court :
a medico-legal casebook for midwifery and neonatal nursing /
Amelda Langslow.

ISBN: 9780992533809 (paperback)
Subjects: Maternal health services—Law and legislation—Cases.
Medical errors—Prevention—Law and legislation—Cases.
Dewey Number: 344.041

Printed by: Ingram Content Group / Lightning Source Australia
© 2014 Amelda Langslow

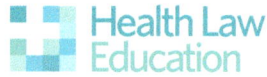

dedicated to midwives and neonatal nurses everywhere

Contents

Disclaimer .... *vii*

Acknowledgements .... *ix*

Introduction 3

Chapter 1   Consent to treatment 11

Chapter 2   Communication 49

Chapter 3   Supervision of junior staff 79

Chapter 4   Malfunctioning equipment 123

Chapter 5   Neurological injury 135

Chapter 6   Shoulder dystocia 169

Chapter 7   Medication 199

Chapter 8   Pain relief 235

Chapter 9   Infection 255

Chapter 10   Postpartum 285

Chapter 11   Nervous shock 323

Chapter 12   Lactation 353

Chapter 13   Resuscitation and withdrawal of treatment 391

Chapter 14   The Neonatal Unit-staff/equipment/monitoring 427

Chapter 15   The Neonatal Unit-times/reporting problems 451

Chapter 16   The Neonatal Unit-medication 467

Chapter 17   The Neonatal Unit-intentional injury 497

Chapter 18   Documentation 511

Conclusion 521

Table and summary of cases *523*

Legal abbreviations *539*

Glossary of legal terms and concepts *541*

Glossary of medical/midwifery terms and concepts *549*

Notes *559*

Disclaimer

The purpose of this casebook is to contribute to the on-going safety of mothers and babies (the patients) in hospital-based maternity services and to lessen the risk of you and your hospital becoming involved in the legal process. Whilst the content in this casebook is written in consultation with a lawyer, it must be used as a general guide and not as the only source of information on this matter. This casebook is neither intended to dictate what constitutes reasonable, appropriate or best care for patients nor is it intended to be used as a substitute for the independent judgment of a physician, senior midwife, neonatal nurse or other qualified health care professional or a lawyer advising you or your hospital. For the avoidance of doubt, the content in this casebook is not to be considered legal or medical advice. You must always discuss any concerns or questions about the health and wellbeing of patients with a qualified healthcare professional. Whilst we undertake to provide accurate and up-to-date information, we do not represent or warrant that the information contained herein is accurate, complete or current. Neither Amelda Langslow nor her writers, contributors and/or other representatives will be liable for loss, injury or damage, of any kind whatsoever, howsoever caused, arising out of or in connection with the use of or reliance on any content in this casebook. It is always your responsibility to make your own decisions regarding the seeking of advice about patients in your care.

Acknowledgements

Discussion of legal cases was central to the monthly article 'Nurse and the Law' that I wrote for many years for the Australian Nurses Journal. I would like to thank the ANJ for that opportunity and to George Thallon and four successive editors for their patience and encouragement. So many nurses and midwives wrote in with their stories and I remember with special affection the long letters from midwives and nurses working in remote areas of Australia. I learned much.

Similar discussions were also central to hospital based classes and the medico-legal workshops I facilitated for nurses in acute, aged, community care and for midwives and neonatal nurses in maternity services. I would like to thank all the clinical educators and conference organizers for inviting me to speak at gatherings – large and small – and for their hospitality. The ANF (as it was then) and Critical Visions provided many of those opportunities. It is from all these events that this casebook has evolved.

Wherever the venue, midwives and neonatal nurses willingly shared their knowledge, and (often very courageously) their experiences - some of which included the courtroom. Their commitment to the safe care of mothers and babies gave direction to this casebook. I thank them all. I have gained much from their resilience and humour.

Anne-Marie Scully, whose skills include midwifery, is a close friend and popular co-presenter at many workshops. As always, she has contributed to my understanding of clinical issues and hospital dynamics.

Vanessa Owen, despite a very busy schedule, kindly read the manuscript and I am really grateful for her constructive comments. I am also very thankful for the care that Susan Seawolf Hayes brought to proofreading the manuscript. To Debra Clay and Judith Parish my gratitude for the time and meticulous care they gave to a final midwifery read. Needless to say – any remaining mistakes are my own. Grateful as well, to Pam Ackland for her helpful suggestions.

Thanks to Samantha Malinay for her help with the cover design and to Joel Ibarra for his formatting work.

Thanks to my husband, David, for the cups of tea and coffee that arrived on my desk; to my family and friends for their encouragement; and especially to my daughter Elizabeth, who has provided her design and publishing skills and so much more. Undeterred by a recent pregnancy, Elizabeth kept us on a steady path. As a bonus, I am holding six-week old Sebastian on my knee as I write this.

A very special acknowledgement to Shaun McCarthy who provided his editorial skills with generosity, support and remarkable patience. That we are talking of another casebook (for operating room staff) and have remained firm friends, says a great deal.

I am grateful to the holders of copyright in material from which excerpts appear in this casebook, particularly to Margaret Puxon, Professor AGM Campbell, Roger Clements, Professor Loane Skene, Patricia Staunton and Alexander McCall Smith.

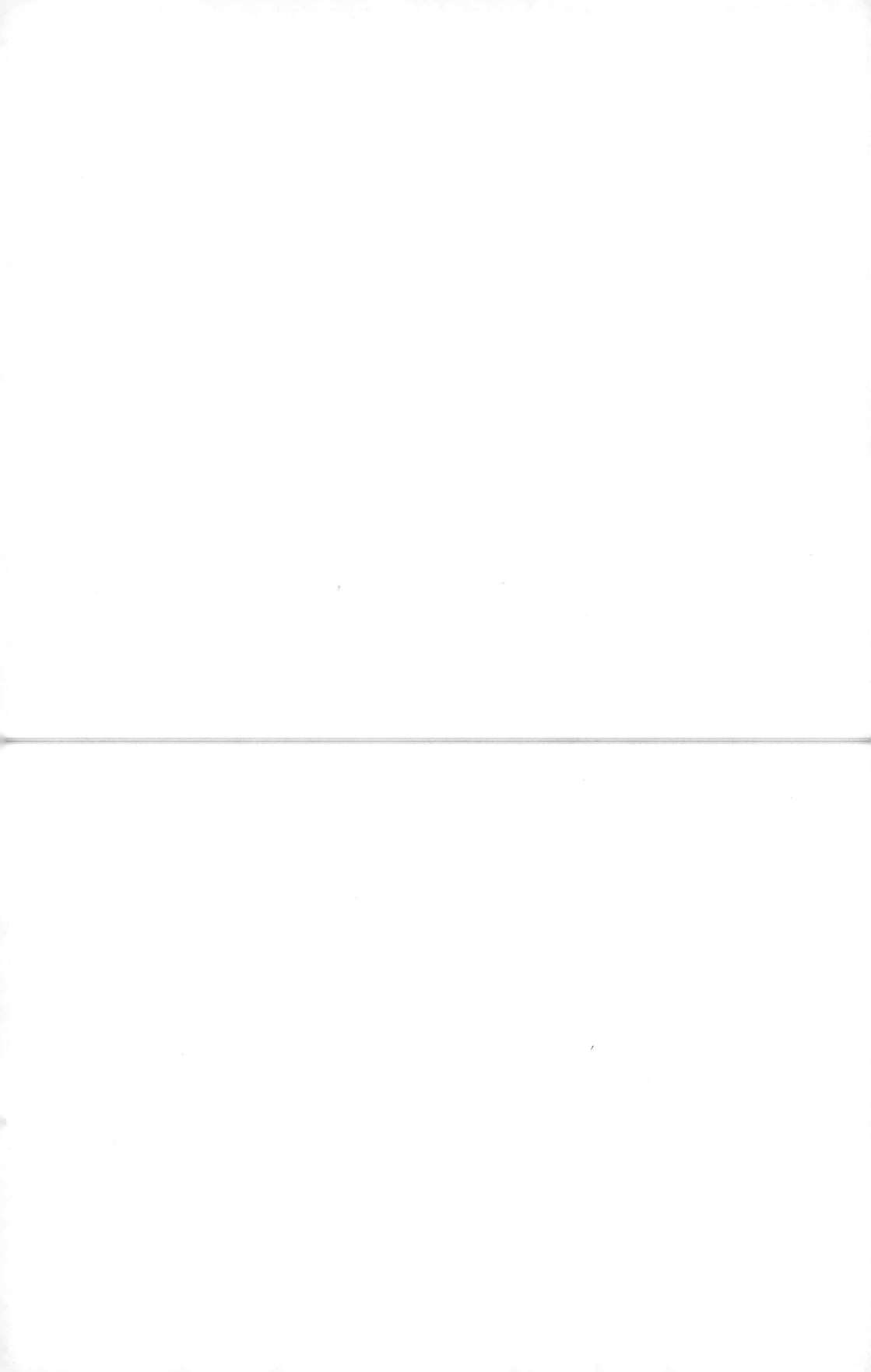

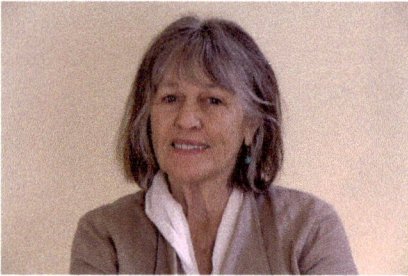

Amelda Langslow studied law at the University of Melbourne and later developed an interest in health law education. She wrote the article '*Nurse and the Law*' (*Australian Nurses Journal*) for many years, lectured in hospitals and facilitated workshops around Australia for midwives as well as nurses working in specialized areas of acute, aged and community care.

Amelda is now writing a series of '*Keep Out Of Court*' casebooks. She lives in Malmsbury, Victoria, Australia.

Introduction

P arents, practitioners and hospitals want uneventful pregnancies, safe births and healthy babies. But against a background of safe and professional care, adverse events in hospitals do occur, leaving mothers, babies and even fathers injured. These events can result in civil litigation, coronial investigations or (on rare occasions) a criminal prosecution. This book is a collection and analysis of such cases from a medical and legal risk management perspective.

The negligence cases relate to decisions of Australian, English, Canadian and United States courts and from a medical board in New Zealand. These legal systems have their roots in the English common law and the same or similar legal principles are applied in each. There are also short reports of cases supplied by United States trial lawyers where agreement (a settlement) was reached out of court. The coronial cases are from Australia. The consistent inquiry is whether care has fallen below a reasonable professional standard and caused foreseeable injury to mothers and babies.

The cases focus on adverse events occurring during pregnancy, admission to hospital, labour, emergency deliveries, postnatal care and neonatal care. One chapter is concerned with lactation issues. A common characteristic of the negligence cases is a considerable time lag between the alleged adverse event and the trial; this is particularly true of the cerebral palsy cases. Civil liability legislation has now tightened the timing and conditions under which negligence actions can be brought. The standard of care applied remains as at the time of the adverse event, not the standard of care prevailing at the time of the hearing.[1]

In addition, there are a number of cases focusing on consent issues, including urgent applications for a court order to override the patient's refusal of consent. Chapter 1, for example, includes a case concerned with the transfusion of blood while another focuses on the need for an emergency caesarean section. The chapters on neonatal care include cases where there is disagreement between parents and doctors about resuscitation and withdrawal of life support. The two criminal cases are concerned with the death of neonates.

The hospital settings and interactions may be familiar, but it is important to understand that each decision has been reached on the basis of its own unique circumstances. That being said, by examining the clinical situations as they develop, the allegations patients and parents make, and the reasoning by which judges and coroners reach their decisions, you will be exposed to a wide range of medico-legal risk management issues.

Consider in each instance whether the central incident (or subsidiary ones) could occur where you work. Put yourself in the shoes of the mother, the baby, or the father. What would you hope a midwife, neonatal nurse, doctor or hospital manager would do? Identify the factors that inhibit or stop you acting in accordance with your standards of safe practice. Check whether the judges' findings or coroners' recommendations could assist in policy development at your hospital.

Each chapter concludes with discussion of key issues raised by the cases in that chapter. Although most of the questions are primarily intended for midwives and neonatal nurses, the issues underlying them are obviously relevant to all members of the obstetric team and to hospital managers seeking to minimize risk and keep a hospital out of court. In a number of chapters, the discussion of key issues includes observations and suggestions raised by midwives and neonatal nurses at medico-legal workshops I have conducted around Australia since the 1980s.

The issues in this casebook focus on communication, documentation, standards of practice and conflict. The cases often describe parental distress and grief but seldom, if ever, acknowledge the pain and trauma of the midwives, neonatal nurses, doctors and hospital management caught up in the legal process and ensuing media attention. You might bear that in mind.

These cases are also part of the history of maternity services. So many midwives, neonatal nurses and doctors found themselves in the witness box being cross-examined about their recall of events, their documentation and their practice.

I hope that by identifying the risks and warning signals, and by facilitating discussion about effective risk management on the labour ward and in the nursery, this casebook will assist in keeping mothers and babies safe and you and your hospital out of the courtroom.

One legal firm[2] lists the type of claims in maternity services that are made in Australia:

- birth asphyxia causing cerebral palsy
- birth asphyxia causing neonatal death
- failure to advise of elective caesarean delivery with anticipated ob-structed labour
- failure to detect fetal abnormalities on ultrasound
- failure to induce labour or expedite delivery causing brain damage and death
- failure to diagnose, monitor and manage pre-eclampsia
- failure to properly test for genetic abnormalities
- failure to perform emergency caesarean delivery
- failure to detect unstable fetal position
- failure to diagnose maternal Haemolytic Group B Streptococcus caus-ing death of baby
- forceps delivery causing skull fracture
- forceps delivery causing spinal cord damage and death of baby
- improper CTG monitoring
- improper ventouse extraction
- improper resuscitation
- improper ventilation at birth
- improper monitoring of fetal kicking behaviour
- improper management of trial of labour
- inappropriate administration of Misoprostol
- inappropriate administration of Syntocinon
- inappropriately prolonged second stage of labour
- inappropriately prolonged pregnancy
- meconium aspiration syndrome
- mismanagement of obstructed labour
- mismanagement of pneumothorax
- mismanagement of breech presentation
- premature labour due to mismanagement of urinary tract infection
- maternal rubella infection in utero leading to brain damage

- shoulder dystocia leading to Erb's palsy
- shoulder dystocia causing brain damage and death of baby

This casebook covers many of the issues listed above, but it is not intended to cover all possible complications that may occur (for example: circumcision difficulties, neonatal abstinence syndrome, Munchausen's Syndrome and failure to detect genetic abnormalities or conditions such as rubella during pregnancy) nor is the casebook intended as a general text on the law. There are excellent books on law and midwifery/ nursing available, a number of which are referred to in the endnotes.

Important points

- A serious adverse event in a hospital can be followed by a number of legal responses and investigations. If you are involved in such an incident, it is important that you protect yourself. Before you make written statements or give evidence that could implicate you, you should contact your professional organization or seek legal advice. This is not intended to impede an investigation, but to ensure that your rights are protected. For the same reason, you should always have legal representation in court.
- The cases, many of which came to trial a number of years ago, have been chosen for the issues they present rather than the date at which an event occurred or the date a case reached court. Recent cases (and they are not prolific) do not necessarily highlight issues more effectively than earlier cases. As the cases originate in hospitals in Australia, U.K, USA, Canada and New Zealand, the delivery of maternity services may differ, or have developed, in certain ways. Nevertheless, the core issues in each case should be familiar. There are complex reasons why monetary damages fluctuate and vary over a period of time and between jurisdictions; for that reason amounts are rarely noted.
- If you are unfamiliar with the law, you will be assisted by first reading the brief notes on negligence and coronial investigations at p. 559. Further explanations are given in the Glossary of legal terms and concepts.
- The ICM 'Definition of Midwife' includes the provision that a midwife may practise in any setting including the home, community, hospitals, clinics or health units. The cases in this book concern midwives, neonatal nurses and maternity services staff working in hospitals, with very occasional references to maternal and child health/community nurs-

es. Research into cases concerning midwives caring for women giving birth in other settings must await another day.

Terminology, Structure and Process

Each case discussed in this book will be treated in the following way:

Use of names. The title of each case uses real names. Pseudonyms are used in the case notes, except in the cases such as *Jones, Wilsher* and *Whitehouse*, which are already very well documented, and *Messenger* and *Miguel Sanchez*, where the case note is a précis of an existing article. Any similarity to real names is unintentional and purely co-incidental.

Judges and coroners sometimes use the terms 'midwife', 'obstetric nurse' and 'nurse' interchangeably. For the purposes of consistency, the term 'midwife' has been used throughout this casebook. 'Obstetric residents' and 'residents' are used interchangeably as are 'mother', 'woman', and 'patient' as well as 'baby', 'infant' and 'child'. Medical terminology may occasionally vary in cases from different jurisdictions.

Citations. In the Table of Cases (and with few exceptions) each case listed has a citation following the names of the parties. This indicates the year, volume, law report series and (where available) page reference for the case. You should be able to locate these cases in university law libraries or be directed to a website.

Structure. Each case will contain a description of key events, a short description of arguments and allegations, and a conclusion containing either the decision of the court or the fact that the parties have 'settled' (reached agreement). However, some case notes will be only brief summaries.

Process. Most cases feature the recollection of witnesses who were there (eye-witness/direct evidence), some will examine how inferences are drawn from circumstances (circumstantial evidence), and the majority will compare the evidence of expert witnesses. Documentary evidence will provide many graphic examples of why documentation is critical to the defence of a hospital and its staff.

Appeals. Many cases are decisions of appeal courts and this will enhance their standing in other courts. Inevitably, there is a certain amount of going backwards and forwards over the issues, as a higher court reviews the lower court's decision.

Legal and medical/midwifery terms. To avoid interrupting the text, definitions of legal and medical/midwifery/ nursing terms are given in glossaries, together with explanations about relevant process – although this list is not exhaustive. Both the legal and medical glossaries are based on definitions from dictionaries referred to in Australian courts. There has been no attempt to duplicate definitions from standard midwifery texts apart from the inclusion of the ICM definition of 'midwife.'

Table and Summary of Cases. A brief summary of each case is provided.

NOTES

1.   In Australia, civil liability legislation imposes conditions, prescribes limitations on time and defines the standard of care to be applied for professionals (but lacks uniformity between jurisdictions):

In Victoria, for example, The Wrongs Act 1958 s 59 states:

(1)   A professional is not negligent in providing a professional service if it is established that the professional acted in a manner that (at the time the service was provided) was widely accepted in Australia by a significant number of respected practitioners in the field (peer professional opinion) as competent professional practice in the circumstances.

(2)   However, peer professional opinion cannot be relied on for the purposes of this section if the court determines that the opinion is unreasonable.

(3)   The fact that there are differing professional opinions widely accepted in Australia by a significant number of respected practitioners in the field concerning a matter does not prevent any one or more (or all) of those opinions being relied on.

(4)   Peer professional opinion does not have to be universally accepted to be widely accepted.

Forester, K. and Griffiths, D., Essentials of Law for Medical Practitioners, Ch. 5, Churchill Livingston (Sydney, 2011).

2.   http://www.mauriceblackburn.com.au/areas/medical/obstetrics.aspx#al

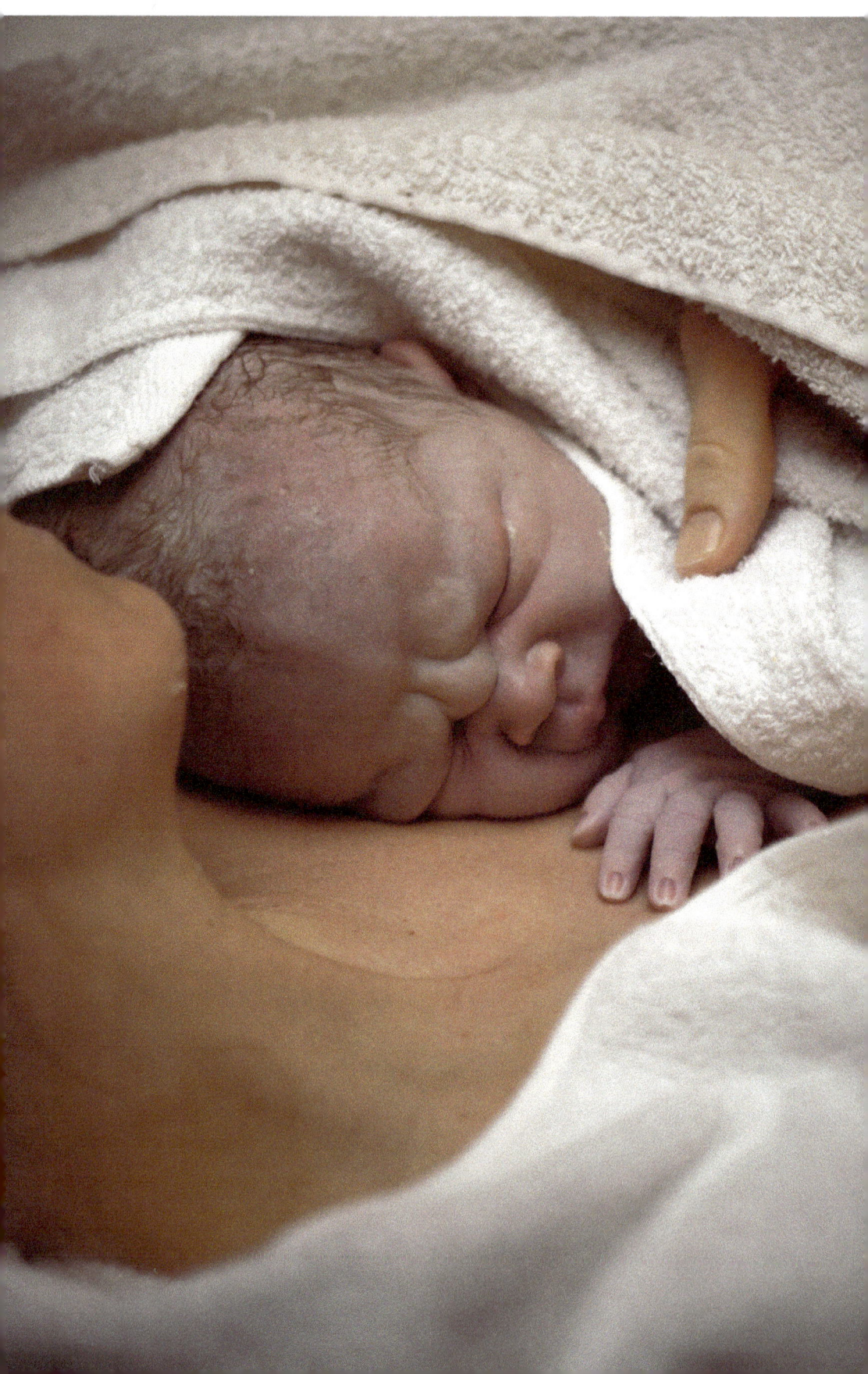

CHAPTER 1

Consent to treatment

'Every human being of adult years and sound mind has the right to determine what shall be done with his or her own body...'.

—Benjamin Cardozo
Associate Justice, Supreme Court of the United States.

Introduction

Most of the chapters in this casebook concern safety issues and the foresee-ability (and management) of risk in the treatment of women and babies in hospital-based maternity services. This chapter addresses the preliminary question of whether that treatment has been consented to. The first group of cases are concerned with the civil action of battery. Battery protects patient autonomy or 'personal space.'[1]

The legal principle that 'every human being of adult years and sound mind has a right to determine what shall be done with his/her own body'[2] is well established. It follows that in the absence of an emergency, any treatment given to a competent adult woman without her consent consti-tutes a battery[3] for which she could receive compensation.

Professor Loane Skene further explains the principle of autonomy:

In a medical context, the principle of autonomy means that pa-tients, not their doctors, must decide about their medical treatment themselves although the patient will obviously consider medical advice in making the decision. Doctors may understand medical issues — the patient's history, the features of the particular medical conditions and treatment, but only the patient knows the patient's own values, which will ultimately determine the treatment the pa-tient is prepared to undergo: the willingness to take risks, bear pain or physical restrictions or the like. Neither the state, 'the com-munity', nor a paternalistic, if well-meaning, health professional is entitled to dictate the medical treatment that a competent adult patient will undertake.[4]

Even if unauthorised treatment results in a successful outcome, a woman can still allege battery — although the amount of compensation awarded may be nominal. A woman's consent to the general nature of the 'touching' will, however, constitute a defence to battery. This reasoning has to be dis-tinguished from the situation where a woman is alleging that had she been properly informed (risks, alternative treatments, outcomes) she would not have consented to the treatment. This is argued in a negligence framework and will be briefly examined later in this chapter. Allegations of failure to inform or disclose risk can be found throughout this casebook.

A mentally competent adult woman who is pregnant can therefore, in the absence of an emergency, refuse treatment even if her health or life is threatened as a result. The law will protect her right to decide what shall be done to her body even though her reasons may be unknown or irrational to others, or even non-existent. The fetus, however, has no legal rights until it is born alive; rights are then retrospective, hence the pre-birth injury cases.

Consent can be written (a usual hospital requirement before surgery), verbal or by implication (arm held out for an injection). It is an affirmative process, not merely the absence of an objection. In whatever form, the validity of any consent is dependent on it being given voluntarily (without force, duress or coercion) by a woman who is competent. The procedure consented to should not be exceeded unless there is a threat (usually immediate) to life or health. If a woman is unconscious, and there is no person authorized to make a decision on her behalf, doctors can lawfully treat in accordance with their best clinical judgment as to her best interests.

....

The following five cases focus on (a) conditions placed on consent, (b) factors temporarily affecting competence, (c) undue influence, (d) exceeding consent and (e) rights of the newborn to receive necessary treatment despite the mother's refusal to consent.

Conditional consent

Sometimes a condition is placed on consent — a not uncommon event in the midwifery/obstetric field, where women hold firm convictions about what they want and do not want. While no strangers to the challenging birth plan, midwives (and doctors) cannot be forced to perform procedures that conflict with professional standards.

....

As risk managers will be aware, consent issues can fuel complaints and possible litigation. In the first case in this chapter, for example, a hospital agreed to respect a woman's religious convictions, then chose to ignore them. Note what the judge says about the lack of an emergency.

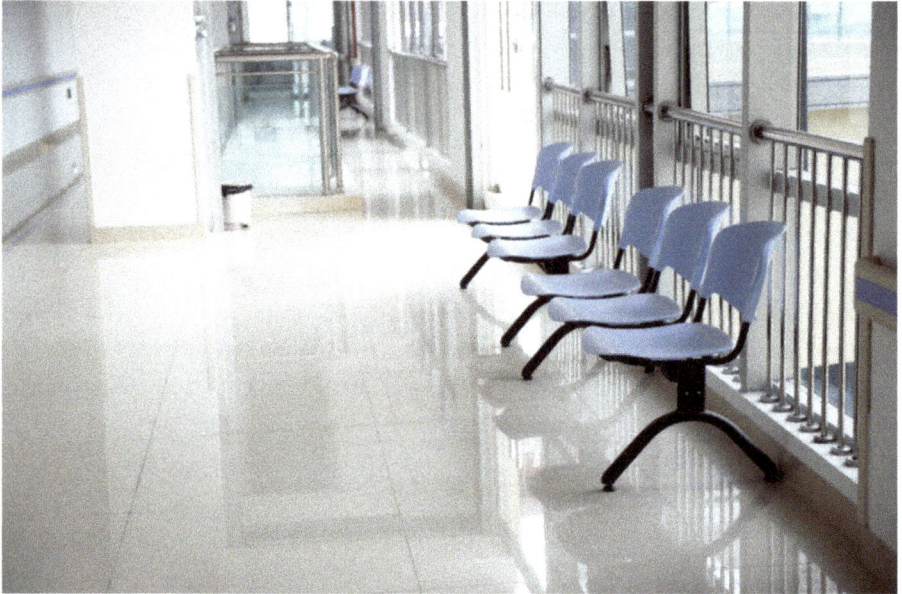

Cohen v Smith [US, 1995][5]

The facts

Alana was admitted to hospital to deliver her baby, but informed after an examination that a caesarean section would be necessary. Alana and her husband told the obstetrician, who in turn advised the hospital, that their religious beliefs prohibited Alana being seen naked by a male. When the obstetrician assured Alana that this religious conviction would be respected, Alana consented.

It was later contended that a male nurse observed and touched Alana's unclothed body during surgery.

Alana and her husband said they had no grievance about how the caesarean section was performed, but argued a fundamental right to refuse treatment that conflicted with their religious views.

When a judge dismissed their action for battery, Alana and her husband appealed.

The appeal

The appeal court emphasised that the protection of physical integrity had always been an important basis for battery, but hospitals could also be liable, not only for contacts that do actual physical harm, but also for contacts which are offensive and insulting.

Nurse informed of condition. The court heard that Alana had been informed by the doctor, through her husband, that the male nurse's presence in the operating room was necessary for the procedure, but that the caesarean section could be performed without him seeing her unclothed. The nurse was told by the doctor who was to perform the caesarean section that Alana had strongly held and deeply ingrained moral and religious views which prohibited her from being seen or observed unclothed by a man.

The decision

No emergency. The appeal court noted that Alana's lawyer had conceded that there would be no battery if she had been placed in the care of the hospital and the nurse in an emergency situation in which she had been unable to inform the hospital of her beliefs.

Knowledge before surgery. However, the fact that the relevant hospital staff had been aware of Alana's religious beliefs before surgery was borne out by evidence that the male nurse had requested a police presence at the hospital. This was to prevent Alana objecting to the male nurse being in the operating room and to physically restrain her husband if necessary.

Right to hold belief protected. The court held that although most people in today's society had accepted the necessity of being seen unclothed and being touched by members of the opposite sex during medical treatment, Alana and her husband had not accepted this. Whilst most people do not share these views, society and courts accept their right to hold those beliefs. They deserved no less protection than more mainstream beliefs.

The choice. The hospital, when informed of Alana's beliefs, had been free to refuse to accede to them. Instead, the hospital had agreed, implicitly at least, to provide treatment with the restrictions imposed by her beliefs, then chosen to ignore them.

Damages awarded.

Temporary factors affecting capacity to consent/refuse consent

....

In the next case, an appeal court in England (convened late at night via telephone links) was faced with the problem of a woman who had consented to a caesarean section but was refusing the prick of a needle to induce anaesthesia. The court recognised that 'temporary factors,' such as panic induced by fear, confusion, shock, fatigue, pain or drugs, can completely erode capacity to make decisions about treatment.

'Fear' as one judge observed 'may paralyse the will and thus destroy the capacity to make a decision.'[6]

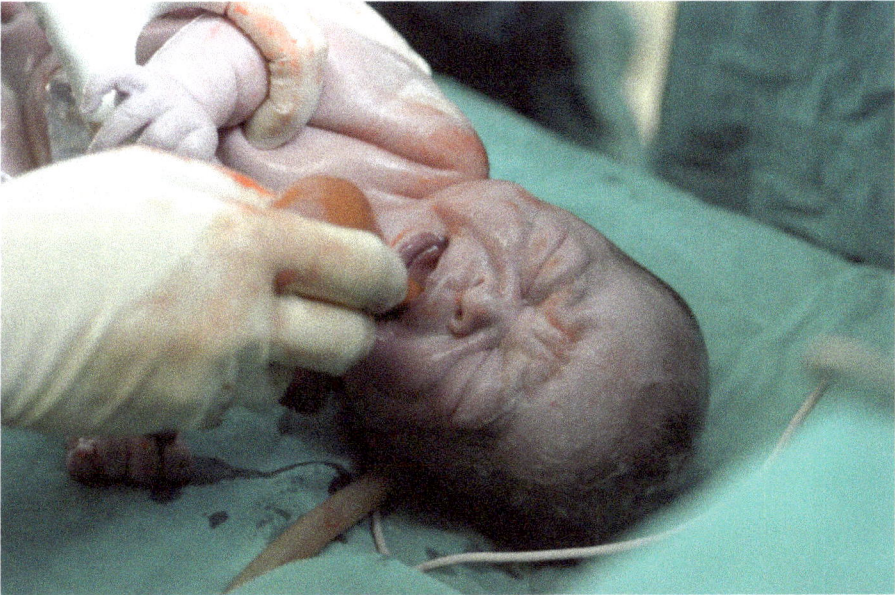

In Re MB [UK, 1997][7]

The facts

Blood refused. Lindy, aged 23, attended an antenatal clinic for the first time during her second pregnancy in December 1996 when she was 33 weeks pregnant. She refused to give blood samples because she was frightened of needle pricks and failed to attend a further three appointments in January 1997.

Breech position. On 3 February, Lindy again attended the clinic, but refused to give blood samples. On 13 February, a consultant obstetrician found the fetus in breech position, which presented an obstetric complication with potentially serious consequences. Although Lindy was in little physical danger, the risk to her unborn child was assessed at 50 per cent.

Alternatives. It was the obstetrician's practice to recommend that a breech presenting by the foot should be delivered by caesarean section. An alternative procedure was an epidural anaesthetic during vaginal delivery to minimize the risk of pushing prematurely, with the possibility of an emergency caesarean section. The obstetrician explained the risk of a vaginal delivery to Lindy, but did not discuss the method of anaesthesia after she agreed to have the operation. Her admission to hospital was arranged for 14 February.

Consent form signed. Hospital records from 14 February showed that Lindy signed a consent form for a caesarean section on admission, but twice refused to undergo venepuncture to provide blood samples. On 15 February, records showed she was requesting a caesarean section but that the hospital required blood samples. On 16 February, Lindy again signed a consent form, but when an anaesthetist attempted to insert the veneflon Lindy refused the procedure. She was not prepared to allow blood samples to be taken nor to undergo anaesthesia by way of injection. Surgery was cancelled.

Surgery again cancelled. Lindy then agreed to anaesthesia by mask (without injection) even though it was explained to her that the dangers of regurgitation and inhalation were increased. The operation was again listed, but cancelled on 18 February when she refused consent. The obstetrician saw her at 3.00 pm, by which time Lindy was refusing to discuss the problem with anyone. He explained the risks to the fetus if she went into labour, noting that she 'does not respond or express any wishes regarding her treatment.'[8]

Pushed mask away. Lindy then went into labour with regular contractions. She was unresponsive towards both the midwife and the obstetrician. Her GP saw her at 7.00 pm, reporting that she was happy to have the operation provided she did not feel or see the needle nor have an IV line or a postoperative catheter. A consultant psychiatrist assessed her at 8.00 p.m. At 9.00 pm, Lindy was taken to the operating room. When she pushed the mask away the operation was cancelled.

Application to court.
At 9.25 pm the hospital sought a court order by telephone; at 9.55 pm, a judge made an order that it would be lawful:

1. for doctors to carry out necessary treatment, including a caesarean section and the insertion of needles for the purposes of IV infusion and anaesthesia;
2. for reasonable force[9] to be used to give appropriate treatment and nursing care to ensure Lindy suffered the least distress and retained the greatest dignity.

An appeal by the lawyer appointed to represent Lindy was dismissed later that night. As she was not in established labour, Lindy returned to the labour ward.

A new morning—a change of mind. The following morning Lindy signed another consent form and co-operated fully with the induction of anaesthesia. A healthy baby boy was delivered by caesarean section.

Because the case raised important principles of law (even though the order was not carried out), the Court of Appeal later gave reasons for its decision on the night of 18 February:

General principles

1. In general, it is a criminal and tortious assault to perform physically invasive treatment (however minimal) without the patient's consent.
2. A mentally competent patient has an absolute right to refuse consent to medical treatment for any reason, rational or irrational, or for no reason at all, even where the decision may lead to death.
3. Medical treatment can be undertaken without consent in an emergency, provided the treatment is necessary and no more than reasonably required in the best interests of the patient.

Capacity to decide

While each case must depend on its particular facts:

4. Every person is presumed to have the capacity to consent to or to refuse medical treatment unless and until that presumption is rebutted.
5. A competent woman who has the capacity to decide may choose not to have medical intervention even though the consequences may be the death or serious handicap of the child she bears, or her own death.
6. Panic, indecisiveness and irrationality in themselves do not amount to incompetence but may be symptoms or evidence of mental incompetence.
7. A person lacks capacity if some impairment or disturbance of mental functioning renders them unable to make a decision about treatment.

This will occur when:

8. The patient is unable to comprehend and retain the information material to a decision, especially as to the likely consequences of having/ not having the treatment in question. The graver the consequences, the greater the level of competence required to make the decision.
9. The patient is unable to use the information and weigh it in the balance as part of the process of arriving at the decision; a compulsive disorder or phobia, for example, may stifle belief in the information presented.
10. The temporary factors of confusion, shock, fatigue, pain or drugs may completely erode capacity, but those concerned must be satisfied that such factors are operating to such a degree that the ability to decide is absent.
11. Another influence may be panic induced by fear. Careful scrutiny of the evidence is necessary because fear of an operation may be a rational reason for refusal. Fear may paralyse the will and destroy capacity to decide.

Best interests. The psychiatrist firmly believed that Lindy's best interests would suffer long-term damage if no operation was performed and her child was born handicapped or dead as a consequence. Conversely, he did not feel she would suffer short-term trauma as a result of a forcible procedure involving a needle prick. When the midwife had described the nature of a caesarean section to Lindy, the psychiatrist noted that she had been interested and not at all distressed.

The decision

The court found that Lindy had consented to the caesarean section but had refused to accept the prick of the anaesthetist's needle.

Immediate fear. The psychiatrist, who had seen Lindy in the presence of her partner as well as the anaesthetist and midwife, believed she clearly understood the reasons for the operation and accepted them without reservation. The only problem lay in the induction of anaesthesia. The psychiatrist believed she lacked capacity to see beyond her immediate fear of needles. He described Lindy as a 'naive, not very bright, frightened young woman, but not exhibiting a psychiatric disorder.'[10] Told that she had pushed the mask away in the OR when confronted by the paraphernalia of anaesthetics, the psychiatrist said:

It seemed to me that at that actual point she was not capable of making a decision at all, in the sense of being able to hold informa-tion in the balance and make a choice. At that moment the needle and mask dominated her thinking and made her quite unable to consider anything else. Her continued refusal to consent to surgery for some time after she had panicked is not in any way inconsis-tent with my view that her refusal was due to a sudden flooding panic. I would expect there to be some difficulty in addressing the subject and balancing the two issues for a period of time after the panic.[11]

The unborn child. The court reiterated the common law principle that the fetus up to the moment of birth does not have separate interests capable of being taken into account by the court. The court also noted the position tak-en by the Royal College of Obstetricians and Gynaecologists, that the child's interests must take second place to the sanctity of the mother's right to con-trol any interference with her own body.

English barrister Margaret Puxon comments:

. . . this right is at the heart of the relationship between doctor and patient, and to make an exception in obstetric cases would not only be anomalous but would take away from mothers' important rights enjoyed by all the rest of the world living in the common law jurisdiction.[12]

Puxon also makes the point that obstetric teams need to recognize potential problems, such as needle phobias, at an early stage so that counselling can be arranged, if appropriate. This saves the stress and confusion of later emer-gency legal proceedings.

The 'forced caesarean' cases. In *Re MB* is one of a cluster of English cases[13] described as the 'forced caesarean ' cases. Professor Loane Skene[14] writes that there have been no 'forced caesarean' cases in Australia. Skene refers to the conclusion of author John Seymour,[15] that the law is unclear in Australia in regard to a court's jurisdiction to make an order authorizing treatment despite a pregnant woman's refusal. Equally unclear, in Seymour's opinion, is the potential liability of a doctor who accedes to her refusal if there is an adverse outcome.

What is clear, is that hospitals should consider seeking legal advice when consent issues arise.

A patient's consent/refusal of consent should be free of coercion or undue influence

The woman in the next case was injured, pregnant and extremely vulnerable when her father sought urgent assistance from a court. Argument focused on whether his daughter's decision to refuse a blood transfusion had been influenced by his ex-wife who was a Jehovah's Witness

Persuasion can slide subtly — and not so subtly - into coercion in hospitals and a relative's religious views can be a powerful influence on a woman's freedom of choice.

Note how Lord Donaldson, in the English Court of Appeal, identifies the central issues:

> *This appeal is not in truth about the 'right to die'. There is no suggestion that 'Anna' wants to die. I do not doubt that she wants to live and we all hope she will. This appeal is about the right to choose how to live. This is quite different, even if the choice, when made, may make an early death more likely. It is also about whether Anna really did choose and, if so, what choice she made.[16]*

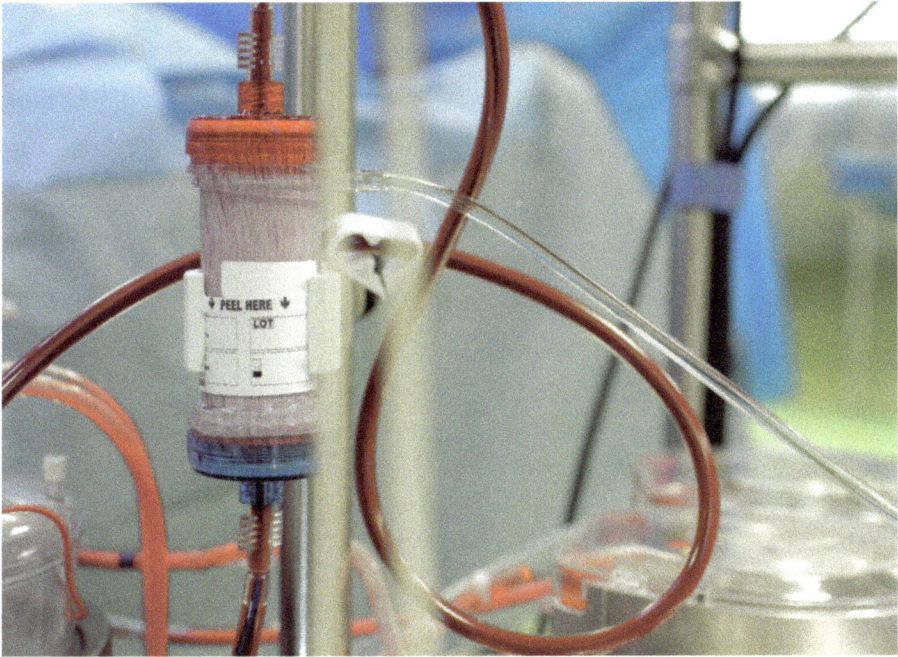

In Re T (UK, 1992)[17]

The facts

Anna's parents separated when she was three years old. Her mother was a Jehovah's Witness; her father rejected that faith. A court order awarding custody to the mother expressly forbade her to bring Anna up as a Jehovah's Witness, the intention being that she should later make her own decision. The mother clearly brought her daughter up with the intention that she would later join the faith, although she was not baptised into it.

Pregnancy. Anna was about 18 years old when she moved away to live with her paternal grandmother. The following year she began living with James and became pregnant. It was during this period that Anna's father said she told him that she was not a Jehovah's Witness. He said there was nothing in her actions which led him to believe that she wished to become one.

The accident. On 1 July, Anna, now 34 weeks pregnant, was taken to hospital after a car accident. She complained of pain in her right shoulder and chest. She was not X-rayed because of her condition and advised to rest and take analgesics. When the chest pains worsened, Anna returned to hospital in the early hours of 4 July. When X-rays showed pleurisy or pneumonia, she received oxygen, antibiotics and analgesics.

Religious beliefs. The hospital's assessment form contained the entry: 'Religious beliefs and relevant practices. Jehovah's Witness (Ex) but still has certain beliefs and practices.' The handwriting of this entry differed from the entry for Anna's name and the name of the consultant (raising a subsequent query as to when the entry was made).

Pneumonia. Anna was admitted to the ward at 6.10 am and received 50 mg of Pethidine, together with antibiotics, at 6.55 am. She was now breathless, expectorating dirty-coloured sputum, and complaining of severe chest and shoulder pains. A lung scan showed a picture consistent with pneumonia. Further Pethidine was administered at 1.00 pm. At 6.30 pm Anna's mother arrived at the hospital, accompanied by James.

Visit by father. Anna's father arrived at the hospital at 8.30 am the following day to find his daughter heavily sedated, with extremely laboured breathing. She was receiving oxygen and had to be raised every 30 minutes to enable her to clear sputum from her lungs. Nurses explained that she was in considerable pain and had had little sleep. The father was anxious about complications that could arise from his ex-wife's religious beliefs. A doctor said that as Anna did not require a blood transfusion there was no need for concern. When her father suggested that she was showing a diminished awareness, nurses told him it was the effect of the drugs.

Visit by mother. At 2.50 pm Anna received a dose of Pethidine. Prior to 5 pm she spent time alone with her mother. At 5 pm a nurse joined them. Anna told her that she used to be a Jehovah's Witness, still maintained some beliefs and did not want a blood transfusion. The nurse later said she thought it strange that this statement should have been volunteered 'out of the blue' moments after Anna's mother arrived. She thought Anna was able to understand what was going on. She had pacified her, believing there was no need for blood to be administered. At 7.30 pm the father returned to the ward. He now felt his daughter's condition was worsening and that she appeared disoriented.

Transfer to maternity unit. Shortly afterwards, Anna went into labour. At 10.45 pm she was transferred by ambulance to the maternity unit a short distance away. During this period she was again alone with her mother. After an obstetric registrar found her to be in a distressed condition with respiratory pain and contractions, the decision was made to deliver the baby by caesarean section. Anna told a midwife that she did not want a blood transfusion.

Blood transfusion discussion. The doctor recalled asking Anna, 'Do you object to blood transfusions?' and that she had replied, 'Yes.' The doctor: 'Does that mean that you do not want a blood transfusion?' Anna: 'No.' She had then asked 'You can use other things though, can't you, like sugar solutions?' The doctor said he could not remember the exact conversation that followed. 'But essentially I said that we could use other solutions to expand the blood, but they were not as effective as blood at transporting oxygen. I also tried to reassure Anna and her father that blood transfusions were often not necessary after a caesarean section.'[18]

Refusal form signed. As the doctor was leaving, a midwife produced a Refusal of Consent to Blood Transfusions form, which Anna signed. The midwife then countersigned. This form contained a space for an obstetrician to countersign, but this was not done. Contrary to what was stated on the form, the provision 'that it may be necessary to give a blood transfusion so as to prevent injury to my health, or even to preserve my life'[19] was not explained to Anna, nor was the form read to her.

Deterioration. A stillborn baby was delivered by caesarean section early on 6 July. Anna was transferred to ICU when her condition deteriorated further and an abscess was discovered on her lung. The consultant anaesthetist said that at this stage he would have 'unhesitatingly'[20] administered a blood transfusion but felt inhibited from doing so in view of Anna's expressed wishes. She was put on a ventilator, remaining in a critical condition throughout 7 July. Some slight improvement followed.

Application to the court. On the evening of 8 July, Anna's father and James sought a declaration from the court that it would not be unlawful for the hospital to administer a blood transfusion in the absence of consent.

Not fully rational. Late night telephone calls were exchanged between the hospital and a judge. Evidence was taken from the doctor who had spoken to Anna. The judge concluded that because of her condition and the effect of the narcotic medication Anna had not been fully rational when she signed the refusal form. The judge granted the order and directed that a further hearing on full evidence take place. Although a blood transfusion was immediately given, we are given no further information about Anna, other than she remained critical throughout the course of the legal proceedings.

The hearing

At the subsequent hearing, the judge now found that Anna's capacity to make a rational decision was unimpaired. This decision was based on what the judge described as 'the unhappy fact that the doctor had changed his evidence completely' as to Anna's mental capacity. The doctor (contrary to his evidence given over the telephone), now maintained that although her conscious level had been 'somewhat clouded', she was fully orientated, with appropriate verbal responses and had made no inappropriate comments. There had been no sign of hallucinations and no signs of hesitation about questions relating to blood transfusions.[21]

The judge also found that Anna's refusal of the transfusion was voluntary.

> *I cannot find that it was the undue influence (of her mother) which sapped her will and destroyed her volition, but I am satisfied that the pressure of her mother, the very presence of her mother, the mother's fervent belief in the sin of blood transfusion, the patient's desire to please her mother despite their troubled relationship, all of this contributed to the focus of attention being drawn to blood transfusion before anyone else had ever contemplated its need.[22]*

The judge rejected the midwife's evidence that she had read the form to Anna, finding that the midwife had given no explanation at all.

The appeal

Refusal not effective.   A government solicitor who was appointed to represent Anna's interests appealed.

The appeal court found 'abundant'[23] evidence that the refusal of treatment was not effective. This decision was based on a review of Anna's mental and physical state when she signed the form, the pressure exerted on her by her mother, and the misleading response to her enquiry as to alternative treatment by the doctor and nurses. In these circumstances the doctors were free to treat her on the principle of necessity in the emergency that had developed.

Lord Donaldson included this warning:

I was surprised to find that hospitals appear to have standard forms of refusal to accept a blood transfusion and was dismayed at the layout of the form used in this case. It is clear that such forms are designed primarily to protect the hospital from legal action.

They will be wholly ineffective for this purpose if the patient is incapable of understanding them and there is no good evidence (apart from the patient's signature) that they had that understanding and fully appreciated the significance of signing it.

. . . such forms should be redesigned to separate the disclaimer of liability on the part of the hospital from what really matters, namely the declaration by the patient of their decision with a full appreciation of the possible consequences, the latter being expressed in the simplest possible terms and emphasized by a different and larger typeface, by underlining, the employment of coloured print or otherwise.[24]

Lord Donaldson formulated the following guidelines to assist hospitals and doctors in similar circumstances:

Although an adult patient is entitled to refuse consent to treatment irrespective of the wisdom of that decision, the effectiveness of such a refusal is dependent on doctors being satisfied that:

1. At the time of the refusal the patient's capacity to decide has not been diminished by illness or medication or by false assumptions or misinformation.

2. The patient's will has not been overborne by another's influence.
3. The patient's decision has been directed to the situation in which it had become relevant.
4. Where a patient's refusal is not effective, doctors are free to treat in accordance with their clinical judgment as to the patient's best interests.
5. In cases of doubt as to the effect of a purported refusal of treatment, where failure to treat threatens the patient's life or could cause irreparable damage to health, doctors and health authorities should not hesitate to apply to the courts for assistance. *[Author's note: In this regard Lord Donaldson praised the initiative shown by Anna's father and partner and criticized the hospital for not making the application.]*
6. Forms of refusal should be redesigned to bring the consequences of a refusal forcibly to the patient's attention.[25]

Treatment consented to should not be exceeded unless there is a risk to life or health

In the next case, the court found that an immediate risk to life *had* developed in the operating room.

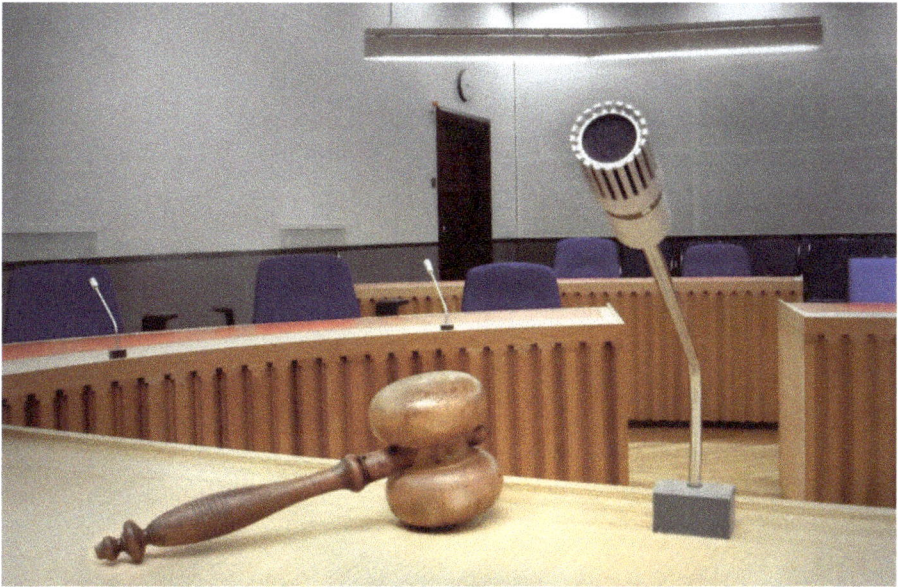

Davidson v Shirley, 616 F. 2d 224 (1980)[26]

The facts

Before her admission for caesarean delivery of her second child, Bernadette, an RN, had requested a tubal ligation. On admission, she signed a consent form authorizing a caesarean delivery, tubal ligation and any other operations or procedures deemed therapeutically necessary on the basis of findings during the course of the operation.

Blood loss. A healthy, but large, baby was safely delivered by caesarean section; however, the uterus contracted at a slower than normal rate and blood loss was occurring. The obstetrician then discovered and removed a large tumour. This necessitated the severance of additional blood vessels - and further blood loss. When IV oxytocin proved unsuccessful, the obstetrician, fearing Bernadette could die, removed the uterus.

Bernadette later alleged that she had not authorized the hysterectomy and brought an action in battery.

The decision

The court found that prior to the caesarean section, Bernadette had consented to any procedure that became therapeutically necessary and had read and understood the language used on the consent form. In the court's view, the removal of a large tumour, and the consequent hysterectomy to halt a life-threatening flow of blood, were therapeutically necessary procedures covered by her consent.

....

Common law rights of the child

If the interests of the fetus take second place to the mother's right to control any interference with her own body — the child, once born alive, comes under the full protection of the law, as the following Australian case illustrates.[27] At common law, a child is 'born alive' when it has a separate and independent existence from its mother.[28]

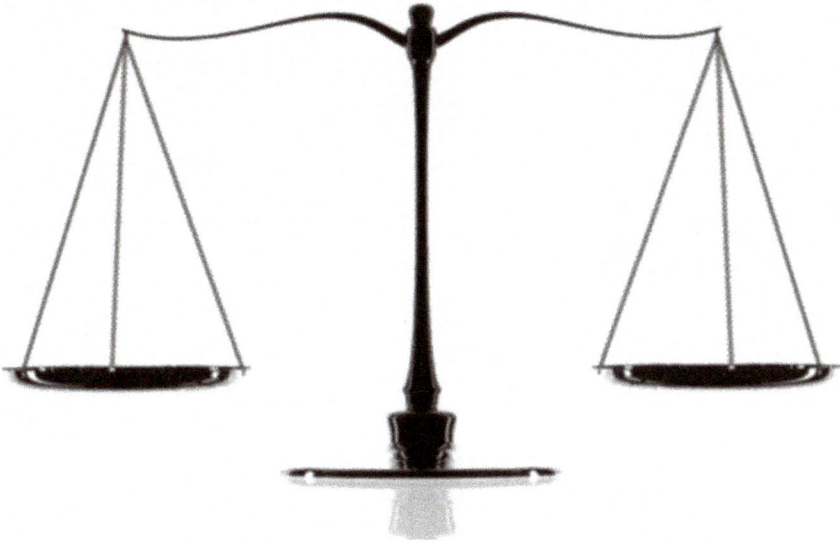

In Re Elm [2006] NSWSC 1137[29]

The facts

Illya arrived in Australia from a refugee camp in Africa in 2002. She later became pregnant, tested positive for HIV and was due to give birth on 22 September 2006. Illya initially agreed to take medication but ceased doing so in March, believing that God had cured her and would protect her child. An interview with community services officers established that Illya did not know who the father of the baby was, appeared to have limited social networks, was on social security payments and had no family in Australia. It was also unlikely that she would be able to continue in the accommodation she shared with a male friend after the baby was born.

During a further interview in September, Illya maintained that she would not agree to either herself or her baby taking anti-HIV medication, nor would she undergo a caesarean section. She did not intend to breast-feed and did not believe that the baby would require on-going medical treatment and monitoring. Illya did not appear to have made arrangements about the baby's needs or alternative accommodation after the birth. She maintained that God had healed her and would continue to protect her.

In 2007, the Department of Community Services in New South Wales (the department) commenced urgent proceedings eleven days before the baby was due to be born. Orders were sought that (a) the baby be separated from its HIV infected mother immediately after birth, (b) that the baby be treated against the mother's express wishes and (c) that the mother not be allowed to breastfeed. This application was made in Illya's absence (ex parte). Doctors feared that if she were aware of the orders, she would not come to the hospital (or any hospital) for the birth and necessary drugs would not be available to treat the baby. Instead, Illya would be notified of the orders shortly after giving birth.

Medical history. The judge found that Illya, despite her belief to the contrary, was still HIV positive. Her blood viral load had risen from a low 49 copies/ml on 6 March 2006 (shortly before she ceased taking medication) to more than 100,000 (the highest that can be reported) on 30 March. By 27 July she had a low CD4 count of about 270/ml, and a high viral load of about 83,900 copies/ml. Given her refusal to take anti-HIV medication or to permit her baby to do so, there was a serious risk that the baby would contract HIV from her at birth. This risk would be reduced if she did not have a vaginal birth and/ or consented to the baby receiving anti-HIV medication at birth and for the following four weeks.

Risk element. Having regard to Illya's high viral load and low CD4 count, as well as her refusal to undergo an elective caesarean section, the risk to the baby of contracting HIV was about 50-70 per cent if no anti-HIV treatment was given at birth nor breast milk given. If anti-HIV treatment was commenced as soon as possible after the birth and maintained, the risk would fall to about 10-15 per cent. If the baby received breast milk from the infected mother, that risk would double, to about 20-30 per cent. Given that Illya intended to bottlefeed the baby but refused to undergo a caesarean section (unless there were obstetric complications), there was the potential for a risk of HIV infection in the baby being reduced from as high as 70 per cent, to as low as 10 per cent, if appropriate medical treatment was commenced promptly after birth.

Treatment of baby. The judge heard that the director of the NICU, at the hospital where Illya was to give birth, had sought advice from an expert in the area of mother-to-child HIV transmission, and developed a protocol. The protocol provided for the baby to be washed thoroughly in the delivery suite, commenced on lamivudine syrup and nevirapine syrup, then admitted to NICU where an IV line would be introduced for a blood test as well as the administration of zidovudine and vitamin K. The baby would then be transferred to the special care nursery and was not to receive breast milk. A second blood test would be performed 48 hours after birth. These steps were to begin as a matter of urgency as soon as possible after the birth, to reduce the risk of serious damage from HIV infection.

Common law rights

The judge found that as the right of a competent adult to refuse medical treatment (whether the reasons for doing so are rational or irrational, unknown or even non-existent)[30] is not diminished by pregnancy, an unborn baby's need for medical treatment does not prevail over the rights of the mother.[31] In these circumstances a court could not order Illya to undergo treatment necessary to save the life and health of the baby. However, the baby, once born, was a separate entity and entitled to the full protection of the law.

Statutory authority. The judge found sections of the Children and Young Persons Care and Protection Act 1998 (NSW) were relevant in that they:

- authorized a doctor to carry out necessary and urgent medical treatment on a child without parental consent in order to save that child's life or prevent serious damage.
- authorized the director general of the department to (a) assume the care and responsibility of a child at risk of serious harm and (b) consent to medical treatment on the advice of a medical practitioner (notwithstanding that any other person who may have parental responsibility for the child does not consent, or refuses to consent).

Orders. The judge authorized the director general of the department to assume the care responsibility of the baby, including the authority to consent to medical treatment on the advice of a doctor (the director of NICU). The treatment was urgent. It was to be instituted immediately after the birth and administered continually for the following four weeks.

The judge further ordered that after the birth of the baby, the mother be prohibited from (a) breastfeeding (directly or indirectly) or (b) removing the baby from the hospital or any other hospital in New South Wales where she gave birth, without written approval of the director general. There is no further information (at the time of writing) about this case other than an anecdotal report that 'Illya' and her baby were cared for at a NSW hospital.

Failure to disclose risks

At the beginning of this chapter, the reasoning in relation to battery/unauthorised treatment was distinguished from the legal principles governing the giving of information, advice and the disclosure of risks of the treatment

These issues are argued in a negligence action. The patient will have to prove that they suffered damage as a result of the health professional breaching their duty of care to properly present information and warn of the material risks and likely outcomes of the proposed treatment.

A *material risk*[32] is one:

- which a reasonable person in the patient's condition would be likely to attach significance;
- which the health professional knows, or should know, the particular patient would be likely to attach significance; or
- where questions asked by a patient reveal their concern.

Courts have held that doctors must use due care in answering questions where the patient, to the knowledge of the doctor, intends to rely upon that answer in making a decision. Information about risks should only be omitted where the risk is too remote, or for therapeutic reasons if it is judged on reasonable grounds that the patient's physical or mental health might be seriously harmed by the information.

....

In the final case in this chapter, the judge explains that when parents have to make a decision, it needs to be an informed decision. This does not mean overloading the parents with technical medical information, but rather a simple explanation of what the possibilities are. In this instance the issue was whether to continue with the trial of labour or proceed to a caesarean section.

The judge also questioned the wisdom of seeking consent from a woman who is in the rigours of labour.

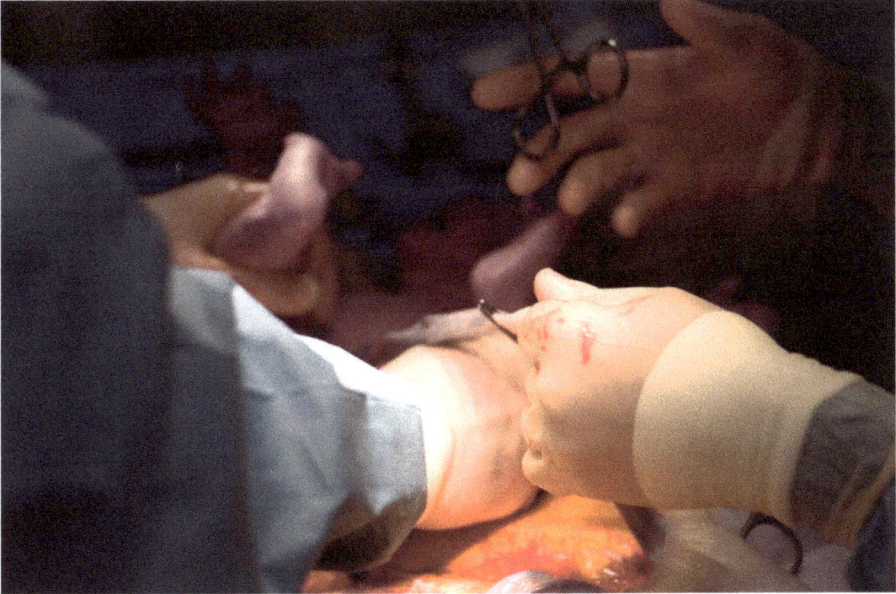

Khalid v Barnet & Chase Farm Hospital NHS Trust, [UK 2007][33]

The facts

Falia was admitted to hospital for the birth of her second child. She had a scar on her uterus from the previous caesarean section that carried a small risk of rupture in the subsequent labour. The parents had been advised during the pregnancy of the options between vaginal delivery and elective caesarean section. The 'overwhelming recollection'[34] of the parents was that it was safe to proceed with a vaginal delivery, and that additional care would be put in place. None of the doctors had wanted to unduly alarm Falia, who was keen to have a vaginal delivery, and so they did not over-emphasise the risk of scar rupture.

Her doctor's instruction four days prior to admission included:

For trial of labour. Once in established labour, i.e., regular contractions and cervical effacement from 3 cm dilatation, must have 2-hourly vaginal examinations. Can have Syntocinon as per primips regimen. However, must progress 1 cm with Syntocinon. If not, for caesarean section.

Plan: Assess vaginally on 28/10. If cervix closed, for caesarean section after discussion with mother. . .

The hospital protocol for the trial of scar included:

Registrar involvement/review re management of labour and action plan to be documented', 'Record of maternal and fetal condition as per partogram', 'Progress of labour to be closely monitored and recorded and registrar to be informed of findings: (i) Record nature of contractions (strength and frequency); (ii) 2 hourly vaginal examinations ... to assess progress after cervix is 3 cm or more dilated or contractions established...;(iii) Monitor position and descent of the baby's head abdominally and by (vaginal examination); (iv) Continue trial of labour if progress is being made with no adverse features. CTG monitoring — continuous.

These plans were designed to ensure safe delivery and to avoid an outcome where the baby was delivered too late in the event of scar dehiscence (splitting open) and uterine rupture.

The following is a sequence and summary of events including direct notes by the midwife and comments from obstetrics experts who later reviewed the CTG/documentation.

1.45 am	Admission noted 'Trial of Scar'.
2.15 am	CTG disconnected, contractions noted as mild to moderate and irregular.
3.40 am	CTG recommenced, stronger pain.
4.00 am	Stronger pain relief asked for.
4.10 am	Midwife performed vaginal examination; noted that mother asked for epidural.
4.45 am	Epidural performed.
5.00 am	First epidural top-up.
5.15 am	Midwife noted: FHR down to 60. Registrar called. Mother turned on left side. Registrar said he gave clear oral advice that he was to be called if any repetition of abnormal fetal heart rate. Reassured parents there was no problem. (Midwife did not recall this.) Registrar signed trace but no further documentation.
5.22 am	Fetal heart recovering.
5.45 am	Midwife noted : CTG now reactive, fetal tachycardia base 155 — 170. CTG 'suspicious.'

5.50 am   Later noted by obstetricians giving evidence that this was the start of one and a half hours of pathological trace.The partogram recorded contractions increasing from medium strength every two minutes to fairly strong every three minutes.

6.15 am   Early decelerations down to 80 baseline 160. (Experts agreed (a) that midwife at this stage (06.15 – 06.20) should have called for medical assistance because of persistent tachycardia and variable decelerations; and (b) that the CTG between 05.57 and 06.30 indicated a change /increase in the level of risk of scar dehiscence. Registrar later put risk at 50 per cent.) Mother put on left side and CTG noted as 'pathological'. Trace did not recover.

6.45 am   Midwife noted : Still having early decelerations – bladder visible.

6.50 am   Following catheterization bladder no longer visible. CTG remained pathological.

7.15 am   Midwife called registrar.

7.20 am   Registrar arrived in room. Discussion between registrar and parents in which caesarean section mentioned – decision made that labour should continue and a fetal blood sample be obtained.

Issue as to frequency of contractions:

Midwife and later, obstetric experts, agreed they were less strong and reduced to one in ten during this period.

Registrar said CTG showed five contractions between 7.00 am and 7.20 am.

It was later common ground that the trace did not show those five contractions, but did show the contraction the registrar said he had felt.

7.30 am   Registrar took three fetal blood samples timed on CTG as 7.30 and as being put into blood gas analysis machine at 07.44, 07.45, and 07.47, each being printed a minute later.

7.47 am   CTG trace showed fetal heart rate down to 80. Experts later agreed that during period 07.00 to 07.47 contraction rate had decreased to around one in ten minutes from one in three in the previous period.

Bradycardia. A question arose as to what happened when the registrar returned to the room. There was no argument that he had told the parents that the news was good; the sample showed normal. The midwife noted further loss of contact in relation to fetal heart rate and contraction rate, and that contractions were now mild and irregular. Almost immediately there was prolonged fetal heart bradycardia.

It was unclear whether (as the midwife said) the registrar applied the fetal scalp electrode before or, (as the registrar said) after the bradycardia commenced. The registrar later said it would be insane to put in a fetal scalp electrode knowing there was a terminal bradycardia. The midwife said she had 'put the mother's leg down - that was how I noticed the CTG. When the FSE was on and it still stayed down, the registrar said they would do a caesarean section and started to talk to the parents.'[35]

Persuasion. The registrar confirmed that when he realized there was prolonged bradycardia he had informed the midwife that they needed to do a crash caesarean. She had left the room to make arrangements and returned a few minutes later to find the doctor 'trying to persuade'[36] the parents of the need to do the procedure. The registrar said he had a prolonged argument with the parents for some nine minutes (the judge found this would have been a shorter time)) during which he finally resorted to saying that the baby could be born brain damaged or dead. The mother then agreed and signed the consent form. This argument was relied upon by the hospital, when delay was in question, as indicating a general reluctance for the mother to consent to a caesarean section at 06.30 or any time thereafter.

7.50 am	Registrar wrote his note. Second midwife took over, wrote her first note at 7.55.
7.59 am	Emergency caesarean section commenced.
8.16 am	Baby delivered, with severe brain damage.

Hypoxic ischaemic stress. Paediatric neurologists concluded that the baby was exposed to 27 or 29 minutes of profound hypoxic ischaemic stress before birth and less than five minutes after birth; the onset of hypoxic ischaemic insult was either at 7.47 or 7.49 and ended at 8.12 or 8.20. In their opinion, had the baby been born prior to 7.57 or 7.59, she would have been born unharmed.

Negligence was alleged.

Arguments and allegations

In the trial that followed in 2007, it was conceded that the midwife was negligent in not calling the registrar by 6.20 and agreed by all sides that the baby would not have suffered injury if she had been delivered 20 minutes earlier.

Delay. As soon as the emergency was recognized, the registrar had arranged for theatre to be opened but argued that it had taken time to persuade the parents to agree to the caesarean section.

Reconstruction. In a reconstruction of events the judge found that had the registrar been called at 6.20, he would have suggested a caesarean section at about 6.30, but the parents would have decided to continue with the labour. It would have been proper for the registrar to allow the labour to continue at that time, subject to close monitoring, and to take a fetal blood sample.

True rate of contractions. Thereafter, the registrar would probably have called to see the parents a second time. Attending for the second time in an hour, he would, more likely than not have discovered the true rate of contractions, which would have been an important sign in addition to the pathological CTG trace.

Stronger advice. Consequently, stronger advice would have been given to the parents to stop the trial of labour, including the risk of harm to the baby. The court heard that in a 'trial of scar' or 'trial of labour' the risk of scar rupture during the subsequent labour is very small — in the region of two per cent at most. Some 70 per cent of trials are successful. Expert medical witnesses agreed that, nevertheless, the possibility of scar rupture remains a substantial risk, involving the potential for a catastrophic result. No responsible obstetrician would ignore the risk because if it does materialize the baby can be brain damaged or die, and the mother put at risk.

Key to choice. In the judge's view, the key to the choice depends, from the obstetrician's point of view, on the degree of his suspicion of the risk of scar dehiscence, and from the mother's point of view on her knowledge of the risk. The pregnancy is regarded as high risk.

Fetal blood sample. Evidence was given that although doctors may regard the offer of taking a fetal blood sample as an alternative to a caesarean section, the judge believed that the true options were either a caesarean section or allowing the trial of labour to continue. The fetal sample, can only reassure if normal, that the baby is not yet acidotic, or, if not normal (showing the baby is acidotic), then it will indicate that caesarean section is the only safe course.

*A **false sense of security.*** The judge could not see the problem in simply indicating this much to the parents. The problem of not doing so meant that, at best, they did not have a clear understanding of the significance of the blood sample and, at worst, they would be given a false sense of security when the known risk of scar dehiscence and uterine rupture remained, and could materialize at any time.

Earlier advice. This advice, had it been given earlier, and even though not in as strong terms as the registrar had used at 07.30, would have been sufficient to lead the parents to consent earlier to the caesarean section. The judge found that once the parents became aware of the seriousness of the situation they had no hesitation in agreeing to the operation. Consequently the baby would have been born more than 20 minutes earlier.

Duty to warn. There was no doubt as to the doctor's duty to warn of the risks. The rationale was clear: to enable adult patients of sound mind to make decisions for themselves which intimately affected their own lives and bodies. The parents in this case did not have sufficient information until the registrar finally spelt out the risk of damage to the baby.

Consent under pressure. In the judge's opinion, once an emergency situation that both mother and baby are in danger is recognized, there is something wrong in seeking consent in the pressure of the circumstances. It is important to make clear from the outset the recognized risks of not stopping the trial of labour when advised and the consequent need for a caesarean section when it (the trial of labour) has to be stopped, particularly in an emergency.

Misinterpretation. In addition, the actual misinterpretation by the registrar of the contraction rate at 7.20 am (from three to four in ten minutes before 7.00 am to only one in ten after that time) was in itself a failure to exercise the ordinary skill of a doctor specializing in obstetrics. Had he recognized this significant sign, his suspicion of possible scar rupture would have been heightened to the extent that he would not have wanted to waste time taking a fetal blood sample and would have advised the parents that caesarean section was really the only safe course.

Scar rupture at 7.00 am. Expert medical witnesses agreed that the scar rupture had in fact begun by 7.00 am. An accurate interpretation would have resulted in the caesarean section being carried out sooner and the baby being born more than 20 minutes earlier.

The decision

Both the midwife and the registrar were in breach of their duty of care, and both breaches were the cause of the baby's injuries.

The judge described the case as 'a true tragedy.'[37] On the one hand, the mother had plainly set her heart on a normal delivery for her second child. On the other hand, the hospital and its medical staff had both the mother's and baby's welfare in mind throughout, desiring the best outcome for this pregnancy. In spite of apparent conflicts of fact, both parents and, in particular, the midwife and registrar obstetrician on duty that night plainly thought they were doing their best for the child about to be born.

The judge in *Khalid* made the following statement which, in general terms, could be applied to many of the parents and hospital staff you will read about in this book.

It is tempting to adopt a simplistic approach to the credibility of the witnesses and to resolve the main issues on the basis that some are telling the truth and some are not. Having heard all the witnesses and considered all the documentary evidence available, I do not think that such an approach would do justice to the respective cases. I formed the view that the Khalids were essentially honest people. They gave their evidence in a straightforward manner, but in their written statements and oral evidence they had no contemporaneous documentation on which to rely and were having to recall events which were catastrophic to them at the time, which happened in unfamiliar and emotional circumstances, which happened in a relatively short time and which happened at a time when (the mother) was in pain and frightened. It is small wonder that they cannot recall events with great accuracy.

On the other hand, both the midwife and registrar were anxious quite understandably to justify their own actions or inactions that night so far as possible in retrospect. I formed the view, neverthe-less, that they were essentially honest. So it is that I have (had) to assess the reliability of each witness's evidence rather than their honesty.[38]

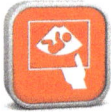

Discussion of Key Issues

The doctor in *Cohen* gave an assurance that Alana would not be seen un-clothed by a male nurse during a caesarean section. A male nurse both saw and touched the patient during the non-emergency operation. The case is concerned with a 'conditional consent'.

- What does your hospital's mission statement say regarding the hon-ouring or observing of religious/cultural beliefs?
- When patients place conditions on treatment based on cultural and re-ligious beliefs, is it always possible, practical or safe to give effect to these?
- Are these conditions compatible with hospital policy? If not, what is the process you follow?
- Is there adequate time spent considering religious and cultural 'differ-ence' in midwifery and obstetric education?
- Should religious convictions override discrimination issues regarding gender and staffing?

....

In Re MB. Lindy consented to a caesarean section but refused any needles because of her needle phobia. The appeal judge found that 'temporary fac-tors' of confusion, shock, fatigue, pain, drugs and panic induced by fear may erode capacity to make treatment decisions.

- How involved are you in the assessment of these temporary factors when dealing with pregnant women?
- British barrister Margaret Puxon comments that problems such as Lin-dy's should be identified at an early stage in antenatal care so that coun-

selling can be arranged if appropriate. After a request to take blood was made, Lindy did not attend another antenatal session.

- Would this have indicated a problem to you?
- If a problem arises and a woman does not attend a further antenatal session, do you have a follow-up plan to make contact?

What constitutes a 'reasonable' follow-up will depend on the circumstances.

- Would your documentation provide evidence of a reasonable follow-up?

....

In *In Re T,* Lord Donaldson was critical of the refusal of consent process at the hospital and found that Anna came under pressure from her mother. The judge found that the 'effectiveness' of a refusal is dependent on doctors being satisfied that:

1. The patient's capacity to decide is not diminished by illness or medication or by false assumptions or misinformation.
2. The patient's will has not been overborne.
3. The patient's decision had been directed, or drawn, to the specific situation. (For example, in Anna's case, that she was in an emergency situation and could die if not transfused.)
4. In life threatening situations, hospitals should not hesitate to seek the assistance of courts.
5. Note particularly the judge's observation that Refusal of Consent will be ineffective if the patient cannot understand the consent form or the form has been clearly designed to protect the hospital from legal action (a disclaimer): 'What really matters is the declaration by the patient of his/her decision with a full appreciation of the possible consequences'.[39]
   - Compare your hospital's Refusal of Consent form with these guidelines. Does your current documentation accord with these guidelines?

The patient's record (if accurate and contemporaneous) will reflect the patient's mental and physical state around the time of any purported refusal. Records constitute important evidence for this reason.

....

The women in *In Re T* and *In Re MB* were both stressed, frightened and in pain.

- Discuss how you would have supported them.

One test used by courts for assessing competence involves assessing whether the patient is:

1. comprehending and retaining treatment information,
2. believing it,
3. weighing it in the balance to arrive at a choice and
4. communicating that choice.

Note the judge's comment in *In Re MB,* that a compulsive disorder or phobia may 'stifle belief' in the information presented. The patient simply does not believe what she is being told.

- What other factors could stifle belief in information given to patients by midwives and doctors?
- What factors could stifle belief in information given by midwives to doctors? For example, one midwife at a workshop I facilitated cited a situation where an overseas doctor came from a culture in which the opinion of women was not given much weight. She felt her clinical opinion was disregarded or not believed for that reason.
- Discuss this issue in terms of risk to the patient. How would you or your organization manage this? Do orientation programmes for overseas doctors address this difference in attitude?
- On the other hand, what factors could stifle belief in information given by doctors to midwives?
- Apart from the issues of competence and emergency, do you agree with the proposition that a woman's right to determine what shall be done with her body should prevail over the interests of her unborn baby?

....

Davidson raises questions about consent and consent forms in the operating room.

- In your experience, can such issues pose difficulties for midwives caring for patients post- operatively?

In *In Re Elm,* the judge heard detailed evidence of a care plan for the baby.

- Discuss a care plan for a mother who has just given birth and whose baby is now being treated without her consent, taking into account her religious values.

....

Khalid. The judge said that once it is recognized that both mother and baby are in danger, there is something wrong with having to seek consent in the pressure of the circumstances. This becomes an important reason for making clear from the outset the recognized risks of not stopping the trial of labour when advised and the consequent need for a caesarean section when the trial of labour has to be stopped, particularly in an emergency.

- Is information given 'at the outset' (during consultation with doctors/ antenatal education) in your hospital — or can consent often be sought during the pressure of labour?

Having heard expert evidence, the judge concluded that if normal, the fetal blood sample can only reassure that the baby is not yet acidotic, or, if not normal (showing the baby is acidotic), then it will indicate that caesarean section is the only safe course.

- Do you agree? Give reasons either way.

NOTES

1. P. Staunton, *Nursing and the Law,* Churchill Livingston (Sydney, 2006), p.103. (Battery can also constitute a criminal offence.)
2. *Schloendorff v Society of New York Hospital,* 211 N.Y. 125, 105 N.E. 92 (1914).
3. Staunton, p.103.
4. L. Skene, *Law and Medical Practice,* Butterworths (Sydney, 1998), p.76.
5. *Cohen v Smith,* 69 Ill. App.3d 1087, 1094, 648 N.E.2d 329, 334 (1995).
6. *In Re MB,* 8 Med LR 217, 224 (1997).
7. Ibid.

8.   Ibid., p.220.

9.   ***Reasonable force.*** The Court of Appeal stated that health professionals can only judge the extent of force or compulsion which may become necessary in each individual case. It may become a balance between continuing treatment which is forcibly opposed and deciding not to continue with it. All that was involved in this case was the prick of a needle to enable the first part of the anaesthesia to be given.

10. Ibid.

11. Ibid., p.221.

12. Ibid., p.228.

13. For further reading of the 'forced caesarean' cases:

In Re S (adult: refusal of treatment) WLR 806 (UK);
   Competent patient's refusal on religious grounds overruled; both mother and baby at immediate risk of death from ruptured uterus; ruling that surgery with necessary postoperative treatment would be lawful; now, not considered good law.

In the Interest of Baby Boy Doe v Mother Doe (No. 1-93-4322 Ill. App.2d) (1994) (US);
   Doctor believed baby not receiving sufficient oxygen; immediate delivery by caesarean section or induced labour recommended; competent patient refused; patient's common law right to refuse invasive medical treatment upheld; baby delivered safely by vaginal delivery.

Tameside v Glossip Acute Services, 31 BMLR 93 (1996) (UK);
   Patient schizophrenic; disturbed, over-aroused, paranoid, delusional; fetus 'small for dates'; patient lacked capacity to consent/refuse medical treatment; surgery authorized; caesarean performed.

Wolverhattom Metropolitan BC v DB (a minor), 37 BMLR 172 Fam D (1996).
   Drug addicted mother; no antenatal care until 33 weeks; fear of needles; eclampsia fits; dangerously hypertensive; order that caesarean section was lawful; reasonable force with least distress.

St George's Healthcare v NHS Trust v S, CCH Australian Health & Medical Law Reporter, paras. 77-144 (1998).
   Patient 36 weeks pregnant; no antenatal care; severe pre-eclampsia; refused treatment; depression diagnosed; mental health admission; caesarean section performed against will at second hospital; court held there was a failure to distinguish need for treatment from whether mental con-

dition warranted detention and assessment; patient found to be wrong-fully detained.

14. Skene, pp.91, 92.
15. J. Seymour, *Fetal Welfare and the Law,* Australian Medical Association (1995). See also: *Journal of Law and Medicine,* Vol. 2, 'A Pregnant Woman's Decision to Decline Treatment: How Should the Law Respond?' p. 27 (Aug. 1994).
16. *In Re T (adult: refusal of treatment)* (CA) WLR 782, per Lord Donalson at 786 (1992).
17. *In Re T.*
18. Ibid., p.789.
19. Ibid., pp.789, 790.
20. Ibid., p.790. No explanation why anaesthetist thought blood transfusion neces-sary.
21. Ibid., p.791.
22. Ibid., p.792.
23. Ibid., p.803.
24. Ibid., p.798.
25. Summary by Lord Donaldson, p.799.
26. *Davidson v Shirley.,* 616 F. 2d 224 (1980).
27. *In Re Elm* is also included in Chap. 12 Lactation.
28. *R v Hutty,* VLR 338 ALR (1953).
29. *In Re Elm,* NSWSC 1137 (2006).
30. *In Re T (adult: refusal of treatment)* 4 All ER 649 at 664 (1992).
31. *St George NHS Trust v S,* 3 All ER 673 at 691 (1998).
32. The High Court of Australia quote with approval the reference of CJ King in F v R, 33 SASR 189 at p.193 (1983); Rogers v Whitaker (1991); on appeal (1992) 175 C.L.R 47. (1991); on appeal (1992) 175 C.L.R 479; 109 ALR 625 (HCA) examines the concept of 'material risk'.
33. *Khalid v Barnet & Chase Farm Hospital NHS Trust UK,* 97 BMLR (2007).
34. Ibid., p.89.
35. Ibid.
36. Ibid.
37. Ibid., p.84.
38. Ibid., p.87.
39. *In Re T,* Lord Donaldson, op.cit., p.798.

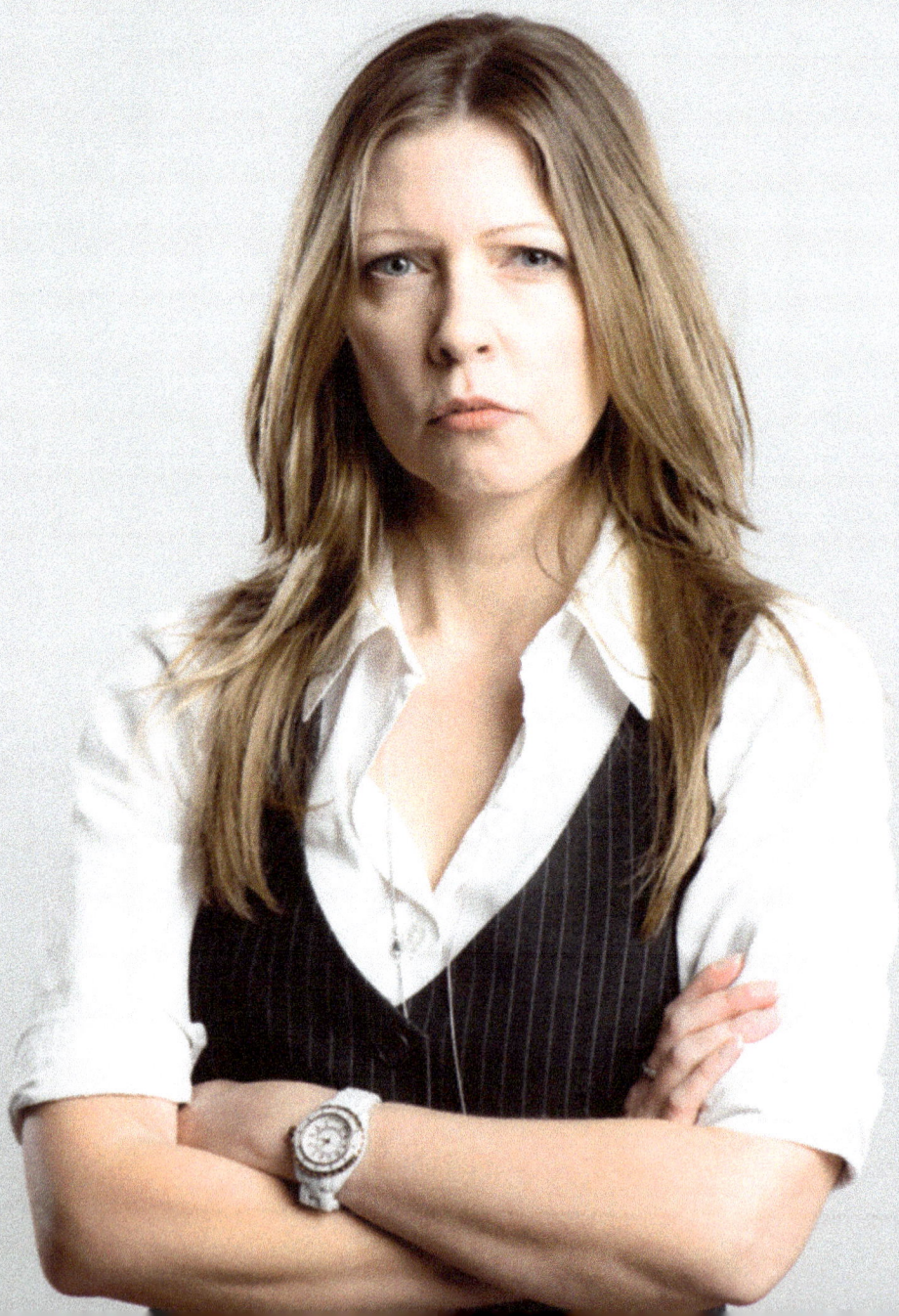

CHAPTER 2

Communication

'The mother told me that she had passed "some blood" and I interpreted this to mean merely "spotting." I believed there was no need to ask further questions concerning the extent of the bleeding.'

—A midwife.

Introduction

Litigation and coronial inquests are replete with examples of communication breakdown in hospitals. Whether communication is made in writing, over the telephone, or face-to-face, misunderstandings and misinterpretations occur, assumptions are made, concerns are ignored. But, suddenly, and maybe not so unexpectedly, there is an adverse outcome for the patient. In the following cases doctors and midwives respond (or fail to respond) to what they are being told by each other, or the patient. There is much to learn in this chapter about the management of risk and avoidance of litigation as a result of 'hearing but not listening.'

....

The first case identifies the risk of a midwife neither listening to nor exploring a patient's history over the telephone. In this instance the patient was anxious about vaginal bleeding.

McCrystal v Trumbull Memorial Hospital [US, 1996][1]

The facts

Bronwyn's three pregnancies were carried to full term with caesarean section births. After re-marrying, Bronwyn discovered she was pregnant again, in December 1989. She told her obstetrician at St J's Hospital that she wanted a tubal ligation after the birth. The obstetrician said she would again need a caesarean section but that St J's did not permit tubal ligation on its premises. She could be seen instead at the Women's Care Clinic at the Memorial Hospital, near to her home.

Cramping. Bronwyn had no major problems during the pregnancy, but on 10 May 1990 experienced cramping. Thinking labour may have commenced, she went to the emergency department at Memorial Hospital. A bladder infection was diagnosed, so she went home. Four days later Bronwyn had a regular check-up with the obstetrician. He said both she and the baby were fine and that he did not need to see her until her next regular appointment.

Vaginal bleeding. But on the morning of 16 May Bronwyn again experienced cramping and went back to the emergency department. After being reassured that she was not going into labour, Bronwyn went home. At approximately 1.30 pm she went back to the hospital. A specific test to determine whether contractions had started proved negative, so she went home again, only to find she was bleeding vaginally.

Telephone advice. This time instead of going back to the emergency department Bronwyn telephoned the Women's Care Clinic at the Memorial Hospital and spoke to a midwife. Based on the midwife's advice, Bronwyn stayed at home, waiting to see if the bleeding would stop. When it persisted, she telephoned the obstetrician, leaving a message on his answering service. The obstetrician returned her call at approximately 5.30 pm, advising that she stay at home and try to relax.

Ruptured uterus. Over the next few hours Bronwyn attempted to rest but on three occasions had to get up to vomit. She was still experiencing vaginal bleeding. At approximately 11.00 pm, while sitting on the couch, she felt a 'lot of fluttering'[2] in the stomach. Her husband took her back to the emergency room at Memorial. The obstetrician performed emergency surgery, finding the uterus had ruptured along the scar of a previous caesarean section.

Cerebral palsy. Despite a fairly heavy blood loss, Bronwyn recovered quite quickly and was discharged within a week. But the baby girl, who had been without oxygen for a sustained period, suffered from cerebral palsy. Twenty-four hour care was required and she died nine months later.

Negligence was alleged against the obstetrician and the Memorial Hospital. After a pre-trial settlement was negotiated with the obstetrician, the case proceeded against the hospital. The trial court found for the hospital and the parents appealed.

The appeal

Bronwyn alleged that the midwife had not handled the telephone call properly. She said she had specifically said that she was bleeding to such an extent that the blood was clotting. The midwife had not asked specific questions concerning her condition, but said to call back if the bleeding got heavier.

Nature of bleeding. The midwife said that Bronwyn only told her that she had passed 'some blood' and that she had interpreted this to mean merely 'spotting.'[3] She believed there was no need to ask further questions concerning the extent of the bleeding. She had spoken to her supervisor before speaking to Bronwyn. The supervisor explained that it was not uncommon for a woman to bleed slightly after the vaginal examination that Bronwyn had just received in the emergency department. Based on this information, the midwife told Bronwyn that she only needed to come back if the bleeding persisted.

The decision

The court found both the midwife and her supervisor negligent. They had failed to make a correct assessment, believing Bronwyn was only having some minor spotting as a result of the examination in the emergency department. Neither midwife had listened to her complaints nor explored her full history. The advice to stay home and wait and see was completely incorrect and had been a direct cause of the baby's brain damage.

A new trial was ordered.

....

In the next case the patient (later described as high-risk) queries whether a midwife listened when she said that 'something had moved or come out'[4] after she came back from the toilet. The coroner commented on a number of issues in this investigation, including: the appropriate level of supervision at consultant and managing clinician level, the adequacy of information about the risk factors of a caesarean section versus a vaginal delivery, and the hospital's internal review process following the baby's death. The coroner's recommendations in relation to the last item should assist most hospitals in the management of risk.

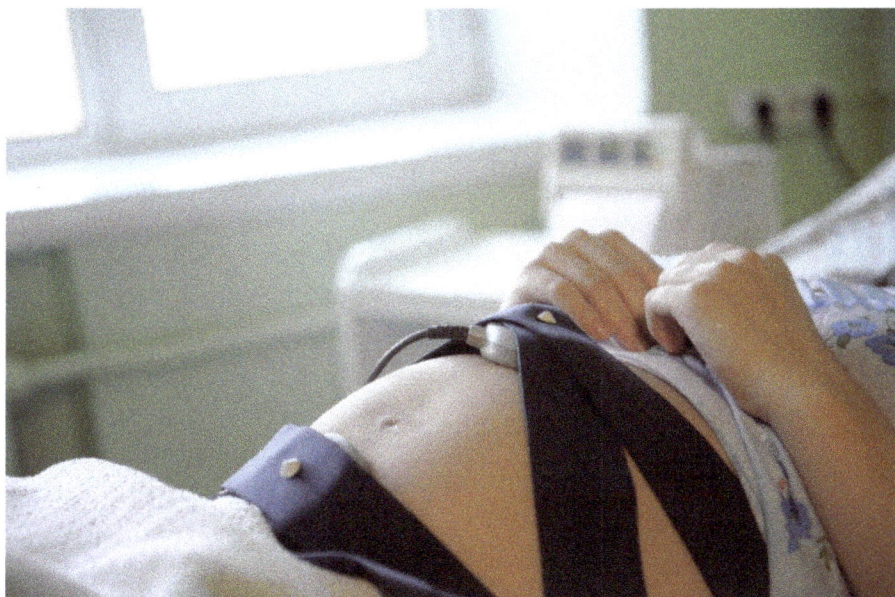

Coronial Investigation
[Aus, 1996]5

The facts

Julie's three children had all been vaginal births. Now 40 years' old, she was due to give birth again. The baby was in the transverse lie position. Julie was told at the hospital that a caesarean section would be performed. Four days later, on 24 September 1996, when she went to hospital for the surgery, midwife James told her that she was not on the operating list, but would be reviewed by the obstetric registrar. The midwife explained that there must have been a breakdown in communication. After some discussion, Julie was admitted. An ultrasound showed a vertex presentation plus an estimated fetal weight of 4.143 kg. No abnormalities were evident.

Midwife James said she saw Julie the next morning:

The obstetric registrar had asked if it would be suitable, workload wise, to induce Julie as she was term. Her baby was now cephalic and had remained cephalic overnight. I said this would be fine and I transferred her from Post Natal Ward back to the Delivery Suite. She stated she was happy that her baby was head first and that she was going to be induced.[6]

Documentation did not show a change to cephalic presentation.

The midwives

Meconium staining heavy. Midwife Evans said that Julie was to have an Artificial Rupture of Membranes (ARM) at 9.15 am. When she arrived on duty on 25 September the obstetric registrar had already started to pierce the membranes. She had applied fundal pressure. The liquor was heavily meconium stained, appearing to contain a moderate amount of blood. The registrar had applied a scalp electrode, commenting that the blood may have been due to an acute partum haemorrhage (APH).

A CTG trace was performed until 10.30 am. The liquor continued to be meconium stained, but only small amounts of showlike blood were seen. The scalp electrode remained connected. The CTG tracing was within normal parameters.

Walk to toilet. At 11.30 am, Julie said she wanted to go to the toilet. Midwife Evans palpated the head, which she said was immobile in the pelvis. Given this immobility, she allowed Julie to get up to go to the bathroom. On her return, observations of the fetal head remained within normal parameters. (The midwife said if the head was not fixed there might have been problems with the cord when the patient was moving about.) As Julie's contractions remained mild, Syntocinon was commenced. A scalp electrode had been connected for the entire shift, except during the trip to the toilet.

Labour more established. Monitoring continued, with labour becoming more established. Midwife Evans handed over to the afternoon shift at 2.00 pm saying that there had been no indications of fetal distress, nor any instructions from the registrar that Julie should not walk about. At about 2 pm, the CTG was re-commenced. A midwife said that at that time the head was 3/5 down. Julie had not been assessed per vagina since the commencement of labour.

Later visit to toilet. Shortly after 3 pm, Julie said that midwife Smith checked the notes and asked if she had been to the toilet recently. 'At approximately 3.30 another midwife came into the room and checked the notes then asked if I had been to the toilet recently. I said I hadn't and was told to get up and go to the toilet before she checked me.'[7] Midwife Smith made no contemporaneous note of the abdominal examination, but a retrospective note at 8.00 pm stated: 'On coming....shift abdominal palpation commenced however patient had felt bladder ... Patient up to toilet with scalp electrode remaining in situ.'[8]

Something had moved or come out. Julie said she had told midwife Smith that she felt something had moved, or come out when she went to the toilet shortly after 3.00 pm.

When I was passing urine I had a desire to push, and felt something had moved or come out. When I got back to the room I said to the midwife the same thing. She then indicated to me I probably had pushed the monitor things out and to get into bed. I said it didn't feel like that, although I knew it wasn't the back passage something had come out, still no examination vaginally.[9]

Midwife Smith did not give evidence on the grounds of illness. She said in her statement that Julie had opened her bowels. Julie disputed this and said that the midwife had not performed an examination.

Prolapse. After 3 pm, midwife James reviewed the CTG readings. She found the fetal heart rate 'was initially at 60 beats per minute but quickly recovered to 111 beats per minute.'[10] Julie had then wanted to push. Midwife James told midwife Evans to take Julie to the labour room as she considered her ready to deliver. Julie walked there. On arrival, there was some difficulty recording a fetal heartbeat. It appeared there was a problem with the scalp electrode. Midwife James took a fetal heart rate with a probe and got 60 beats per minute. She instructed midwife Evans to page the doctor. It was during an examination that a large loop of umbilical cord was discovered between Julie's legs.

Delay. The obstetrician did not respond to her pager, which was later discovered to be malfunctioning. She was then paged over the intercom system. This led to a delay of nine minutes. On examining Julie, the obstetrician considered the delay too great to undertake an emergency caesarean section to save the baby.

The inquest

Cause. The fetal death was found to be caused from the prolapse and compression of the umbilical cord. The prolapse was believed to have occurred in the bathroom.

The coroner noted that, according to midwife James, midwife Evans had not told her that Julie had a feeling that something had come down after she returned from the toilet.

Fetal heart low. Midwife James told the court that a routine four-hourly internal examination is the best way of discovering the condition of the mother and baby. There had been no measure of descent of the head after 11.30 am. She said she would not have turned the tracing off and that a monitor should be used with a risky patient.

Outside normal limits. The coroner heard that the CTG trace started at 3.09 and at 3.21 (am/pm not specified) it was outside normal limits of 100 to 120 at the bottom of the range. Midwife James said she was concerned when the fetal heart rate was low. She considered that something was wrong.

Variations. The coroner found the patient had been monitored with only one abdominal palpation being performed and only one inspection of the presenting part, which occurred earlier in the day. In addition, the monitor had no alarm to assist detecting variations and no one had been there to detect movements.

Findings and recommendations

When Julie was first examined on 24 September the clinical presentation was a transverse lie. A later ultrasound showed a vertex presentation 'with back to the maternal left and an estimated foetal weight of 4.143 kg. The placenta was fundal, liquor volume normal and no foetal abnormality was present.'[11]

Management plan. After discussions with a consultant, the obstetrician had discussed the management plan with Julie and said they would aim for a vaginal delivery. The obstetrician did not tell Julie that some doctors would have conducted a caesarean section at an earlier time.

Managing the risk factors

The coroner found that having made the decision to induce the labour, the relevant hospital staff's management of the risk factors could have been better. Julie was regarded by all medical experts as a high-risk patient because of:

1. maternal age (40),
2. history of unstable lie,
3. breathing problems,
4. meconium,
5. antepartum haemorrhage,
6. maternal weight (difficult to do abdominal palpation),
7. weight of baby 4.3 kgs, (risk assessment requires consideration of a variation of plus or minus 10 per cent in weight, baby's weight could have been higher than 4.3 kgs and surgical intervention was probably required),
8. high position of head in pelvis and
9. problems with achieving induction of labour.

Julie had received one-to-one midwifery supervision. But the problems that arose during her care indicated she was not managed with the degree of attention required for a high-risk patient:

1. The CTG monitor did not have a chart running for most of the monitored period to enable comparisons of the fetal heart rate to be made, even where physical observations were not carried out.
2. There was no abdominal examination by the doctor after induction (although the doctor relied on the examination of a midwife).

3. Once the fetal heart was noted as having dropped to 68, a physical examination should have been immediately performed prior to Julie being asked to walk to the birthing suite.
4. Once Julie told the midwife of her difficulties after having gone to the toilet, there was no requirement that she be confined to bed and an immediate physical examination carried out.

Greater level of supervision. The coroner commented that in this type of case it may be necessary to provide a greater level of supervision at consultant and managing clinician level. It was a question of directing a greater degree of clinical and midwifery attention to managing the risk factors.

Need to inform. Julie said that if she had been properly informed of the risks of induction of labour, in comparison with the risks of caesarean section, she would have demanded the latter. The obstetrician said she had discussed caesarean section versus induction of labour with Julie, who had seemed happy to proceed to an induction. The obstetrician could not recall telling her about the risk of cord prolapse in connection with induction of labour. The obstetrician did not accept that it was a very significant risk, given that the lie had stabilized.

Risk of prolapse. An obstetrician giving expert medical evidence for Julie considered she should have been advised about the relative risks. In particular, she should have been warned about the risk of cord prolapse, which was one in 40 or one in 50.

In the coroner's view Julie received less than adequate information on the risk factors of the respective procedures to enable her to make an informed decision.

Internal hospital review. A midwife (who had been involved in Julie's care) told the court the case was discussed at the hospital's perinatal meeting:

Q: Were there any suggestions raised in relation to changes in procedures and practices?

A: No

Q: Were the doctors involved in this process?

A: Yes there were.

Q: Did they make any suggestions about changes in procedures and practices either at the midwifery or medical level?

A: No.[12]

A second midwife (who worked regularly at the hospital) gave evidence about discussion by midwives on the incident:

A: I couldn't tell you if minutes were kept, but there was certainly a free conversation with the people involved.

Q: Are you able to recall the outcome of the discussion as to whether there were any concerns or issues that were raised amongst the unit that may be better addressed in the future?

A: It was more a debriefing session on the actual incident and obviously the tragic circumstances and then it was just explained that it would be obviously be brought up at the perinatal morbidity audit to discuss what had happened and that was all.

Q: Are you aware as to what the outcome of the other discussion was?

A: No, I wasn't present.

> *Q: Did this unit receive any instructions in relation to any future management of patients of a similar risk?*

> *A: Not that I know of, more just the case that people were aware that the protocol (for managing a cord prolapse not a high risk patient) was there and that the protocol had been followed.[13]*

The coroner made the following key points:

1. General evidence at the inquest had demonstrated a considerable amount of information about the management of high-risk patients. Effective inquiry during the hospital's perinatal or midwifery debriefing may well have discovered improvements in procedures and practices at medical and midwifery level.
2. Therefore any review meeting (perinatal or midwifery) should not be regarded as a debriefing exercise but as a real opportunity to investigate an incident and examine procedures and practices with a view to identifying any potential improvements in patient safety and care.

If women believed midwives were not listening in the two cases already discussed, in the next case the obstetrician does not seem to be listening to the midwife. In any event, her concerns about pre-eclampsia were not acted upon.

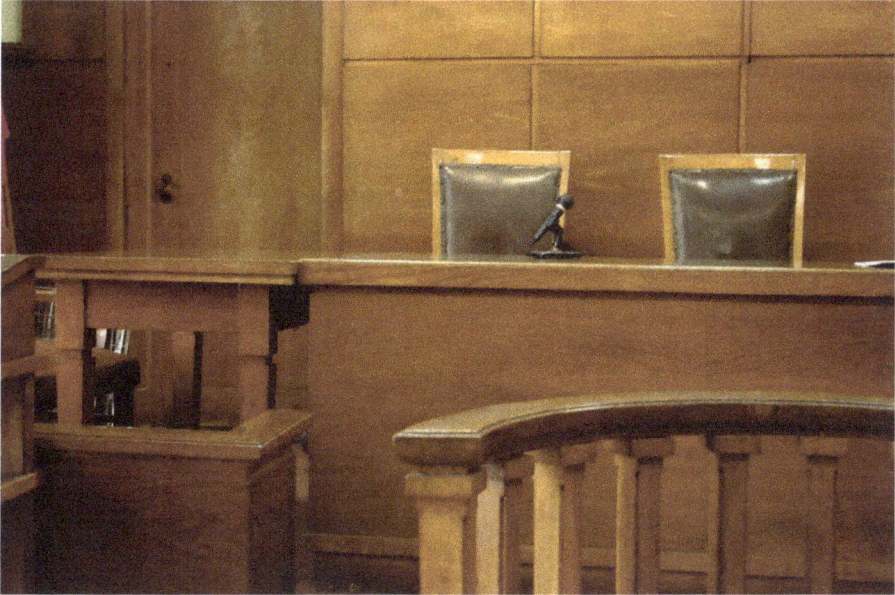

Nguyen v Tamth [US, 1997][14]

The facts

Alice became pregnant in early 1989, seeing the obstetrician in April and May while in her second trimester. During visits on 7 June, and 5 and 25 July, BP was 100/70, urine samples negative for protein, and weight gain was normal. On the last prenatal check on 22 August, BP was 120/86, a 3+ reading for protein in the urine and 4.09 kg had been gained since the previous visit. The obstetrician did not believe these observations required immediate admission and induction of labour.

Edema. On 31 August at 10 am, Alice went to hospital in advanced labour. Midwife Jones admitted her to the labour and delivery unit. At 10.15 am, the midwife noted initial BP as 170/120. The patient was rolled on her left side. BP then read 186/118. The midwifery notes indicated the patient's reflexes were -2. There was 'a large amount of edema noted in the legs.'[15] The RMO did not believe this was normal edema, noting 'massive pitting lower extremity edema on both sides.'[16] Deep tendon reflexes were described as abnormal.

Magnesium sulphate; urine test. When the obstetrician arrived, he was given Alice's records and asked if he wished to administer magnesium sulphate to lower the BP. He did not make an order, nor did he order a urine test for protein.

Stroke. BP was recorded regularly up until delivery by caesarean section at 12.05 pm. The obstetrician co-signed the standard postoperative orders written by the RMO. Recovery room nurses took BPs at 12.45 pm, 1.00 pm and 1.55 pm. There were no recorded BPs between 1.55 and 4.00 pm. At 4.00 pm, midwife Beattie found the patients right arm dangling over the side of the stretcher. Alice had suffered a stroke to the left side of the brain that was to interfere with her speech, render her right arm virtually useless and impair her ability to walk.

The trial

Allegations of negligence were made against medical and midwifery staff during the antenatal period and delivery, but the case proceeded only against the obstetrician. It was alleged his failure to diagnose and treat the pre-eclampsia had resulted in the cerebral haemorrhage, with consequent partial paralysis and aphasia.

Lethargic. Delivery notes indicated that at some point before going to the recovery room Alice 'felt her leg had fallen from the stirrup.'[17] She was observed at the time to be particularly lethargic and drowsy.

The obstetrician had visited after being informed of the paralysis, and attributed the weakness to some cerebral accident. He said during the pre-trial process that someone made a note on Alice's chart that her leg had fallen off the delivery table. Under cross-examination the obstetrician said this was 'obviously incorrect.'[18] He now believed the stroke had occurred in the recovery room.

Pre-eclampsia. The court heard that pre-eclampsia is a fairly common condition of late pregnancy characterised by symptoms not normally present during a pregnancy. These are an increase in blood pressure; a tendency toward excessive weight gain, excessive fluid accumulation; and the presence of protein in the urine.

Medical experts explained to the court that in 1989 (the date of the incident) the exact cause of pre-eclampsia was unknown. It was understood that the condition causes an elevation in BP, which can range from mild to severe or profound. This can cause spasm of the blood vessels and damage to the mother, including strokes, coma, brain haemorrhage or death. Obstetricians normally check for evidence of pre-eclampsia at every prenatal visit.

Checklist. The obstetric department used a standard printed checklist, which was part of the patient's chart. 'Severe pre-eclampsia' was defined as BP greater than 160/110 and a proteinuria greater than 2+ after 26 weeks' gestation. The patient's BP had been as high as 186/118.

Neurologist. A neurologist reviewed Alice's records. He believed the stroke was caused by high blood pressure, which had occurred during delivery, or just afterwards, in the delivery room. The neurologist explained that untreated pre-eclampsia is a known cause of intracerebral haemorrhage. The patient's BP on admission was capable of causing the haemorrhage. If medications had been administered to treat her pre-eclampsia and lower the BP (after it was found to be 186/118), it was more likely than not that the stroke would have been prevented.

Perinatologist. A perinatologist contended that care had fallen below a reasonable standard when the obstetrician:

1. Failed to diagnose pre-eclampsia on the last prenatal visit and did not order a follow-up BP check the next day, or admit the patient to hospital.
2. Failed to diagnose pre-eclampsia prior to delivery. He did nothing to treat it and neglected to address the BP. At this point the obstetrician should have ordered magnesium sulphate to relax the spastic vessels and assess its effect on the BP. Additional anti-hypertensives could then be ordered if necessary.
3. Failed to order frequent BP checks after the delivery.
4. Failed to continue magnesium sulphate for 12-24 hours after the birth.

The decision

The appeal court upheld the trial court's verdict in favour of the patient, finding:

1. Alice had proved conclusively that she suffered from pre-eclampsia.
2. Her expert witnesses clearly established the diagnosis. This had been confirmed by experts called by the obstetrician.

3. The obstetrician should have initially administered magnesium sulphate. If the BP did not come down, other antihypertensive drugs should have been given. He should also have taken a protein reading of the urine, given the findings at the last pre-natal visit.
4. Each midwife had recognised the problem and suggested that magnesium sulphate be administered. Nothing had been done.

....

A strange twist to the *Nguyen* scenario occurs in the next case. Neither the midwife nor the obstetrician appears to be listening to the patient or the paediatrician.

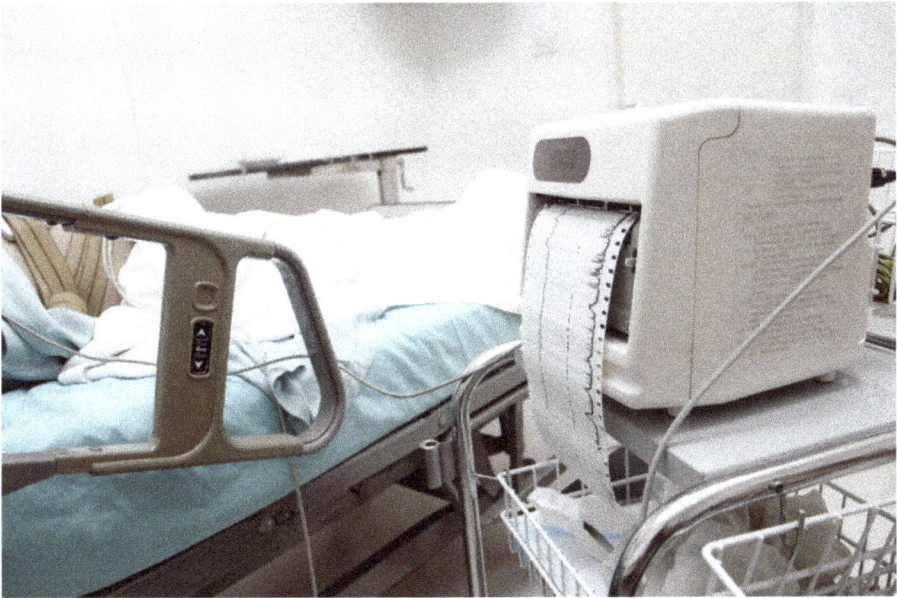

Lopez v Southwest Community Health Services [US, 1997][19]

The facts

Heather was admitted to hospital, 28 weeks pregnant and complaining of abdominal pain. She insisted she was not in labour. The midwife told her she was wrong, that she was in fact dilated to 10 cm and ready to deliver. A paediatrician was sceptical. The fetal heart monitor was registering a normal beat with no contractions; Heather did not seem to be in labour.

Obstetrician. An obstetrician reviewed the midwife's assessment, examined the patient, and said not only was Heather in labour but she had a prolapsed uterus and the baby was in the transverse position. The obstetrician broke the amniotic sac and delivered a baby who was found to be at least 10 weeks' premature.

The parents alleged negligence against the obstetrician and the hospital. At the time of the trial, the child was a severely disabled 14-year-old.

The trial

The obstetrician said that he alone determined that the patient was in labour. He also believed that the baby would die if not delivered. But an expert witness told the court that doctors were 'primed', partly by what midwives and other people tell them. It was contended that the obstetrician might have been influenced by the midwife's faulty assessment.

The decision

The jury found the child's injuries had resulted from the negligence of both the obstetrician and the midwife. Both appealed. The obstetrician then settled out of court.

The appeal

The appeal court upheld the jury verdict. There was enough evidence for the jury to find that despite the obstetrician's insistence to the contrary, the midwife's faulty assessment had influenced his decision to deliver the baby.[20]

....

In the next case, midwives listen with growing concern to what a GP is telling an obstetrician over the telephone. But as the coroner was later to observe:

This was not a case where hindsight dramatically altered one's view of anything. The C.T.G. tracings were there for anyone competent to read from the start.[21]

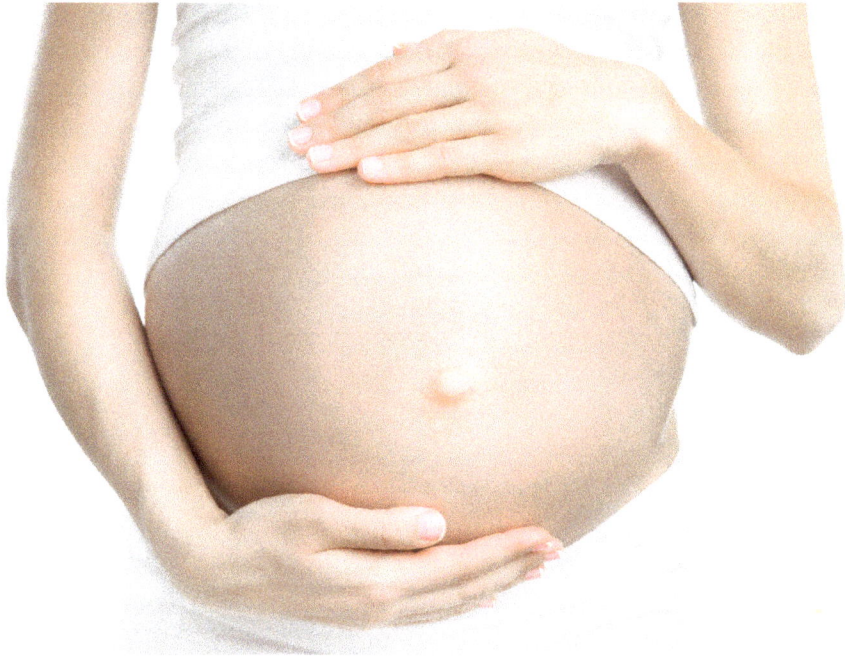

Coronial Investigation
[Aus, 1993][22]

The facts

Paula was admitted to hospital in October, 1992, under the care of a GP who held a diploma in obstetrics. The GP arranged to consult with an obstetrician if there were any complications. At approximately 8.00 pm, CTG monitoring of the baby commenced. At about 8.30 pm, midwife Allan observed the CTG to be abnormal. She consulted midwife Coates, who agreed. Both believed the CTG showed poor beat to beat variation and before type 1 or type 2 dips. (Type 1 dips are now referred to as 'early decelerations' and type 2 dips as 'late decelerations'.) Type 2 dips suggest fetal distress and/or compromise. An examination at about 8.30 pm revealed the baby was still a considerable time away from birth.

GP called. Midwife Coates asked Paula not to eat or drink in case a caesarean section was needed. Both midwives believed the CTG tracings called for immediate attention. Midwife Coates telephoned the GP at about 8.30 pm. When the GP came to the hospital at 9.00 pm, the midwives expressed their concern. The GP telephoned the obstetrician. Midwife Allan heard the GP report that the CTG showed type 1 dips only. Midwife Allan later gave evidence that she was surprised at this. Having spoken to the obstetrician, the GP ordered Stemetil and an analgesic and gave instructions for monitoring the mother and baby.

Fetal bradycardia. Midwife Allan remained on duty until approximately 10.00 pm, then handed over to midwife Smith and midwife Dowdie. At about 11.15 pm, the membranes broke and Paula was transferred to the labour ward. CTG monitoring recommenced. At about 11.30 pm, midwife Smith telephoned the GP, advising her of the ruptured membranes and status of the CTG tracings. The GP said to continue monitoring. By about midnight the CTG revealed fetal bradycardia down to 80 beats per minute for approximately eight minutes. Midwife Smith called the GP and asked her to attend.

Deterioration. At 12.10 am, the GP examined the CTG tracings and assessed and examined the mother. Midwife Smith later gave evidence that in her opinion not only was the CTG abnormal in showing type 2 dips, but that the beat to beat variability was not satisfactory.

At 12.19 am, midwife Smith overheard the GP telephone the obstetrician to say the CTG showed type 1 to type 2 dips. The GP then ordered Pethidine and Stemetil.

Between 4.15 am and 5.15 am, midwife Smith went for a break. Charge nurse Dowdie took over. Midwife Smith returned at 5.15 am and was still very concerned that the CTG tracing was abnormal. The trace showed the 'fetal heart rate continuing to dip, baseline getting higher, and beat to beat variability less'.[23] At this time, the cervical dilation was only 1 cm; the baby's head was still high.

GP does not attend. By this stage midwife Smith believed a caesarean section was a real possibility. She prepared accordingly, contacting the GP at 5.30 am to request attendance. The doctor did not come in. At approximately 6.34 am, she called again requesting immediate attendance. (The GP later gave evidence that she may have inadvertently drifted off to sleep after the first phone call, as she was attending to her own child.)

Syntocinon. The GP then came to the hospital, examined the CTG tracings, had a discussion with midwifery staff and called the obstetrician. Syntocinon was prescribed. The staff, particularly midwife Smith, were alarmed that Syntocinon would be prescribed when the CTG was showing fetal distress. She queried this with the GP, who replied that it had been approved by the obstetrician. When midwife Talbot came on duty at about 7 am, her first reaction was to halt the Syntocinon.

Caesarean futile. The baby's condition deteriorated from the time Syntocinon was administered. A subsequent caesarean section proved futile.

The inquest

The obstetrician died prior to the inquest, but had made a statement (which the coroner accepted as truthful) that he had relied upon the information given by the GP.

Traces grossly abnormal. A consultant obstetrician was asked by the coroner for an independent opinion. The obstetrician said the CTG tracings were 'abnormal in their entirety'[24] and presented a terminal tracing of the baby's heartbeat. An early caesarean section would probably have saved the baby's life. The obstetrician found it 'almost unbelievable'[25] that a doctor could sit on the information being printed out of the CTG and was 'astounded' the baby had lasted as long as she had. Urgent medical attention was required at the start of the CTG monitoring, at approximately 8.30 or 9 pm.

All type 2 dips. There had been no type 1 dips shown around midnight on the CTG. They were all type 2 dips. The obstetrician said the CTG in its entirety showed no type 1 dips but only type 2 dips. Syntocinin should not have been administered, as it was contra-indicated where signs of fetal distress were present.

The findings

The GP. The coroner found any competent reading of the CTG tracings up to midnight should have produced 'a high state of alarm immediately requiring medical attention.'[26] The GP was found to be principally, if not totally, responsible for the death of the baby. She had not been a credible witness and had demonstrated a high degree of incompetency.

The midwives. Criticisms were made that the midwives had:

1. Not reported the matter to the director of nursing (DON) that night or in the early hours of the morning to indicate their concern that totally inappropriate action was being taken by the GP.
2. Failed to continually call the GP throughout the early hours of the morning to attend.

An unenviable position. The coroner heard evidence that if a midwife formed a view, in an exceptional case, that the doctor's treatment of the patient was totally inappropriate, she could report the matter to the DON. On the evidence before the coroner, no midwife, including those with 20 years' experience, had ever gone behind a doctor's back and appealed to the DON. The midwives had found themselves in an unenviable position in nearly all respects.

Not acted unreasonably. Because of the long and deeply entrenched doctor/midwife professional relationship, the midwifery staff had not acted unreasonably by failing to go to the DON to complain of the doctor's treatment. On several occasions the midwives had brought their concerns regarding the CTG printouts and administration of Syntocinon to the GP's attention.

The midwives. The midwives had also been in a difficult position in trying to get the GP to attend. They had called her twice and received instructions. Nothing new had really changed since her previous two visits. The printouts were the same. They were still 'deplorable'[27] and continued to be so. The midwives had twice referred the GP to these printouts. They had observed her examine them, heard her consult with an obstetrician and then received their instructions.

The coroner concluded that the midwives had not contributed to the baby's death.

....

In the final case in this chapter the coroner found that a clear error in communication had occurred. A midwife's evidence about a forceps delivery led the coroner to conclude that she was not sure whether the obstetrician was attempting to rotate, or, having successfully rotated, was attempting traction on the baby during the second attempt.

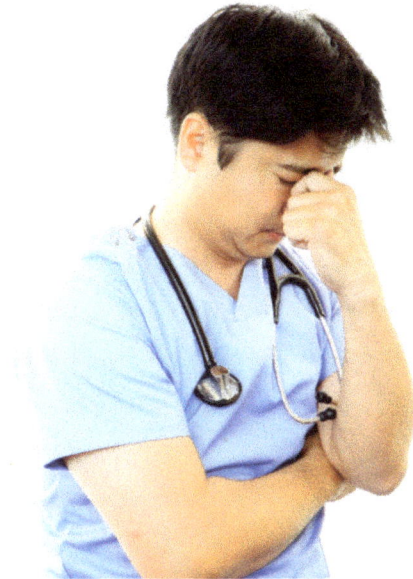

Coronial Investigation
[Aus, 2000][28]

The facts

After spontaneous rupture of the membranes, Jane was admitted to the delivery suite, in labour, during the evening. The obstetrician reviewed her at about 10.30 pm, finding the cervix fully effaced and 3-4 cms dilated. CTG was commenced at about 12.00 pm, and an epidural administered by an anaesthetist at about 1.30 am. A midwife did a vaginal examination at 4.30 am, finding the mother now fully dilated and wanting to push. The obstetrician, who had slept at the hospital, reviewed Jane at about 5.40 am, finding the baby in right occipito posterior position.

Trial by forceps. The obstetrician decided to undertake a trial by forceps in the delivery suite after discussing with the midwife the length of time it would take to organize a theatre. He said that the midwife told him that it would be quite inconvenient and expensive to get staff in at that early hour on Sunday morning.

Moderate rotation. The obstetrician said that he had encountered a moderate resistance to further rotation at about the midpoint of the rotation distance. Jane was distressed and had screamed at him to stop. He had done so, leaving the forceps in situ. He then asked the midwife to organize a theatre and she went to do this. He again attempted the rotation, altering the angle of the Keilland's blades. After moderate rotation force the fetal head had appeared to rotate the rest of the way to direct occipito anterior position. He waited for a contraction, then delivered the baby with one pull, using moderate traction.

Irreversible damage. The baby had low Apgar scores and was transferred to another hospital, where a decision was made that an MRI scan be done at a third hospital. The results were consistent with extensive, probably irreversible, damage to the upper spinal cord. After 48 hours of intensive care, there were no signs of improvement. The parents agreed that active treatment be withdrawn and the baby died soon after.

The findings

Confusion. The coroner found there was no way of knowing whether the baby's injuries were sustained during the first or second attempt with forceps. Failure to deliver by caesarean section in theatre after meeting the first resistance would not necessarily have resulted in a different outcome. In the coroner's opinion, the application of forceps, after directing the midwife that a theatre be organized, had led to some confusion.

Error in communication. The midwife, who had been present during the first and second attempt, seemed to have been confused as to what the obstetrician had actually done. Her evidence led the coroner to conclude that she was unsure whether the doctor was attempting to rotate, or, having successfully rotated, was attempting traction on the baby during the second attempt. The coroner was not satisfied that the midwife had been telling the obstetrician when a contraction was starting and when one was easing off. A clear error in communication had occurred.

Decision and comment

The coroner found the obstetrician was primarily responsible for the management of the baby's delivery. It was therefore his responsibility to direct the midwife in such a way that she would provide him with the relevant information for a successful procedure.

The coroner concluded that:

Ritualised checking and communicating is the best way to avoid human error and misunderstanding and to determine adverse consequences that might otherwise flow.[29]

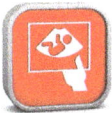

Discussion of Key Issues

In *McCrystal* a pregnant woman and two midwives had differing versions of a telephone call in which the severity and significance of the patient's bleeding (later resulting in a ruptured uterus) were discussed.

If your telephone advice about blood loss is later queried, would your records show:

- the date and time of the call
- the mother's name, UR number, address and telephone number (early in the call in case of disconnection)
- what the mother said, in her own words, using abbreviations and terminology approved by your hospital
- the questions you asked about her presenting problem and medical history
- whether you matched this to an appropriate protocol or
- why you deviated from a protocol
- who else you spoke to
- what advice was given and by whom
- what other action was taken
- that the mother was asked if she had any further questions
- that the mother was asked what she planned to do at the end of the call
- any other information you thought relevant

- the contact details of an interpreter or anyone else providing information
- the time(s) and name(s) of any doctors contacted and whether a sense of urgency was conveyed
- the time the call finished
- your signature, designation and printed surname

- What difficulties can arise if the caller is not the pregnant woman but, for example, a husband, child or neighbour?
- Discuss how difficulties could be compounded by language or cultural differences
- Is there anything you would add or subtract from the above checklist? If so, give reasons.

....

Coronial investigation. (1) The coroner found that any review meeting (perinatal or midwifery) should not be regarded as a debriefing exercise, but as a real opportunity to investigate an incident and examine procedures and practices, with a view to identifying any potential improvements in patient safety and care.

- How would you describe the outcomes from similar meetings at your hospital?

....

In both *Nguyen* and the second coronial investigation midwives are concerned at the lack of response by doctors to the midwives' clinical concerns.

Hospitals should have procedures for midwives to take patient care issues up the hospital's chain of command until they get appropriate results.

- Discuss differences between the public/private hospital in this regard. If there are differences between the two settings, why is this so?
- It is foreseeable that professional differences of opinion will occur in the obstetric/midwifery team. Is there a process at your hospital for resolving such differences?

....

In *Lopez,* the patient, nurse, obstetrician and paediatrician all had differing views as to whether or not the patient was in labour.

- Discuss the merits of the reasoning (limited though it is) preceding each decision.
- What more would you have wanted to know in similar circumstances?
- Do you agree with the finding of the appeal court that, despite the obstetrician's insistence to the contrary, the nurse's faulty assessment had influenced his decision to deliver the baby?

Coronial investigation. (2) The midwives in this case were very concerned at a GP's lack of response to CTG readings indicating fetal distress. They did not believe the GP's telephone conversation with a consultant obstetrician reflected the true position.

The coroner found that the GP had contributed to the death by not responding to what one witness described as 'terminal tracings.'

It is not unusual for differences of professional opinion to occur between doctors and midwives:

- How would you record such differences?
- What resources could you call upon in similar circumstances?

Coronial Investigation. (3) In this case an apparent miscommunication was found to have occurred between an obstetrician and midwife during a forceps delivery. The coroner commented that 'ritualised checking and communicating is the best way to avoid human error and misunderstanding . . .'[30]

- Discuss this comment in relation to the management of forceps deliveries in your unit.

NOTES

1. *McCrystal v. Trumbull Memorial Hospital,* 115 Ohio App.3d 73, 684 N.E. 2d 721, (1996).
2. Ibid., p.723.
3. Ibid., p.724.
4. *Record of Investigation into Death,* Case No. 2896/96 State Coroner's Office (Victoria, 1999), p. 4.

5. Case No. 2896/96.
6. Ibid., p. 2.
7. Ibid., p. 4.
8. Ibid.
9. Ibid.
10. Ibid.
11. Ibid., p.5.
12. Ibid., p.11
13. Ibid.
14. *Nguyen v. Tama,* 298 N.J. Super. 41, 688 A.2d 1103 (1997).
15. Ibid., p.1105.
16. Ibid.
17. Ibid.
18. Ibid.
19. *Lopez v Southwest Community Health Services,* 114 N.M. 2, 833 P.2d 1183 (1992).
20. Midwives have suggested that this limited case note does not answer such questions as: (a) did the obstetrician do an ARM which induced labour, or was Heather already dilated? (b) How long between ARM and delivery? (c) Why would an obstetrician do an ARM if the baby was in transverse lie ? (she should have had a LUSCS) and (d) Did the obstetrician do an ARM and internal podalic version to be able to deliver the baby vaginally?
21. *Record of Investigation into Death.* Case No. 3480/92 State Coroner's Office (Vic), 1993. p4.
22. Case No. 3480/92.
23. Ibid., p.3.
24. Ibid., p.1.
25. Ibid., p.7.
26. Ibid.
27. Ibid.
28. Both the case number and page references to this coronial investigation (Vic, 2000) are unavailable at the time of writing as are the details of a legal article on the case headed: *'Coroner finds forceps communication crucial.'*
29. Ibid.
30. Ibid.

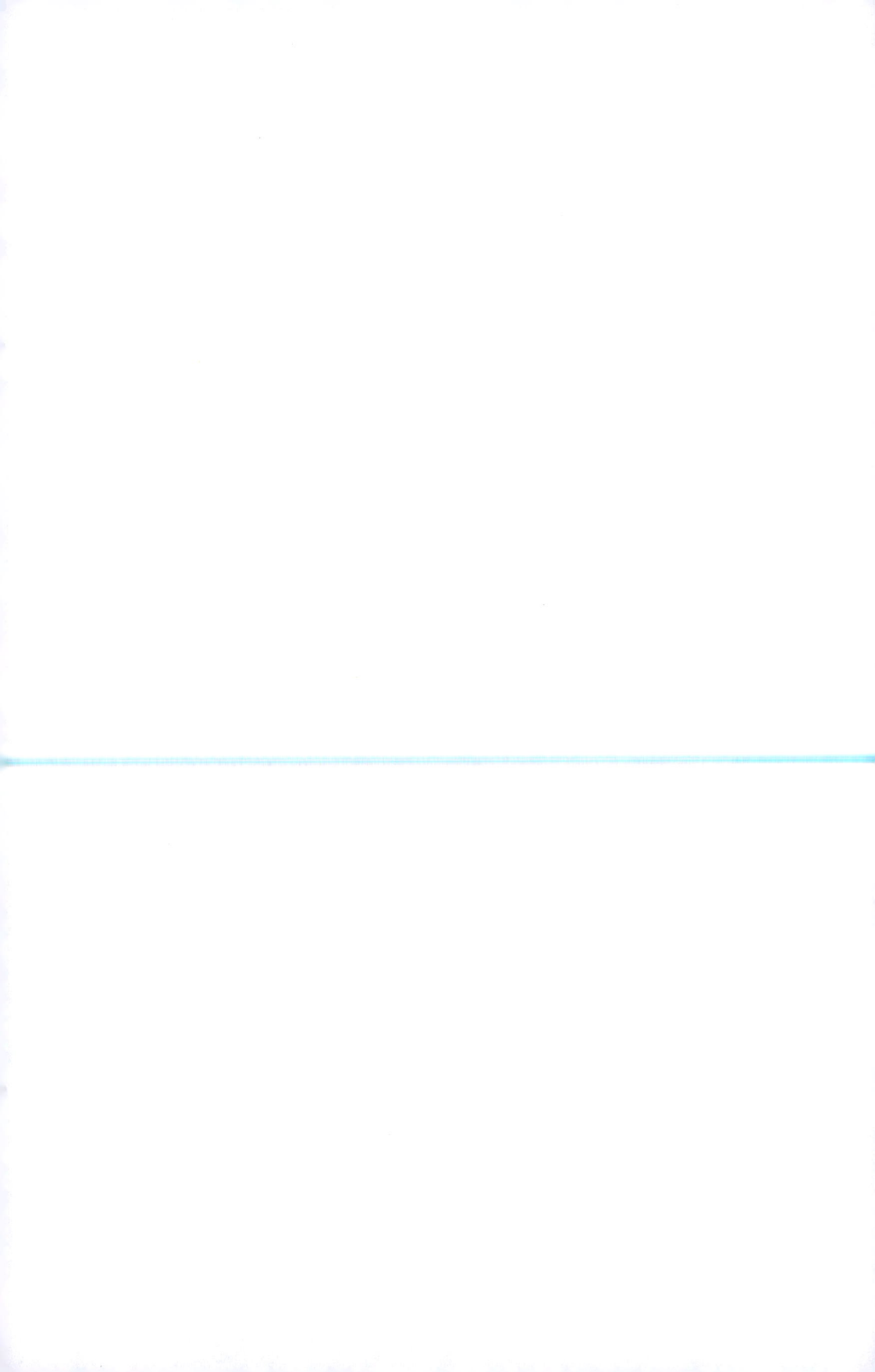

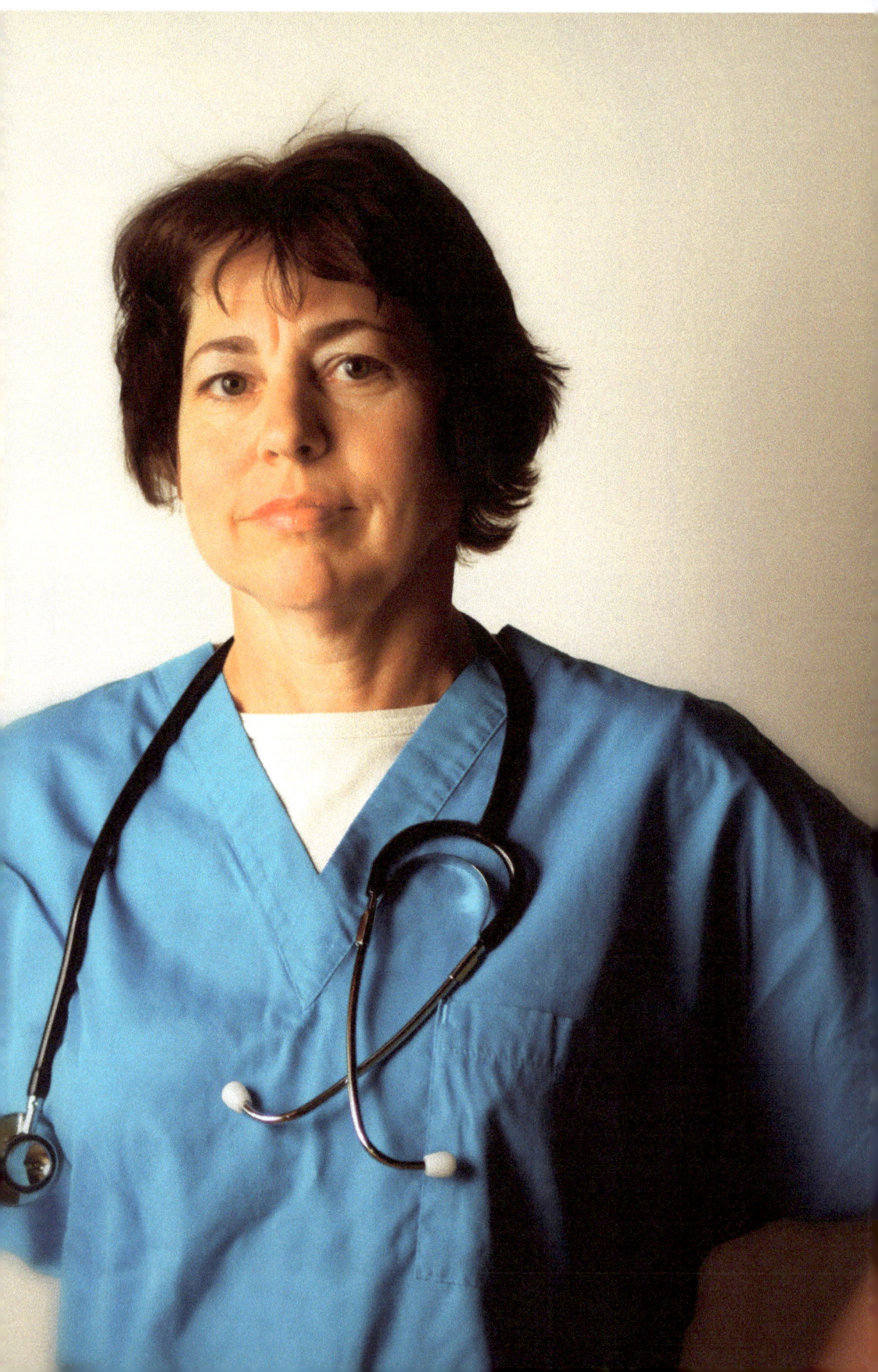

CHAPTER 3

Supervision of junior staff

'Ideally junior doctors should only carry out tasks within their competency, and have a responsibility to contact senior staff if they get out of their depth. Unfortunately, due to their lack of experience, junior doctors may fail to recognise when they are out of their depth.'

—Ron Paterson
New Zealand Health and Disability Commissioner

Introduction

If poor supervision is suspected of contributing to the injury or death of a mother or baby, supervising doctors, midwives, junior staff members and the hospital could all become involved in the legal process. This chapter contains cases concerned with supervision and on-call issues as well as guidelines from a number of sources on the supervisory process. Knowing the level of competence of junior staff being supervised, training juniors to seek help 'sooner than later', making sure that lines of communication are known (and open) and that no stigma attaches to seeking help or querying orders will all assist in the management of risk.

Common concerns of midwives about RMOs, for example, have included their inexperience in:

- telephone advice,
- IV cannulation,
- insertion of speculum,
- vaginal examination,
- interpretation of CTGs and
- suturing perineums.

One midwife who attended a workshop I facilitated suggested new RMOs need to 'double up' and be taken through many facets of labour and delivery, so they are not thrown in at the deep end, especially on their first night.

A Victorian coroner identified a further risk when he recommended that a tertiary hospital examine the culture that had developed where junior medical staff, despite the urging of nurses, were often fearful of ringing a consultant at 3 am.[1] New Zealand Health and Disability Commissioner Ron Paterson makes the same point when he cautions that the expected response of a specialist to calls for advice profoundly affects the behaviour of junior staff, who are far more likely to contact specialists who are available and approachable.[2] None of this will be news to midwives, RMOs or consultants who remember the rigours of their own training.

The Douglas Inquiry into obstetric and gynaecological services at the King Edward Memorial Hospital[3] in Perth, Western Australia in 2001, addressed a number of the key concerns about supervision.

Recommendations from that inquiry included:

- The introduction of on-site, 24 hours a day, 7 days a week obstetric cover by senior doctors to ensure supervision of junior doctors.
- The consultant rostered to the Delivery Suite on a weekday was not to be rostered to any other area in order to provide direct and indirect teaching and supervision of junior medical staff.
- Clear policy statements to ensure fail-safe lines of communication when a midwife or nurse holds concerns for patient safety or comfort that have not been addressed by the junior medical staff.
- Residents and registrars to be certified as competent before interpreting CTG traces and managing a non-reassuring trace.
- A senior clinician, competent in perineal repair, to be responsible for the training of registrars and residents, who are to be assessed as competent before performing a perineal repair on patients without supervision.

What is 'supervision'?

Two cases (one not concerned with maternity services) make important legal points. The first case arose out of a death under anaesthetic at an English hospital in the 1950s.

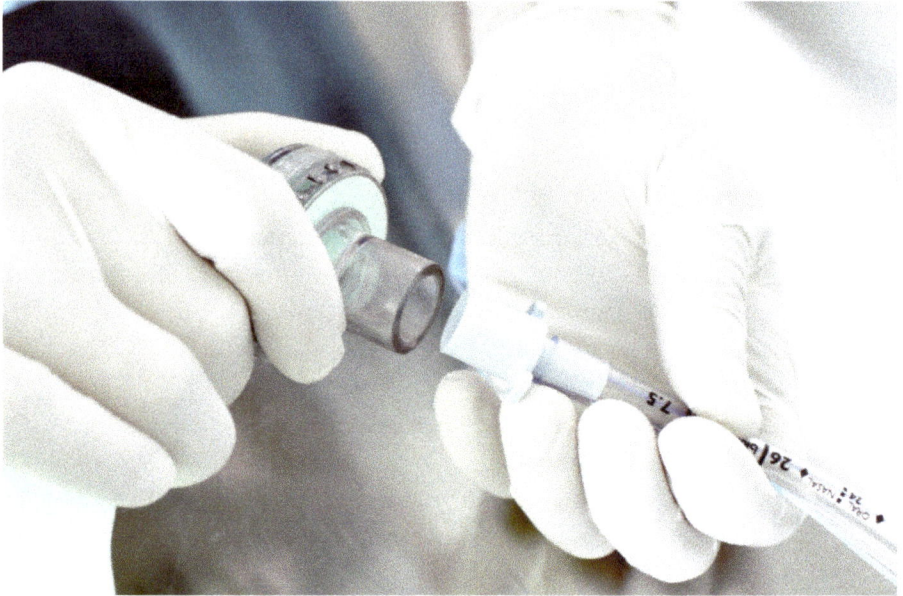

Jones v Manchester Corporation [UK, 1952][4]

The facts

Mr Jones was brought to casualty with facial burns. A house surgeon of two years' standing was in charge of cleaning the facial area and decided to anaesthetise the patient with nitrous oxide. A junior house surgeon (of five months' standing) acted as anaesthetist and commenced administration of the gas. When the patient was either unconscious or semiconscious, it was discovered that the mask covered some of the burned areas. The two doctors then decided to administer Pentothal. The junior doctor administered a full dose to Mr Jones, who died as a result.

The trial

The trial judge held that the junior doctor was negligent, not only in administering a full dose of Pentothal to an already anaesthetized patient, but also in the method of administration - too swiftly and without watching the patient's condition.

The appeal. In the Court of Appeal, Lord Denning was of the view that the senior doctor was also negligent. He was in charge of the operation; he had decided to use the nitrous oxide; the two doctors had then decided to use Pentothal. If the administration of pentothal needed special care and skill, then the senior doctor should have been consulted. The junior doctor had administered the pentothal 'under his very eyes and to his entire approval.'[5] The senior doctor therefore had a greater share in the responsibility.

Jones stands for the proposition that the right of a senior doctor (or, as matter of principle, any senior health professional) to rely upon junior assistants is never an absolute one. Where the junior is known to be inexperienced, the senior comes under a duty to exercise more detailed supervision. This will also be the case where the senior doctor has no previous experience of a 'team' and no first-hand knowledge of their capabilities.

....

The second case questions whether a consultant (in this instance, a gynaecologist) is entitled to assume that a trainee who is allowed by a hospital to continue in a training programme has in fact passed the earlier stages of that programme, having achieved an appropriate level of competence.

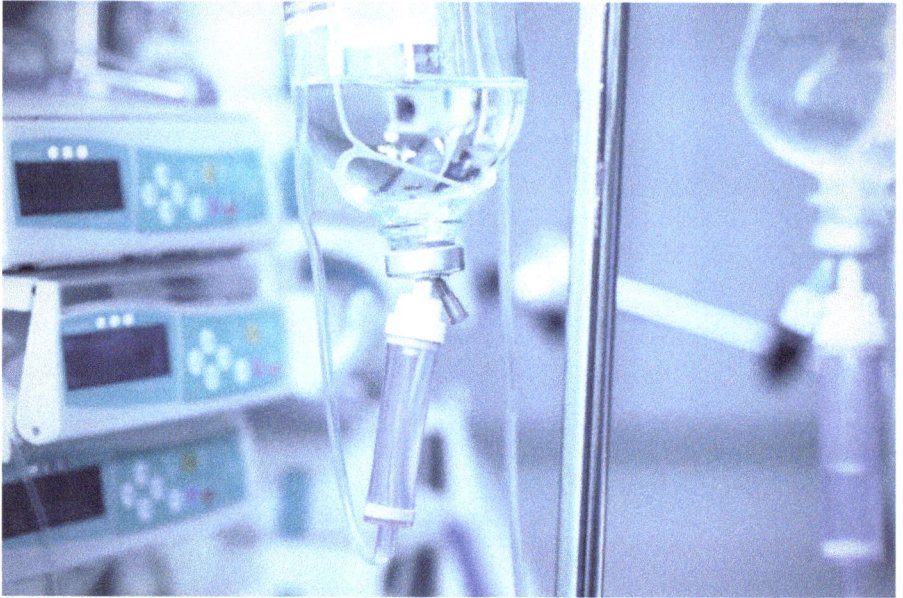

Brus v Australian Capital Territory [Aus, 2007][6]

The facts

Kay was admitted as a public patient in September 1998 for a vaginal hysterectomy. The consultant obstetrician had previously delivered her children under private health cover. When Kay continued to complain of pain and discomfort post discharge, it was discovered that her right fallopian tube had prolapsed into her vagina.

Negligence was alleged.

The trial

The court heard that the vaginal hysterectomy had been carried out by a surgical registrar, under the consultant's supervision. While an experienced consultant obstetrician would have performed this routine procedure in less than 40 minutes, the registrar had taken an hour.

Kay said that the consultant had told her that he would personally perform the surgery. She said that had she known the surgery was to be performed by a registrar, she would have declined the procedure. She alleged negligence against the consultant and the hospital because it:

- permitted a registrar to perform the procedure.
- failed to inform her that the operation was to be performed by the registrar and
- failed to inform her of the registrar's qualifications and experience.

The consultant said that he always told his public patients they would be admitted as his patients. The surgery would be performed under his list, but he might be assisted by, or would himself assist, a registrar.

No guarantee given. The judge found that Kay was mistaken in her recollection. An experienced surgeon, familiar with dealing with both private and public patients, would not have given a guarantee to a public patient that they would be treated as a private patient, so guaranteeing his individual services. The admission form (signed by Kay) acknowledged that the hospital would make the decision as to which doctor would perform the procedure:

Most people would say, as the plaintiff has said in this case that, given the choice between an experienced consultant surgeon and a registrar, who is a qualified medical practitioner undergoing a training program to qualify as a specialist, they would choose the experienced consultant. This would have two effects if such a duty existed. The waiting list for procedures would clearly expand significantly, but more seriously, registrars would not be able to perform the procedures, under close supervision, that they need to qualify as specialists, resulting eventually in a dearth of suitably trained specialists.[7]

Fallopian tube caught. In this case, the negligence occurred when the registrar caught the fallopian tube within the suture line as she was closing the incision in the vaginal vault. This occurred on the internal side, and could not have been observed by the consultant.

Qualifications. The judge accepted evidence that it was appropriate to permit a level-three registrar to undertake a vaginal hysterectomy under close supervision, but it would never be appropriate to permit a level-two registrar to undertake such a procedure. In this instance, the hospital was negligent in holding the registrar out as a level-three registrar, in good standing, capable of performing the procedure. The hospital was, in fact, in possession of adverse assessment reports showing that the registrar had been rated unsatisfactory for surgical skills as a level-two registrar.

The judge found that had the consultant been properly informed he would have simply taken over and performed the procedure himself:

A consultant is entitled to assume that a trainee who is allowed to continue in the program has passed the earlier parts of the program at a satisfactory level, and is entitled to assume that a registrar at a given level holds the appropriate skills for that level.[8]

The consultant said that when he was supervising a level-three registrar:

If I perceive that they are not competent or technically there's a difficulty beyond their level of expertise then I'll relieve them of that duty and I will take over the surgery.[9]

The decision

1. There was no general duty of care on a public hospital to provide public patients with a choice of doctor or to inform them as to the academic standing of a registrar.
2. A hospital has a duty to ensure that it provides patients with suitably qualified staff. (In this instance, the rigorous training programme of The Royal Australian and New Zealand College of Obstetricians and Gynaecologists ensures that, at each stage of their training, a registrar in good standing is suitably qualified to perform the range of procedures commensurate with their training.).
3. The registrar, known by the hospital to have major deficiencies in surgical techniques for a level-two registrar, was held out to the consultant

as a level–three registrar, and he allowed her to perform a procedure that he would not have allowed a level-two registrar to perform.

Damages awarded against the hospital.

....

In the following case, the court hears a number of doctors attempt to explain what supervision entails in obstetrics. Note that although the two supervising doctors gave evidence of their usual practice of touring the labour wards, hospital records did not contain any notation that either doctor had seen the patient.

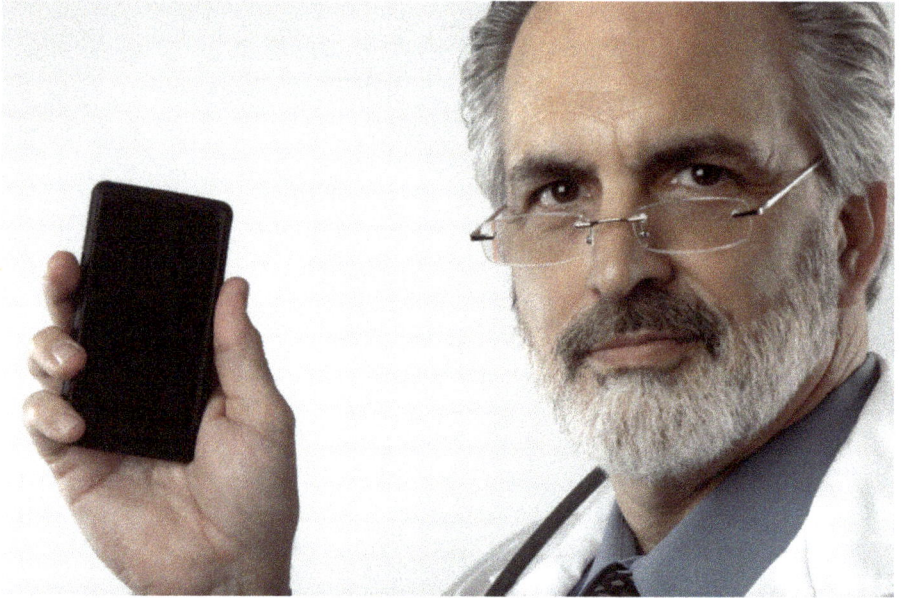

Rouse v Pitt County Memorial Hospital, Inc [US, 1994][10]

The facts

Elise's pregnancy presented a risk. She was obese, suffered from chronic hypertension and had a family history of diabetes. It was alleged that two doctors had been negligent in their supervision of residents who failed to monitor her labour properly or recognise that her son was in fetal distress. Though no details of care are given, this judgment notes that labour and delivery records demonstrated that junior doctors were 'not able to give, and did not give'[11] obstetric care that complied with appropriate standards.

The trial

Expert evidence. The court heard evidence that hospital policies do not usually require supervising doctors to personally examine each patient admitted while they are on-call, nor are doctors required to review all medical charts. On-call doctors are permitted to provide cover by being present or, unless a problem develops or is specifically anticipated, being available by telephone if needed urgently.

Duty to know competency. Medical experts told the court that it is the duty of supervising doctors to know the competency level of the residents they supervise. This duty to know competency is not only necessary but essential in order to provide safe and adequate care.

One of the defendant doctors said he understood that supervision can vary depending upon the extended training of the residents:

At times, I think supervision can be actually doing a task in the form of teaching. I think supervision could be holding someone's hand while they do something. I think supervision could be observing them while they do something and commenting about their performance. I think supervision could be saying please don't do that; let me do that. I think supervision could be a combination of all these things, but basically I think supervision involves being able to respond when called on to help. Supervision involves being certain that the patient is being cared for well.[11]

Calling the hospital. One doctor said a supervising doctor should call in at the beginning of a shift and periodically thereafter to check on the condition of patients. Another doctor told the court attending doctors should 'tour' the wards with residents to assure themselves that patients were receiving satisfactory care. Both defendent doctors explained that each time they were on-call they would make rounds with the residents to assure themselves that things were under control and to address any problems.

The decision

The court was guided by the principle that supervising doctors who, as attending doctors, accepted responsibility to supervise resident doctors, and who were aware when they accepted such responsibility that the residents were actually treating patients, owed a duty to the patients to exercise reasonable care in supervising those resident doctors.

Usual practice. Despite the fact that the supervising doctors presented evidence of usual practice, there was no evidence that either supervising doctor had actually toured the wards on the day the patient had given birth. Her records revealed no notations by either doctor that might indicate they had seen her.

Judgment given originally in favour of the defendant doctors, reversed.

While doctors struggled somewhat to explain supervision in *Rouse's* case, New Zealand Health and Disability Commissioner Ron Paterson, writing on supervisory responsibilities of specialists, cuts to the chase:

Ideally junior doctors should only carry out tasks within their competency, and have a responsibility to contact senior staff if they get out of their depth. Unfortunately, due to their lack of experience, junior doctors may fail to recognise when they are out of their depth.[13]

Paterson recommends:

1. Junior doctors should participate in an orientation program whenever they move to a new speciality or a new hospital. Such a program should include information on how the consultant likes things done, with a clear indication of the consultant's expectations.
2. Junior doctors should be informed about lines of communication with their specialist during normal working hours and on-call hours. Ground rules for communicating with other team members should also be set out and house officers clearly directed that if they are not satisfied with their registrar's response, they should contact the specialist directly.
3. Specialists should have a regular and well-understood timetable so that junior doctors know where and how to contact them. Junior doctors should be encouraged to make contact early, rather than 'battle on alone' until the situation is irretrievable. Junior doctors should also be encouraged to preface phone conversations with clear indicators of why they are calling — for approval of a management plan, advice or active assistance.

4. The expected response of a specialist to calls for advice profoundly affects the behaviour of junior staff, who are far more likely to contact specialists if they are available and approachable.

5. Clear clinical notes, including comprehensive management plans, help to ensure the patient is treated in accordance with the specialist's wishes. These can include parameters clarifying when specialist involvement is required for that particular patient — and can serve as an aid to, rather than substitute for, the junior doctor's clinical judgment.

6. Junior doctors should have regular feedback and specialists should seek the opinion of other ward staff, particularly the charge nurse, on the junior doctor's performance. Poor performance should not go unaddressed.

7. Written policies/guidelines based on established professional standards help to protect the patient, the specialist and the junior doctor. At Rotorua Hospital in New Zealand, for example, standing orders state that it is the duty of the house surgeon to examine all patients coming under his/her care immediately after they have been admitted. The house surgeon must, as a minimum, notify his or her senior officer of all emergencies, unforeseen complications and cases where the question of surgery arises. The timing of this can be varied by agreement, depending on the experience of the junior doctor, but, once notified of a problem, the senior medical officer becomes responsible.

....

Paterson cites the following case that came before the Medical Practitioners' Disciplinary Tribunal in New Zealand. On appeal, the judge warned that: 'It cannot be right that supervision can be relaxed for the benefit of the junior doctor's progress, if this poses a risk to the patient.'

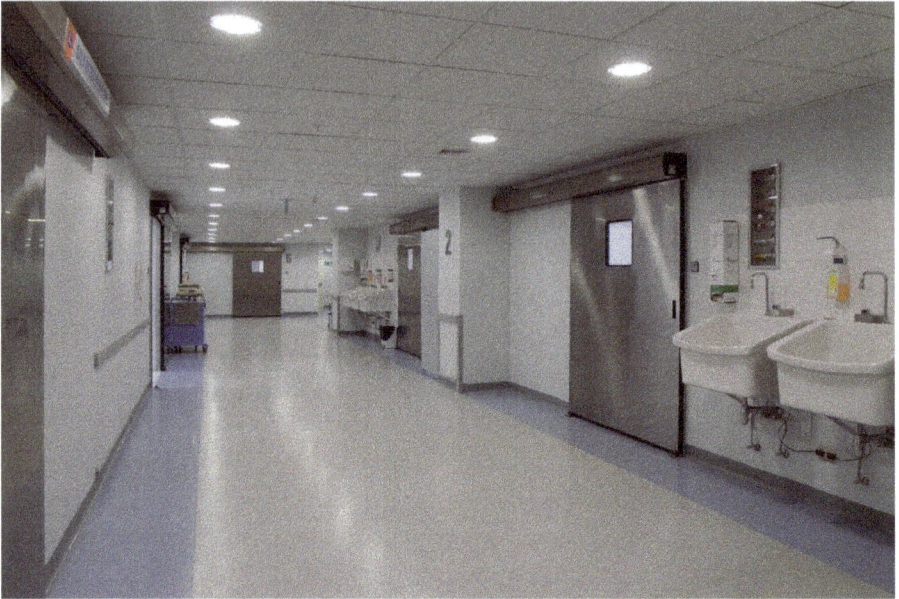

Director of Proceedings (Mrs V) v Dr Mc [NZ, 2001][14]

The facts

Theresa, aged 42, was admitted to hospital for delivery of her seventh baby. She was obese, with high blood pressure, and had a history of large babies. A previous emergency caesarean section had been performed for fetal distress. The registrar on-call delegated management of Theresa's labour to a senior midwife and to a senior house surgeon from overseas. The registrar had never worked directly with the senior house surgeon, but had been told that he was a very experienced doctor, soon to be considered for a registrar's position.

During the labour, the registrar relied on reports from the midwife and the senior house surgeon. She did not personally assess Theresa until urgently summoned when the CTG indicated the baby's heartbeat had ceased. The senior house surgeon appeared to have departed from the agreed management plan and missed warning signs of fetal distress. The baby was born without a heartbeat and could not be resuscitated.

The decision

The Tribunal found that the registrar had failed to take responsibility and fulfil the role expected of a registrar when supervising junior staff, but that her conduct did not fall so far short of acceptable standards as to warrant an adverse disciplinary finding.

The Director of Public Prosecutions appealed successfully. During the appeal, the judge commented:

A doctor supervising junior staff must be expected to make reasonable observations of their competence and draw reasonable conclusions on what is observed. The judgment so formed will in turn form still further judgments as to how great the degree of delegation to those staff members should be ... But delegation, while permissible, cannot be at the expense of the patient's well-being. It cannot be right that supervision should be relaxed for the benefit of the pupil doctor's progress if such a course carries a risk for the patient.[15]

Paterson notes that the registrar had appealed to the High Court.

Acceptance of responsibility. Consultant obstetrician and gynaecologist Dr Roger Clements[16] writes that whatever their attitude to delegation of care, consultants have a duty to provide a reasonable standard of treatment for the women for whom they have accepted responsibility; and believes they need:

1. To satisfy themselves that the person to whom they delegate a particular task or responsibility is competent to carry it out safely and properly, having generally observed the abilities and skills of their junior medical staff. Generally, it would be wrong to assume by reference to their past anecdotal experience, the recommendation of others or the mere possession of paper qualifications that the person concerned is either sufficiently skilled or competent to carry out the duty assigned.
2. To provide guidelines in principle for their junior staff, including nurses, midwives and doctors.

3. To leave explicit instructions in individual cases to warn of foreseeable difficulties, to call for advice and to ask for more experienced skill.
4. To ensure that nurses and midwives know they can obtain consultant advice directly to override the decision of junior medical staff.
5. To be ready to attend in person, or know that there is a named deputy of equivalent rank experience who can be called in their stead, whenever complications demanding their presence arise.

Clements, commenting on labour ward organization, maintains:

Nowhere is communication between various levels of staff more important. The chain of command is often difficult. The judgment of the senior midwife is often superior to that of the inexperienced SHO (or even the registrar). In every labour ward, the senior midwife should have the authority to go over the head of the junior doctor if she feels that decisions are not being taken appropriately.[17]

Should an order be followed?

Whether or not a junior member of staff is obliged to follow an order of a senior doctor was addressed in the English case of *Junor v McNicol*[18] (a case concerned with the amputation of a child's arm). The House of Lords held that as a general principle, where instructions were manifestly wrong, 'duty and common sense combined to say they must not be followed.'[19] (The Oxford Dictionary defines 'manifest' as clear, obvious to eye or mind.) Whether or not an order is 'clearly wrong' will be a question of fact to be determined by the court.

There is no reason why, as a matter of principle, this reasoning should not apply to midwives. A number of courts have acknowledged that nurses, for example in medical surgical wards, are highly skilled professionals who frequently hold the life and death of patients in their hands. Because of the nature of this close relationship, nurses have a duty to query orders if they know, or should know, that the order is placing their patient at foreseeable risk. If not professionally satisfied by the response, the nurse's duty to the patient is to refer the matter to management as soon as possible, so that appropriate action can be taken.

Good risk management will therefore need to recognize that:

- Some midwives and junior doctors are more experienced and assertive than others.
- Disagreements will occur over clinical care.

Hospital policy should provide clear guidelines for managing these predictable disagreements about clinical care. Underpinning such policy is the acknowledgement that in the delivery of safe midwifery, obstetric and neonatal care, the welfare of mothers and babies should not be dependent on who is on duty.

....

The next four cases further explore the concepts of supervision and being 'on-call.' In the first case the question before the court was specific: Did the obstetrician on-call have a responsibility to call the hospital and ascertain the condition of patients, to formulate plans of management and to call periodically to check their status?

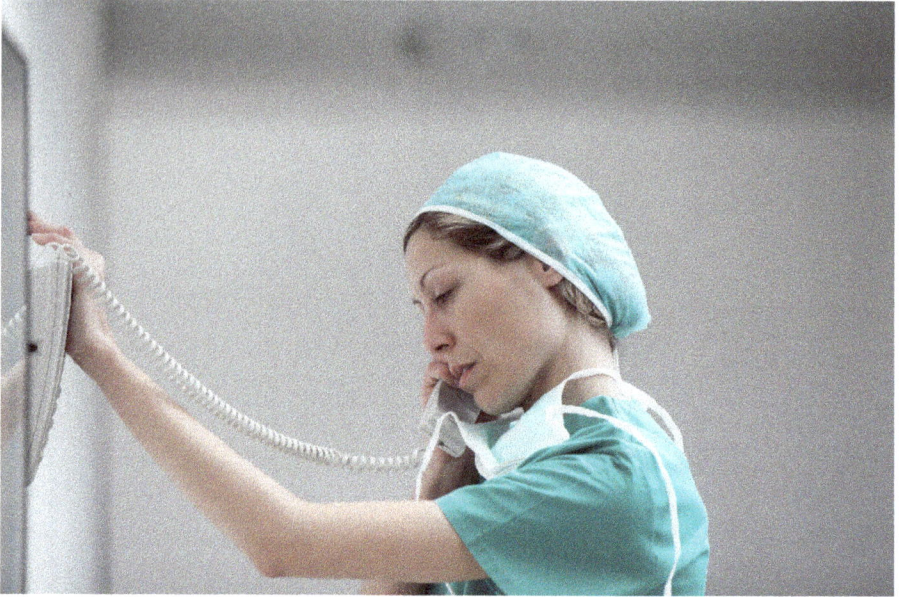

Mozingo v Pitt County Memorial Hospital, Inc. [US, 1992][20]

The facts

Kirsten was admitted in the afternoon for the delivery of her second child. At 5.00 pm, the obstetrician began his on-call coverage for the obstetrics residents at the hospital. The obstetrician had remained at home available to take telephone calls from the residents until shortly before 9.45 pm. He then received a call from an RMO saying there was a problem with Kirsten's delivery. The obstetrician immediately left home, but when he arrived at the hospital the baby, already delivered, had suffered injury.

The trial

Specific claim. It was alleged that the obstetrician had negligently supervised the residents who cared for the mother and baby during the birth.

There was no argument that the obstetrician was negligent in responding to the telephone call or in anything he did, or failed to do, after receiving the call. The claim was specific. As the supervising doctor, the obstetrician had a responsibility to call the hospital at the beginning of his shift to ascertain what obstetric patients had been admitted and their condition, to formulate plans of management, and to call periodically to check on their status.

No direct contact. The obstetrician argued that he was never in direct contact with Kirsten, nor was he consulted by the treating residents or in any way involved in her care.

Decision. Acknowledging that the modern provision of medical care is a complex process, the court nevertheless upheld the patient's claim that negligent supervision had been the cause of her child's injuries.

Damages awarded.

....

The second case concerns an on-call issue in a New South Wales hospital. The incident occurred in 1995 and was settled in 2003 for $7.5 million plus costs. The health service then commenced proceedings against the VMO who had been on call at the time, to claim contribution to the damages.

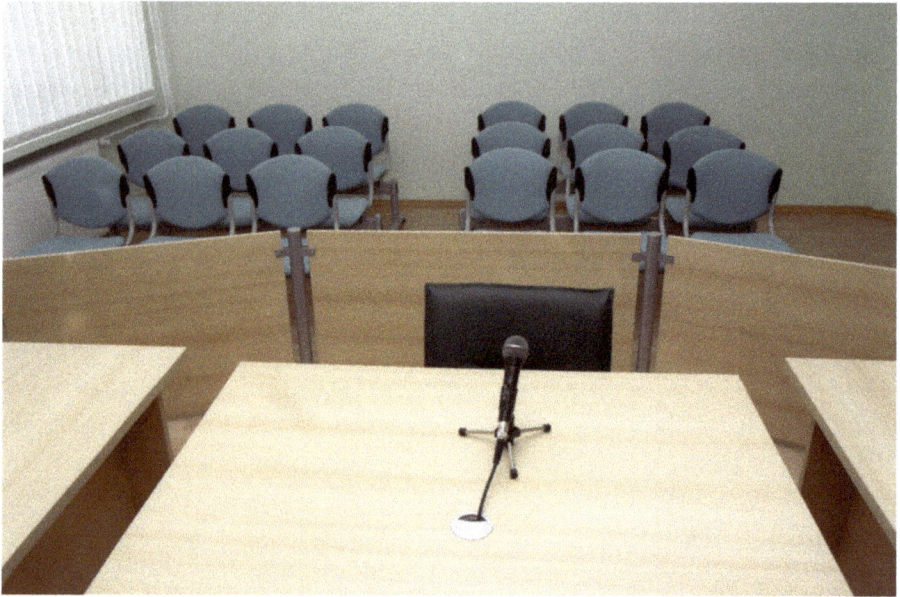

Greater Southern Area Health Service v Angus [Aus, 2007][21]

The facts

On 25 September 1995, an obstetrician was on-call at the hospital every one week in five; the on-call period was for one week. There was no dispute that he was responsible for the proper care and management of all patients admitted under his care. A junior registrar in obstetrics at the hospital, with 15 months' experience in that position, was under the supervision of the senior registrar in obstetrics and of the VMOs who specialized in obstetrics, including the obstetrician in question.

No abnormalities. The junior registrar saw Kerry in the antenatal clinic on 5 September 1995, detected no abnormalities and assessed her for continuing management in the midwife's clinic. On 19 September, Kerry was admitted to hospital and the junior registrar saw her at about 12.20 pm. He noted that she was thirty-eight and a half weeks' gestation, the membrane had ruptured spontaneously at 7 am and she was not distressed. Blood pressure, pulse and temperature were unremarkable. On palpation, the fetus was found to be lying in a right occipito-transverse position.

The junior registrar noted in the progress chart:

Plan

1. Await events
2. I will D/W (discuss with) (the obstetrician), re Syntocinon if not contracting
3. (CTG) good.[22]

Birthing suite. The junior registrar, who was working a day shift, next saw Kerry between 9.15 am and 9.20 am the following morning in the birthing suite, which was located in the labour ward. His note of the examination was started at 9.35 am with the date and time and his name but no more. The rest of the note was made at 9.55 am. (Later accepted by the judge as the time the note was made, not the time of attendance.)

Slow progress. The junior registrar noted that there had been slow progress in the labour since the cervix had dilated to 6 cm and contractions had eased over the previous three quarters of an hour. Kerry was pushing. The fetal heart rate, assessed by a midwife using a Dopplor, was satisfactory. The junior registrar found that the cervix was fully dilated and the head of the fetus was in occipito-transverse lie. There was moulding and mild caput. His assessment was that Kerry had either a deep transverse arrest or incoordinate contractions, with partial rotation from the occipito-posterior position.

The junior registrar noted :

Plan

1. Syntocinon
2. R/V [review] after 30-60 minutes of good contractions.[23]

Midwifery notes. Irregular contractions had been recorded from 9 am. The partogram record noted that a student midwife made a vaginal examination at about 9.15 and that her findings were confirmed by the junior registrar. Syntocinon was administered at 9.45 am. An inconclusive (non-reassuring) CTG trace was obtained at 9.59 am. Intermittent ascultation was used to monitor the fetal heart rate. The partogram noted that between 10 am and 10.15 am contractions were becoming regular. The Syntocinon rate was increased from twenty to thirty ml/hour at 10.15 am.

Midwifery staff telephoned the junior registrar when the baby's head was on view and were instructed to continue.

Delivery. The midwifery note: 'Progressed to a difficult delivery of head by (senior midwife) and head easily rotated manually ...'.[24] When Kerry was unable to deliver the shoulders, the midwife discovered the umbilical cord was tightly wrapped around the neck. The midwife cut and clamped the cord, but was still unable to deliver the shoulders. Kerry was taken off the bed and, while squatting, the baby was quickly delivered at 10.58 am by the midwife pulling firmly on his head, and taken to the resuscitation table. The junior registrar was paged (sometime between 11.05 am and 11.10 am) and returned in haste to the birthing suite about five minutes later.

Emergency. The baby was born clinically dead, with no fetal heartbeat. The emergency button was pressed moments after the baby was being bagged and masked and (probably) before cardiac massage was commenced. Apgar scores were zero at one and five minutes and 3 at ten minutes, with a score of 1 for heart rate and 2 for colour. Somewhere between one and five minutes there was a sub-optimal fetal heart beat.

Injury. The brain damage suffered during the labour and delivery resulted in a number of disabilities, including cerebral palsy, epilepsy and moderate intellectual disability.

The trial

The claim that there had been negligence in the management of the labour and delivery having been settled, the health service now claimed financial contribution from the obstetrician who had been on call.

The crucial questions were :

1. Was the obstetrician consulted by the junior registrar in connection with the augmentation of labour by intravenous Syntocinon?
2. If so, should the obstetrician have ensured that certain procedures were put in place as precautions against the risks to the mother (and particularly the baby) associated with such augmentation? It was not

suggested that administration of Syntocinon was inappropriate or negligent. It was argued that augmentation posed certain risks and that had monitoring been undertaken, intervention in the delivery would have occurred which, in all probability, would have resulted in the baby being born uninjured.

Move from birthing suite. It was also argued that Kerry should have been moved out of the birthing suite into a labour room bed since, once her labour had been augmented by Syntocinon, she was no longer a low-risk patient. Being in a labour ward made certain delivery procedures easier.

Concession. The health service conceded that if the obstetrician was not informed of the proposal to administer Syntocinon, then there was no basis of claiming contribution.

The junior registrar

No recollection. The junior registrar admitted that he had no recollection of speaking to the obstetrician, but believed he had done so. This was based on his belief that he was not sufficiently experienced at the time to make such a decision without speaking to the obstetrician. There was also a strong likelihood that the obstetrician was in the labour ward at the time and the junior registrar said that he would usually accompany the obstetrician on his rounds.

The obstetrician

Identifying problems. The obstetrician agreed that he had been on-call and had done ward rounds between 8.30 and 9.30 am. He said that, unless he had been asked to visit patients for a specific reason, it was likely that he commenced his round on the labour ward and then went down to the maternity and other wards. The senior medical officer or the registrar in obstetrics would usually accompany him. The obstetrician said it was his practice on arrival at the labour ward to go to the nurses station, where the senior registered medical officer (in this case the junior registrar) or registrar would identify any patients about whom there were concerns. Where the registrar had not performed the check, the obstetrician assumed that a member of the midwifery staff would alert him to any issues that might have required his attention.

Hospital records. Relying on his records for the day, the obstetrician believed that he had completed his rounds by 9.30 am and left the hospital. On the other hand, he was due at another hospital (a five-minute drive away) at 9.15 am and there was no note on his copy of the list for the day at that hospital of any delay, although it was his nurse's practice to make a note if this occurred. The hospital records showed (the obstetrician thought mistakenly) that the junior registrar's decision to augment Kerry's labour was made at about 9.45 am.

No specific recollection. The obstetrician was in no doubt that he was not involved in Kerry's labour as the VMO, but admitted he did not have a specific recollection one way or the other. He would not have expected to have been consulted about a decision to augment labour after the commencement of the second stage of labour by someone like the junior registrar, who was near the end of his training and in whom he had full confidence, unless there were particular reasons giving rise to a concern. If he had been asked whether Syntocinon should be used, then he would have been involved

The decision

The judge found:

1. The junior registrar did not consult the obstetrician about whether Syntocinon should be administered.
2. The omission to monitor by CTG or monitor by auscultation with sufficient frequency (both issues canvassed at length in the judgment) made no material contribution to the baby's injuries.

The obstetrician received judgment in his favour.

Associate Professor Thomas Faunce, writing in 2008 in the *Journal of Law and Medicine*,[25] comments that the Angus case raises particular issues about the responsibilities of on-call VMOs. The practice of the VMO in question seemed to be to rely on registrars and midwifery staff to alert him to any problems with any of the patients. Faunce queries whether the specialist college concerned or the hospital produced a guideline about on-call responsibilities and whether the doctor had consulted it.

Note the recommendation in the Douglas Report on the O&G unit at King Edward Memorial Hospital, Perth, that the morning and evening rounds in the Delivery Suite are to be attended by the on-call consultant, an anaesthe-tist (or registrar) and neonatologist (or registrar) in addition to the Delivery Suite midwife co-ordinator, Delivery Suite registrar and resident. The on-call consultant is to be informed of all new admissions of women in high-risk categories and is to approve the care plan. Further, all these actions are to be documented.

....

In the next case, a Canadian court marks the need for close scrutiny and su-pervision of an inexperienced midwife, and defines a number of roles within the obstetric team.

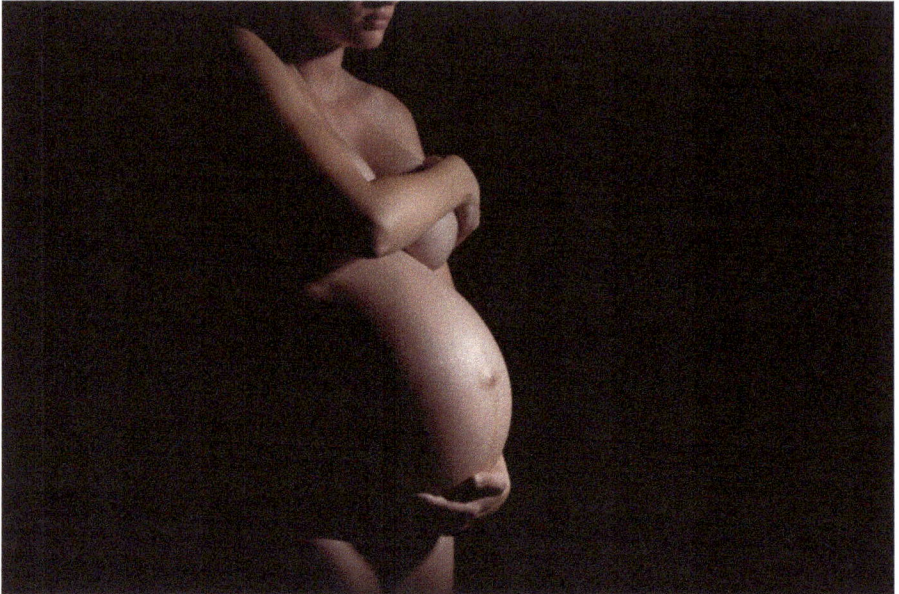

Grainger v Ottawa General Hospital [Canada, 1996]²⁶

The facts

Jessica was in active labour when she arrived at the hospital. Monitoring indicated true labour, with no complications. After artificial rupture of the membranes, a fetal monitor was applied by the student midwife. This showed deep severe decelerations, indicating oxygen deprivation for the entire period (no times noted in judgment) the monitor was on. The baby, delivered by emergency caesarean section, suffered severe brain damage.

The trial

The court found that the student midwife was in breach of the standard of care. A competent midwife would have assessed the strip and alerted the doctor after 20 minutes. Had the doctors been properly alerted, surgical intervention would have saved the baby from irreversible brain damage.

Failure to supervise. In addition, the supervising midwife had completely failed to perform her assigning and supervisory duties in accordance with appropriate standards. If she had done so, there was a chance that she or other midwives might have picked up the severe decelerations.

The decision

The court held that the hospital had clearly breached its duty to ensure a 'minimum level of competency' of midwives in the obstetric unit. The hospital was responsible for the training of the student midwife, and for ensuring that she was subjected to 'close scrutiny and supervision' once she was assigned to the obstetrical unit.

Damages awarded.

....

The last case in this chapter again makes the point that inexperience (in this instance of two midwives new to the birthing suite teamed with an inexperienced resident) can put a baby at risk if staff are not clear as to their roles and responsibilities, particularly as to who is acting as supervisor.

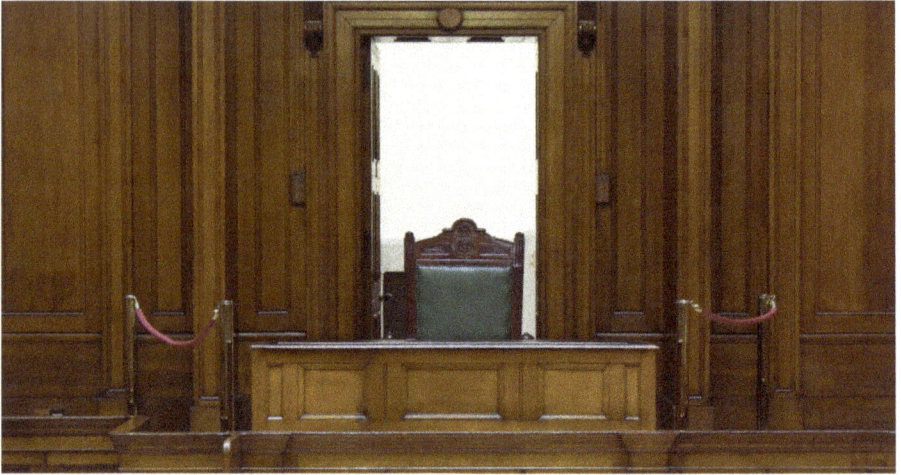

Coronial Investigation
Case No: 0057/2007 [Aus, 2009][27]

The facts

Valerie saw midwives for most of her pregnancy, then moved closer to her family and had one visit to the antenatal clinic at the hospital in that area. When she was 35 weeks' and six days' gestation (considered premature), her waters broke at 3.40 am. Valerie went to the hospital and, though not in active labour, was admitted to the delivery suite to see if labour progressed.

Junior staff. Early in this period, a junior male midwife asked if he could be involved and wanted to feel Valerie's stomach. She agreed at first, but then formed the view that he had 'no idea'[28] and told staff that she did not want junior staff involved. She was told this might not be possible but that she would be informed of the level of experience of those caring for her.

Active labour. Valerie went into labour early the next morning. At 3 am, a vaginal examination showed she was 4 cm dilated and in active labour. An IV cannula was inserted and IV antibiotics started; a partogram and CTG were commenced at around 4 am. At 7.20 am, the cervix was still only 4 cm dilated. An epidural was performed at 9.35 am.

Midwifery roster. The roster provided for a team leader (with a supervisory role) and two other midwives on the birth suite. The team leader was midwife S and midwife H was the midwife allocated to Valerie.

Obstetric roster. This roster provided for a consultant, registrar and resident. At 8.50 am, Valerie was reviewed by the medical team. The resident, who was doing his GP Diploma,[29] had done 10 out of the 25 required deliveries. He was under the supervision of the midwife and stayed with Valerie most of the day.

Syntocinon commenced. At 10.50 am, Syntocinon IV was commenced. (Evidence was later given that this drug, given intravenously, increases uterine contractions. It also increases the risk to the baby as very strong, frequent contractions can cause distress to the baby.)

High-risk. Valerie was in the higher risk category because of the baby's prematurity, the epidural and the Syntocinon drip. Contractions increased to a high rate and a vaginal examination at 11.20 am showed the cervix 7 cm dilated—a rapid progress. The Syntocinon dose was increased. There was no note as to the frequency or regularity of contractions and no indication that the midwife had any concerns. The registrar saw Valerie at 11.30 am and signed the CTG to indicate she had reviewed it. Limited clinical notes were made from this time although the CTG continued and the partogram was completed graphically.

The CTG. While the evidence later showed there were significant concerns with the CTG (with particular concerns at 12.40 pm and 3.20 pm), these concerns were neither recognized nor acted upon by staff. When some decelerations occurred, the midwife wrote 'maternal'[30] suggesting she considered that the heart rate was Valerie's rather than the baby's. (Evidence was later given that the trace was the baby's and, if a fetal scalp clip had been applied to the baby's head, this uncertainty would have been removed.)

Second stage. A vaginal examination conducted by the resident at 3.20 pm showed the cervix fully dilated and Valerie in the second stage of labour. Midwife H was relieved for her lunch break from 1.30 pm to 2.05 pm, but Valerie was not told that the relieving staff member was a student midwife. It was not clear who midwife H handed over to at the end of her shift at 3.50 pm, but at 4.10 pm midwife W took over Valerie's care. The team now consisted of team leader midwife Y, who had taken over at 1 pm, midwife

W, and a student. The resident was still present. The consultant came to the ward and conferred with the midwifery team leader. She did not see Valerie, later saying she had been reassured that things were progressing normally.

Active pushing. Valerie commenced active pushing at 4.30 pm. Midwife W was concerned that Valerie had been in the second stage for 40 minutes. She consulted her team leader about the unit guidelines and was told that until a woman has an urge to push, the second stage can be up to two hours. Once she has the urge, she can push and, if no progress has been made after 30 minutes, then a review is required.

Birth. A baby girl was born at 5.42 pm—72 minutes after active pushing started. The cord, wrapped around her neck and shoulders, was clamped and cut. She did not breathe spontaneously and was pale and floppy. Her very poor condition surprised staff. Because of the pre-term birth, a paediatric resident had been present since 5.30 pm. The paediatric registrar arrived three minutes after birth and commenced resuscitation; this was continued by the paediatric consultant. The baby was transferred to the NICU, where she died the following day.

No autopsy. Valerie was told that the hospital would be conducting an internal investigation into the baby's death and that an autopsy was not necessary as it would only reveal brain damage. She asked why her daughter's death was not being reported to the coroner and was told repeatedly that it was not a reportable death. Valerie pursued the matter and, after making a formal complaint to the hospital, a report was made (some seven months later) on the grounds that the death was (a) unexpected and (b) the result of an injury sustained during labour.

Cause of death

The cause of death was found to be a lack of oxygen during labour (intrapartum hypoxia).

Failure to report the death

Legal requirement—not discretionary. Failure to report the death was of very real concern to the coroner who noted that there appeared to be a widespread belief at the hospital that the reporting of a "reportable" death was discretionary.[31] The coroner emphasized the mandatory requirement under Coroner's Acts to report unexpected deaths, pointing out that it is a criminal offence not to do so. In this case there was clearly a communication issue between the obstetric and paediatric teams, neither genuinely believing that referral was necessary.

Deficiencies in care

Vaginal examinations. Referring to reports from midwifery and obstetric experts, as well as the Critical Incident Report conducted by the hospital, the coroner found that the wait of four hours between the vaginal examinations at 11.20 am and 3.30 was too long. Most women in pre-term labour would progress very quickly from 7 cm to fully dilated, especially with a contraction frequency of 4-5 in 10 minutes. As Valerie may well have been fully dilated when the CTG trace changed at about 12.40 pm, an opportunity was lost to start her pushing much earlier than 4.20 pm. A vaginal examination should have been done at about 1 pm as part of the investigation of why the CTG trace had changed. This may have led to an expedited delivery and a better outcome.

CTG. Expert witnesses in obstetrics who later reviewed the records said the CTG showed problems just prior to 4.30 pm when Valerie started to push. Once active pushing starts it is difficult to read the trace. If a fetal scalp clip had been attached or a fetal blood sample taken to assess fetal ph, this would have indicated whether the baby was distressed. These actions were not taken. During pushing, the CTG showed that the contractions were too frequent and the fetal heart too high for too long. This was not picked up. There was quite a long delay from the point at which the vertex was first visible at 5.00 pm until the baby was delivered at 5.42 pm, a time when the CTG was, at best, uninterpretable. There was evidence of fetal compromise.

The coroner identified a number of significant issues:

1. Lack of supervision of the labour

The resident. The most senior medical input came from the resident who was a junior doctor in training and did not have a supervisory role. The management of the labour had then reverted 'almost by default'[32] to the midwife, who had taken more of a passive approach.

The registrar. Evidence was given that, at a minimum, a registrar should perform labour ward rounds at least every four hours, visiting high-risk patients perhaps every two hours. The registrar described her job at the hospital as 'exhausting.'[33] She was extremely busy, working a 24-hour shift, then ward round, covering antenatal clinics, and had been in the emergency department when called to see Valerie. The coroner found that this work load explained why the registrar did not return to the ward after 11.30 am.

The consultant. The coroner found that it was not workload issues that prevented the consultant seeing Valerie, but a failure to categorize her as a higher-risk labour that required active medical management.

The consultant had written a retrospective note after the baby was born which included:

Seen by me 08.30, 13.30 and 15.40, Satisfactory progress and Clear Liquor, CTG — Baseline 140/m. Variability — 5–15, Clear liquor throughout, Fully dilated at 15.30, I agreed with plan to allow head to descend before pushing.[34]

A later statement by the consultant that she had no contact with the mother between the ward round at 8.30 am and after the baby was born contradicted the above note. The consultant said she was aware that the mother was progressing normally because she was in touch with her registrar and would have checked a whiteboard which charted the progress of each patient and gone through any concerns with a senior midwife. There was a concern not to 'over-medicalise'[35] normal labour so patients were not routinely checked every few hours. Had she seen Valerie, she would have written notes. The consultant said the registrar should have been involved more by invitation.

Lack of senior medical supervision. The coroner found that the consultant had been content to allow the labour to be supervised by the primary midwife. This was reflected in her notes written at the morning ward round, where there was no suggestion that the birth would be medically managed and no plan written down for any medical monitoring. Experts had shared

Valerie's concern that the lack of senior medical supervision was a major contributing factor to her daughter's death.

2. Midwifery supervision and training in the Birth Suite

Interpretation of CTGs. The coroner found that the interpretation of a CTG is difficult and requires interpreting against the background of a particular case. In this instance, it was not reasonable that this responsibility was left to the midwives. However, even had there been closer medical supervision (with four-hourly or two-hourly review), most likely the midwifery team could be expected to pick up the presence of abnormalities in the CTG and alert the medical team. This had not occurred.

New to birthing suite. The two midwives responsible for Valerie's care were extremely new and had very limited orientation to the birthing suite. The midwifery team leaders, senior and experienced, were unable to supervise fully due to combined clinical and governance roles.

CTG not reviewed. The significant delay in reporting the death meant that statements were taken a considerable time after the events and it was difficult to find out what happened in regard to supervision on that day. On the available evidence the coroner found that a team leader did not review the CTG in any detailed manner after 10 am. It was therefore likely that for the following seven hours the only people who reviewed the CTG were two junior midwives and a resident. This was not acceptable for a high-risk labour.

Skill mixes. The coroner heard evidence that concerns existed at the hospital about the lack of experienced staff and inadequate skill mixes. Team leaders often took a caseload and could not easily mentor students; students were counted in midwifery numbers from the first day of recruitment, even though they were not trained. In Valerie's case these factors may have reduced the effectiveness of the team leader supervising the midwives providing primary care in her high-risk labour.

3. Lack of clarity of roles

Who was managing the labour and birth? There seemed a lack of clarity about who was 'managing' Valerie's labour and birth. Both the midwife and resident were in attendance and both were under the impression that the other was unconcerned about the CTG, Valerie's contractions or the length of the second stage. Midwife H assumed the resident had more responsibility than he actually did and that they were jointly sharing care. In fact, the resident was under the supervision of the midwife in charge and had very limited obstetric experience and knowledge. Midwife W believed she was supervising the resident and he was conducting the delivery. They did not establish who would oversee the elements of labour care.

Assumptions. The coroner found it was easy to see that each primary midwife believed the resident had a greater experience and knowledge than he had. They were new to the birthing suite, had received very brief orientations and were unclear about both the respective roles and responsibilities of midwife and resident and the practice guidelines in the Birthing Unit.

4. Documentation
The Critical Incident Review (CIR) conducted by the hospital pointed out numerous deficiencies in the documentation on the partogram :

a. For the 11.20 am vaginal examination there are no records of the position of the presenting part and no corresponding abdominal palpation recorded.
b. The examination record was not signed.
c. When the CTG was recorded as being reassuring at 11.35 am, there was no corresponding breakdown of how this was assessed.
d. There was no subsequent documentation of CTG interpretation (the CIR said the CTG should be reviewed at regular intervals using a template for interpretation).
e. There was a gap in documentation after 2.15 pm.
f. As there was no evidence in the documentation to suggest that review by a senior medical officer was sought or planned for, there was no evidence that planning and review had taken place.
g. There was inadequate evidence of a care plan (documentation that would reflect risk factors, an action plan with time frames for referral, and review/checks and by whom).

The obstetric consultant who reviewed the records found:

h. Minimal recordings of Valerie's last prenatal visit.

i. Limited information in her records as to discussions about the labour/birth/post-natal period.
j. No plan of care documented during the medical ward round on the morning of the baby's birth.
k. Poor documentation on the partogram during the day shift, with no entries made in the plan/comment section after 2.15 pm until midwife W took over at 4.10 pm. When asked about this, midwife H said she was busy attending to various medical and midwifery duties at the same time, and in a workplace that was quite new to her.
l. No documentation that Valerie was to be told (as earlier agreed) about the experience level of staff caring for her.

The coroner reiterated his concern about the inaccuracy of the consultant's retrospective notes and emphasised the importance of good documentation — not only for patient care but for quality, safety and coronial purposes.

5. Communication with the family

The resident said he had explained to Valerie and her family that he had been a doctor for six years, but thought they may have misinterpreted this to mean he had been an obstetrician for that time. He explained that he was the most junior in the team, but believed it was difficult for patients to understand how the team worked. Valerie had found out after the delivery that the resident was unqualified in obstetrics. The coroner described this as 'particularly unfortunate'[37] as Valerie (who did not want students looking after her) had been reassured that she would be informed of the experience level of those looking after her.

After the baby's death, communication difficulties arose with the consultant and organizational difficulties occurred in relation to changed appointments and unavailability of records.

Changes implemented by the hospital

The consultant apologized on behalf of the department of obstetrics and gynaecology for the sub-optimal care received by Valerie. The hospital acknowledged that there were failings in the system and that they had failed in the care of the baby. A critical incident review had been performed, recommendations from the midwifery and obstetric fields had been adopted and the following changes had been implemented:

1. Clear guidelines had been developed (based on the Australian College of Midwives Consultation and Referral Guidelines) about which labours should be primarily managed by a midwife and which should be primarily medically managed.
2. Midwives would continue to care for all women in labour but decisions about the management of labour and care plans (review and management) would be the responsibility of the registrar/consultant for medically managed labours.
3. There was a clear expectation that the registrar would be available for advice and to oversee those labours that are progressing normally.
4. The registrar's workload in the labour ward was to be reduced. (An elective caesarean section list to be performed three mornings a week and other elective caesarean sections were scheduled in the gynaecology theatre list. It was hoped this would reduce the times the on-duty registrar was taken away to perform these operations at unscheduled times on the emergency theatre list.) An extra registrar position had been approved which would reduce the current 24-hour on- call to 12 hours.
5. The Department of Obstetrics and Gynaecology had clarified the roles of health professionals and these would be emphasized at orientation of medical and midwifery students.
6. Practice guidelines had been developed detailing the role of the resident, the requirement for regular CTG monitoring and the required involvement of senior medical input for high -risk pregnancies.
7. CTG training was now mandatory for medical and midwifery staff and part of the orientation program. Steps had been taken to improve the interpretation of CTGs. A rubber stamp had been developed which was to be placed on the CTG hourly in stage 1 of labour and every 30 minutes in stage 2 of labour, and filled in, to comply with best practice monitoring. If any single element was non-reassuring then the CTG must be identified overall as non-reassuring and signed by the midwife, registrar or consultant, and followed up by referral.
8. Obstetric and midwifery staff had been involved in the psychological and social aspects of perinatal bereavement.

The coroner noted conflicting evidence as to whether the midwifery team leader was required to have a caseload. Student midwives were still being counted in the numbers (although not regularly).

Recommendations

1. All staff need to be aware of the policy regarding the reporting of neonatal deaths.
2. Regular senior medical input should occur in the management of high-risk labours. At a minimum, the registrar should be performing labour ward rounds every four hours, or more frequently in individual cases.
3. Mandatory education for all midwives and doctors involved in the application and interpretation of electronic fetal monitoring should be included in orientation programmes.
4. Staffing on the Birth Suite must ensure that the team leader/senior midwife is available to support other midwives and doctors. This midwife cannot also be expected to take a primary clinical load and be responsible for the care of individual women as well.
5. Improved lines of communication between junior medical staff, senior medical staff and midwives in relation to consultation, referral and supervision need to be developed. The lines of accountability and responsibility need to be formalized and an escalation policy developed and implemented.
6. Hospital staff should be reminded about the importance of note taking, both in relation to medical treatment, and in the documentation of requests made by patients in relation to their care.

Finally, advice to supervisors from the *Journal of Obstetrics and Gynaecology*:[38]

- Make sure supervision is available.
- The message is to seek help rather than soldier on alone.
- Cultural blocks against seeking help are a common factor in legal claims.
- Create a guideline setting out the 'triggers' for seeking supervision, with contact numbers for the relevant staff members.
- Emphasise that no stigma will attach to seeking help, but failure to do so will be a problem.
- Training your juniors to seek supervision is probably the single most effective risk management measure, and costs nothing.

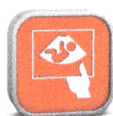

Discussion of Key Issues

Teaching hospitals have a duty of care to mothers and babies to have a policy on supervision and a risk assessment process in place.

The policy should be:

- in accordance with safe practice,
- clearly articulated,
- disseminated to staff (and new staff orientated to its use), understood by supervisors, trainees and nursing/midwifery staff and
- enforced; policies and protocols may be 'state of the art', but a court will hear evidence on what is being practiced (and condoned) on the floor.

Dr Roger Clement writes that consultant obstetricians have a duty to ensure that midwives know that they can obtain consultant advice direct and to override the decision of junior medical staff.

- In your experience are some midwives more experienced and assertive than others in seeking further medical advice ?
- Do you believe the safety/welfare of mothers and babies is dependent on who is on duty ?
- Does your hospital policy address this risk? How?

....

The mother in *Pitt* alleged that her baby's brain damage was due to a lack of supervision of junior medical staff during her high-risk labour and delivery. A lack of evidence that they had 'toured' the wards was the downfall of supervising doctors in this case.

- What documentary evidence exists in your unit that supervising doctors have visited on any particular day?

....

Angus. Associate Professor Faunce comments on the practice of a VMO seeming to rely on registrars and midwifery staff to alert him to any problems with the patients.

- Does this happen in your unit?

....

Grainger. Do you agree with the court's description of the role responsibilities of the student and supervising midwives and the hospital?

....

Coronial investigation. In this case of failure to supervise a high-risk labour by senior medical staff, the coroner emphasized the legal requirement to report 'a reportable' death.

- What does your hospital policy require in relation to the reporting of neonatal deaths to the coroner ?

This case contains many supervision issues. Consider the following:
Who was managing the birth? Both primary midwives (new to the birthing suite) believed the (inexperienced) resident had more responsibility than he actually did, and that they were jointly sharing care. The resident was in fact under the supervision of the midwife in charge.

- Can you understand how these misconceptions could arise?
- Do 'inadequate skill mixes' occur where you work?
- Do you have clear guidelines about which labours should be primarily managed by a midwife and which should be primarily medically managed?

The coroner recommended that staffing on the birth suite must ensure that the team leader is available to support midwives and doctors and cannot be expected to take a primary clinical load and be responsible for individual women.

- Is this recommendation realistic?

- Should student midwives be counted in staffing numbers? Give reasons either way.

The registrar had a very heavy workload (which she described as 'exhausting') and was on 24-hour call. The hospital later reduced the on-call period to 12 hours.

- What is the on-call period at your hospital ?
- Could a registrar's workload (usually) be described as 'exhausting'?

The coroner recommended that as a minimum, a registrar should perform labour ward rounds every four hours, or more frequently in individual cases.

- Is this a reasonable expectation?
- What is the policy where you work?

The coroner recommended that :

(a)   lines of accountability and responsibility need to be formalized between junior medical staff, senior medical staff and midwives in relation to consultation, referral and supervision; and
(b)   an escalation policy should be developed and implemented.

- Are lines of accountability and responsibility formalized with respect to supervision at your hospital?

The Critical Incident Report stated that best practice documentation would reflect risk factors, an action plan with time frames for referral and review / checks, and directions as to who should conduct them.

- Review that Report and discuss whether your partograms/ records (if scrutinized in a court) would reflect similar deficiencies.
- Would evidence of a very busy shift account for some deficiencies?

Following the patient's dissatisfaction with a junior staff member, it was agreed that she would be informed about the level of training of staff providing care. This was neither documented nor implemented.

- Would you have suggested this or agreed to such a request?

....

Junor stands for the principle that where medical orders are 'manifestly wrong,' duty and common sense combine to say they must not be followed.

- Have you been the recipient of 'manifestly wrong' orders from a supervisor?
- What did you do?
- Did hospital policy assist?
- Were there any factors that explained/mitigated the 'wrongness' of the order?

Guidelines

1. For the KEMH Inquiry (the Douglas Report) and its implementation see www.slp.wa.gov au/index.html
   - Discuss and compare the recommendations on supervision in the Douglas Report with the policies in place at your hospital.

2. New Zealand Health and Disability Commissioner Ron Paterson made a number of recommendations about supervision.
   - Does your hospital policy on supervision reflect some or all of Paterson's recommendations?
   - If not, give reasons.

3. English obstetrician Dr Roger Clements described the duties of consultants.
   - Would you add or subtract anything from this list?

4. *The Journal of Obstetrics and Gynaecology* contains the comment that cultural blocks against seeking help are a common factor.
   - Do you agree?

NOTES

1. Reference not available but in workshops I facilitated, maternity service staff readily agreed that this fear was not uncommon.
2. R. Paterson, *'Supervisory Responsibilities of Specialists,'* Journal of Law and Medicine, Vol. 10, pp. 187–97 (Nov. 2002).

3.   *Inquiry into Obstetric and Gynaecological Services at King Edward Memorial Hospital,* Vol.1 (1990-2000) (Final Report, Nov. 2001).

4.   *Jones v Manchester Corporation,* 2 All ER 125, 2 QB 852 (1952).

5.   Lord Nathan, *Medical Negligence,* Butterworths (London, 1957), p.70, citing *Jones v Manchester Corporation,* 2 All ER 125, 2 QB 852 (1952).

6.   *Brus v Australian Capital Territory & Heaton* ACTSC 83; BC 200708690 (2007).

7.   http://www.austlii.edu.au/cases/act/ACTSC/2007/83.ht ml, p.5.

8.   Ibid., p.10.

9.   Ibid., p.14.

10. *Rouse v Pitt County Memorial Hospital., Inc.,* 116 N.C. App. 241, 447 S.E.2d 505 (1994), *rev. granted,* 339 N.C. 615, 454 S.E.2d 257 (1995).

11. Ibid., p.508.

12. Ibid., p.510.

13. Paterson, Journal of Law and Medicine, p.188.

14. Paterson, citing, at p. 190, *Director of Proceedings (Mrs Vinuela) v Dr K McKenzie Medical Practitioners Disciplinary Tribunal.* Decision 177/01/77D (2001).

15. Ibid., p.197.

16. Powers & Harris, *Medical Negligence,* 2d ed., Butterworths, London, p.945 (1994).

17. Ibid.

18. *Junor v McNicol,* The Times (Nov. 1957).

19. Ibid., p.3.

20. *Mozingo v Pitt County Memorial Hospital, Inc.,* 331 N.C. 182, 415 S.E.2d 341, p. 344-5 (1992).

21. *Greater Southern Area Health Service v Dr Angus,* NSWSC 1211 (2007).

22. Ibid., p.3

23. Ibid., p.4.

24. *htpp://www.lawlink.nsw.gov.au/scjudgments/2007nswsc.n sf/2007* at p.22.

25. Thomas Faunce, *Supervising Junior Doctors and 'On Call'Responsibilities: Brus v Australian Capital Terri tory; Greater Southern Area Health Service v Angus,* 15 JLM, p. 513 (2008).

26. *Grainger v Ottawa General Hospital,* 7 O.T.C. 81 (Ont. Gen. Div. 1996).

27. *Record of Investigation into Death,* Case No: 0057/ 2007, Darwin (2009).

28. Ibid., p.3.

29. RANZCOG. 'GP Diploma' is verbal shorthand for the College's Diploma of Obstetrics and Gynaecology. There is a basic Diploma as well as an Advanced Diplo-

ma, the latter covering complex deliveries like a caesarean section, hysteroscopy, miscarriage, termination, first trimester scanning and late pregnancy scanning.

30. Ibid., p.4.
31. Staff perceptions included the following:
    a. A coroner's inquest involves a post-mortem of the baby, which may be stressful for the parents, so care needs to be taken in consideration of the definition of a reportable death;
    b. A post-mortem, a coroner's inquiry, is usually done with a purpose to finding an answer; it was not clear that any answers would be provided by this.
32. Ibid., p.9.
33. Ibid.
34. Ibid.
35. Ibid., p.10.
36. Ibid., p.17.
37. Ibid., p.14.
38. *Journal of Obstetrics and Gynaecology,* Vol. 21, No. 2, pp.114–20.

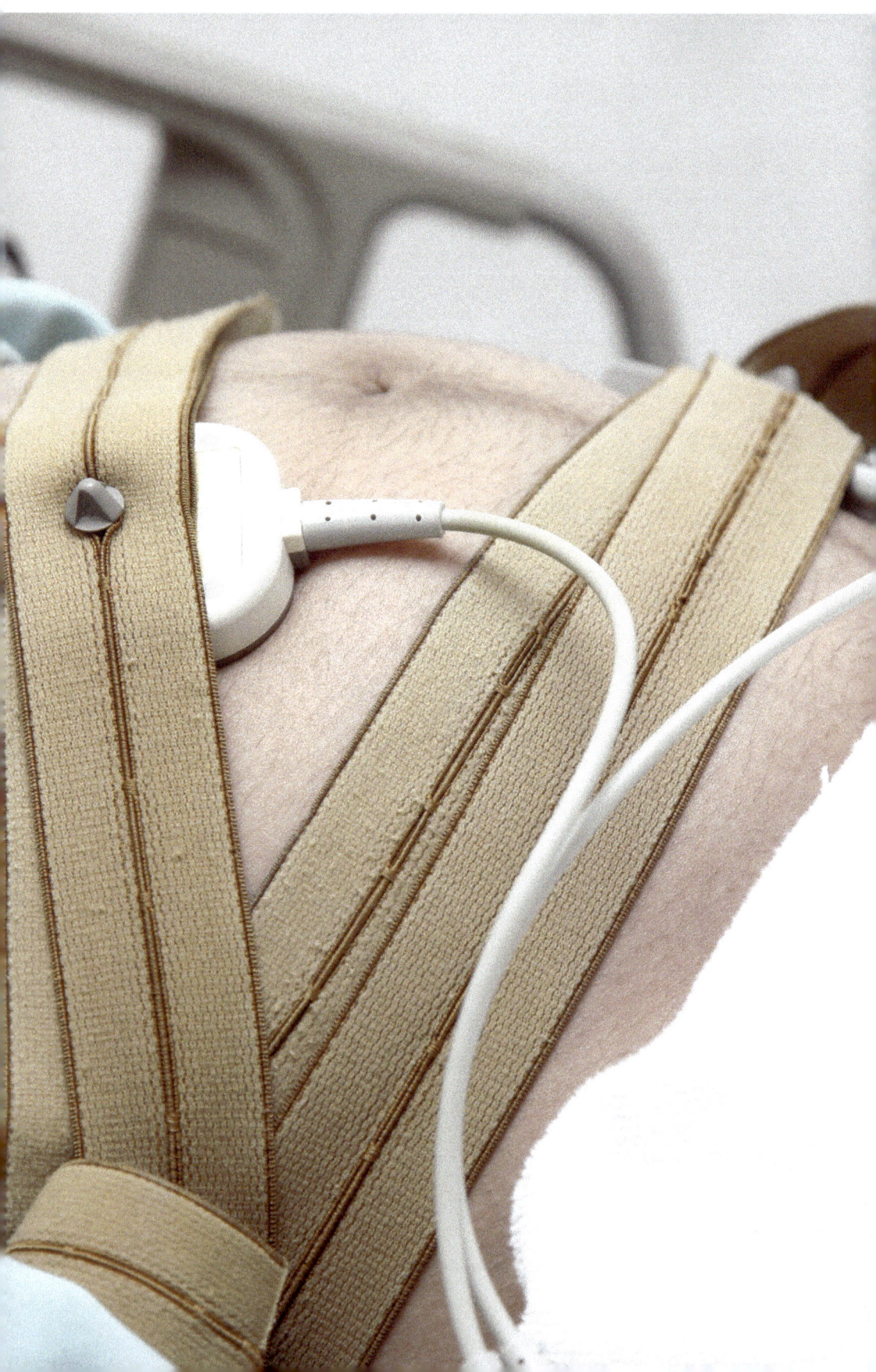

CHAPTER 4

Malfunctioning equipment

'This case serves as a warning against blind acceptance of information given by machines; in the end, it is the clinical judgment used in the whole conduct of the case which is important. The machines are no more than humble (and fallible) servants of the doctors and midwives.'

—Margaret Puxon Q.C.

Introduction

Are clocks synchronised in your hospital? Does equipment work? Can staff use it safely? Serious adverse outcomes from faulty equipment, or the wrongful use of equipment, clearly involve the threat of litigation and can make the defence of a hospital more difficult — for example, the different times recorded by staff (watch, CTG, ward clock, corridor clock, OR clock) when an obstetric emergency is rushed to theatre. A hospital's duty of care requires that equipment comes from a reputable source, is properly maintained, and that staff are competent in its use. Emergency equipment in working order needs to be readily accessible. The chapters on the high-tech area of the neonatal nursery (see Chapters 14, 15) also contain a number of cases where equipment became an issue. The present chapter focuses on two cases relating to the malfunctioning of equipment.

....

In the first case the hospital's paging system malfunctioned. As time is of the essence in midwifery and obstetrics, delay and the reasons for it remain a constant theme in cerebral palsy litigation.

Anderson v Salvation Army Maternity Hospital [Can, 1989][1]

The facts

The baby was in breech position and a vaginal delivery was planned. But, because the obstetrician could not be located at his telephone extension, four to five minutes elapsed between the delivery of the navel and delivery of the head. The baby suffered from cerebral palsy. The parents alleged negligence against the hospital and the obstetrician. The hospital settled out of court and the case proceeded against the obstetrician.

The decision

The court held that the obstetrician had not been negligent in relying on the paging system at the hospital. The system had worked perfectly both before and after this incident. Although the parents failed to prove the delay was the cause of their son's condition, this case underscores a hospital's responsibility to properly maintain its paging system.

....

The second case comes with a clear message from English barrister Margaret Puxon:

An apparently clear case of indefensible delay of 69 minutes in recognising a severe abnormality in the fetal heart action turned out to be a delay of no more than nine minutes which would not have affected the outcome for the child. The huge evidential error was simply due to reliance on the wrong setting of the clock on the CTG machine.

This case serves as a salutary warning against blind acceptance of information given by machines; in the end, it is the clinical judgment used in the whole conduct of the case which is important. The machines are no more than humble (and fallible) servants of the doctors and midwives.[2]

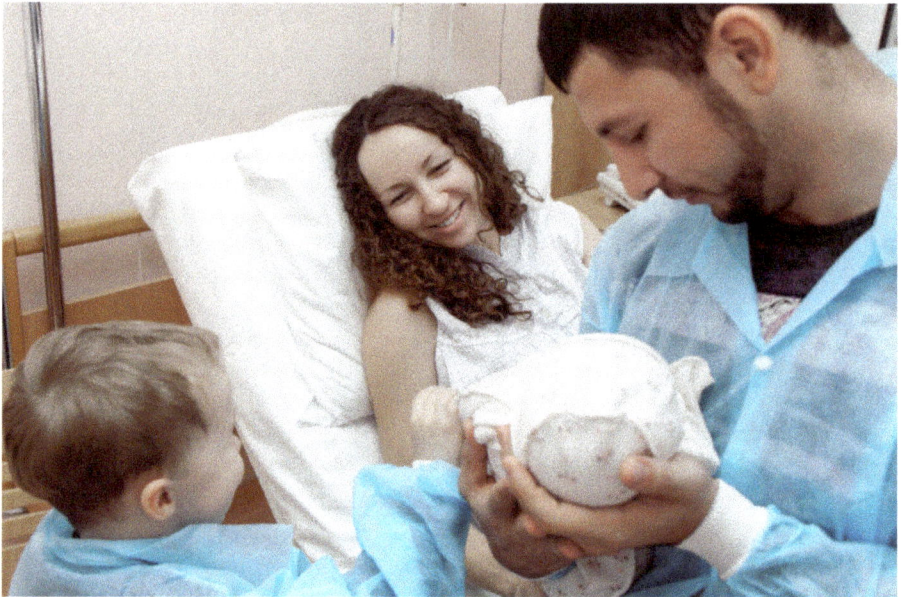

James v Camberwell
Health Authority [UK, 1994][3]

The facts

Nicola's first child was delivered by caesarean section due to fetal distress and failure to progress. Her second child (also a caesarean delivery) suffered from cerebral palsy brought on by hypoxia caused by severe prolonged fetal bradycardia. The obstetrician who had supervised Nicola's antenatal period during the second pregnancy was on holiday and did not perform the surgery. Two years later, during her third pregnancy, Nicola sought an explanation from him about the circumstances of the second birth. Dissatisfied with the obstetrician's inability to provide any information, Nicola alleged negligence against the hospital. The case was heard nine years later.

The trial

High risk. It was contended that while her second antenatal period was uneventful, Nicola was a particularly high-risk patient because of her age (37 years), pelvimetry results, postmaturity of the fetus (term plus eleven days), and obstetric history. At 36 weeks, the obstetrician had noted 'trial of scar.'[4] The labour, it was argued, should have been conducted and monitored with particular care, and a midwife should have been in constant attendance.

Failure to monitor CTG. Hospital records showed that Nicola was admitted to hospital at about 9.45 pm, with a history of contractions since 4.30 pm. A CTG was connected, but discontinued after 40-45 minutes when the trace showed normal.

Re-examination in two hours. At 11.00 pm, a vaginal examination by midwife Neale showed the cervix was only 2 cm dilated and the head still high. A senior house officer (SHO) noted that the mother was in very early labour and should be re-examined in two hours. It was understood this examination would be performed by a midwife.

At 12.45 am, midwife Neale noted contractions were becoming stronger and that Nicola requested analgesia.

CTG recommenced. At 1.00 am, CTG monitoring recommenced, the midwife taking that time from the trace rather than from her watch or a clock.

The following note about what occurred at 2.40 am was written by midwife Neale on information provided by midwife Kemp, who was supervising Nicola's labour during midwife Neale's lunch break:

2.40 am 'called to see. FH 50 bpm; O_2 commenced. Dr Curtis informed.'[5]

Midwife Kemp explained in evidence:

On entering the room, I could see the baby's heartbeat slowing down. I then glanced at the monitor and noticed that the rate was down to 50 beats per minute. I asked Nicola to turn onto her left side, then I went to the door and called the midwife in charge of the labour (midwife Neale).[6]

Dr Curtis said that, on entering the room, he noticed the plateau contractions on the trace. Vaginal dilatation was only 3 cm. He decided a caesarean section was necessary. The registrar was notified and Nicola taken to theatre. Dr Curtis noted: 'Previously 10/10 CTG. Suddenly developed bradycardia and prolonged contraction ... immediate caesarean section.'[7]

The delivery. A baby girl was delivered at 3.04 am in very poor condition, with an Apgar score of 1 at 2 minutes, 6 at 5 and 8 at 10 minutes.[8]

Arguments and allegations

Bradycardia. It was alleged that between 2 am and 2.40 am the severe prolonged bradycardia and reduced baseline variability were not observed or noted by staff and that there had been a 69-minute delay between the onset of fetal bradycardia and delivery of the baby.

Errors in clock. The hospital argued that the time on the CTG trace was approximately 33 minutes slow, so that when the fetal heart went down at 1.55 am (or thereabouts) the real time was 33 minutes later. The caesarean section had therefore been conducted within a reasonable time.

Half an hour discrepancy. Traces relating to patients who were on the same CTG machine before and after Nicola were analysed and cross-referenced to the notes kept by relevant staff. Different discrepancies appeared for that day.

'Flipping.' One midwife referred to the clock as 'flipping'[9] up to a discrepancy of 30 minutes. The court heard that midwives, doctors and consultants were clearly aware of errors occurring in the CTG clock's reading system. Evidence was given that in the context of speed of response to a crisis such variations could be crucial.

Critical period. The judge found that up to 1.00 am there was no indication of anything on the trace that could have caused staff any concern as to the progress of labour. The time of 1.00 am which was taken off the trace by midwife Neale was plainly an error. There was no dispute that the sudden drop in the fetal heart rate (probably the commencement of bradycardia) occurred at 1.55 am. If, in real time, the onset of the crisis occurred at 2.30 am, then the period from onset to delivery was 34 minutes.

Nine minutes. The critical period within which fault could be alleged was then between 2.30 am and about 2.39 am. That time related to midwife Neale's note that midwife Kemp had re-entered the room at 2.40 am. On the basis of those calculations, it was likely the bradycardia had been in place for nine minutes.

Should midwife Kemp have been in constant attendance?
The parents said the midwife was popping in and out. Nicola said: 'She spent very little time with us. She came in from time to time, but very brief visits. There was no support, no dialogue.'[10] Her husband said: 'It would have been comforting to have her in the whole time. She came in to take certain measurements.'[11]

Expert medical evidence of obstetricians

Experts for the baby. One obstetrician described the period in question as 'established labour'[12] and would have expected a midwife to watch the trace most of the time. A second obstetrician said he would expect virtually continuous attendance, subject to staffing levels and patient numbers.

Experts for the hospital. One obstetrician said the extent of midwifery care depended on the stage of labour. From the contemporaneous notes he found the mother was in early spontaneous labour. The 'latent phase' was defined as up to 3 cm dilatation; the 'active stage' was defined as up to full dilatation. He believed that Nicola was in the stage before established labour. Continuous monitoring was not necessary; attendance should be 'from time-to-time.'[13] A period of five minutes would be acceptable, providing there was no warning on the trace.

A second obstetrician said the fetal heart should be checked every 10 minutes, perhaps every 15 at this stage. He would not expect a midwife to be present the whole time until the second stage of labour.

The decision

Wisdom after the event. The judge preferred the opinion of the obstetricians called to give expert evidence for the hospital. They had concluded that midwife Kemp's absence between 2.30 am and 2.40 am did not fall below a reasonable standard of care. From the point of view of providing comfort to the mother, who was experiencing pain, it would have been better if she had stayed. From the point of view of forestalling any risk that might arise from trial of scar, her continuous presence was not medically necessary. The Judge was clear, 'The criticism levelled at her has all the hallmarks of wisdom after the event.'[14]

The causation issue: Would the degree of disability have been less if the fetal bradycardia had been observed earlier?

While five minutes was a reasonable time within which a drop in the fetal heart should have been observed, the judge held that it could not be proved that a reduction of, at most, ten minutes would have materially lessened the baby's disability. Experts explained to the court that there was 'a possibility not a probability'[15] that a reduction of ten minutes in labour time may have led to a sparing of damage. This would have been in relation to cortical, rather than basal ganglia, damage.

The following comments by Margaret Puxon QC on the James case should assist risk managers:

---

1.   It was common knowledge to staff that the clock malfunctioned from time to time and that this was not uncommon. This had not been communicated to, or followed up by, those responsible for investigations at the hospital. If this matter had been attended to, the whole trial and its costs could have been avoided.

---

2.   Why was there no note that the timing of the clock was wrong, and by how much? As soon as staff knew, as they must have immediately known from the state of the child, that there could be a complaint, and possibly a claim, why were the notes not checked with the CTG record? Could this be negligent note-taking and therefore failure to identify and manage, at an early stage, the potential damage?

---

3.   A great deal of public money had been spent 'and perhaps even worse, the wasted suffering of the mother in the protracted wait-

ing, and the prolonged anxiety of the midwives and obstetricians in the eight years that had elapsed between the incident and the hearing.[16]

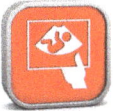

Discussion of key issues

This chapter has been about equipment and times. The story of admission, labour, delivery, inter-hospital and intra-hospital transfer and monitoring in NICUs is chronological.

- Are clocks synchronised in your hospital?

In the Canadian case *Laidlaw v Lionsgate Hospital*[17] the PACU was under-staffed during a coffee break. Patients came back from operating theatres more quickly than expected and an RN's delay in monitoring resulted in a patient's brain damage.

One issue before the court was the time when the RN called the code. Her version was disputed by an anaesthetist in an adjoining theatre, who said that when he heard the code he had checked the time on the wall clock.

Nurses working in OR and PACU say that times are not always synchronised between the two areas. One RN said the times on the four-sided clock in her PACU were all different. Another said it had taken months to re-adjust their clock after daylight saving finished.

- What source do you take your times from before documenting? Check the times on the CTG clock against the wall clock, your watch and other wall clocks in your unit.
- Does this accord with the time in the OR (to which a patient may be rushed and arrival noted in the OR record)? How do these times accord with the hospital mechanism of timing an emergency code?

If you are involved in an incident, raise the possibility of time discrepancy with legal advisers for you/the hospital.[18]

....

Anderson. The court found there was no reason for the obstetrician not to rely on the hospital's paging system working properly.

- Have you experienced problems with paging systems?

....

James. Margaret Puxon makes the point that failure to note the malfunctioning CTG and take appropriate action could be seen as negligent note-taking and failure to identify and manage the damage potential of the incident at an early stage.

- What does your hospital policy require of staff if they notice equipment error?

NOTES

1. *Anderson v Salvation Army Maternity Hospital,* N.S.J. No.339 (Nova Scotia, 1989).
2. *James v Camberwell Health Authority,* 5 Med LR 253 (1994).
3. Ibid., p.257.
4. Ibid., p.253.
5. Ibid., p.255.
6. Ibid.
7. Ibid., p.253.
8. Ibid. Midwives point out that the first Apgar is taken at 1 minute. This judgement, however, records the Apgar score as 1 at 2 minutes.
9. Ibid., p.255.
10. Ibid., p.256.
11. Ibid.
12. Ibid., p.256.
13. Ibid.
14. Ibid., p.257.
15. Ibid.
16. Ibid.

17. *Laidlaw v Lionsgate Hospital,* 70 WWW 727 (1969).

18. Before you make written statements or give evidence that could implicate you, you should contact your professional organization or seek legal advice so that your rights are protected. For the same reason, you should always have legal representation in court.

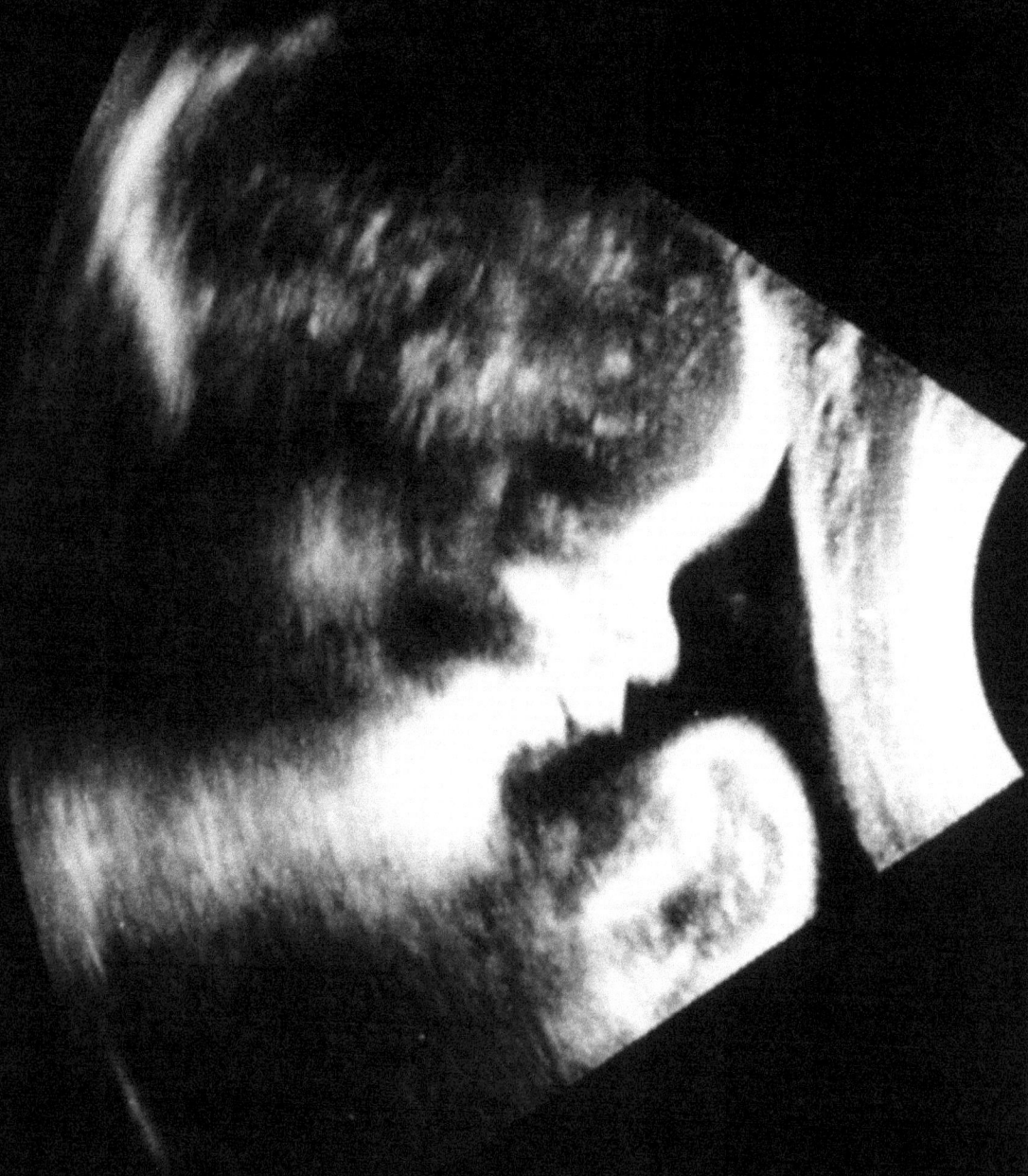

CHAPTER 5

Neurological injury

From the record, the judge determined that Robyn arrived in theatre at 1.30 pm; a spinal anaesthetic was administered at 1.45 pm; the surgeon put knife to skin at 1.58 – 1.59 pm. Baby Ned was born at 2. 05 pm with cerebral palsy.

Introduction

The Australian and New Zealand Perinatal Societies maintain that the origins of cerebral palsy are usually hidden and almost always occur during pregnancy, only to become apparent after birth.[1] While existing neurological problems may result in the fetus showing signs of distress during labour, existing brain damage may not be prevented or reversed by earlier delivery or by caesarean section.

It is believed that the frequency of cerebral palsy has not changed over the last 40 years, despite a four-fold decrease in both perinatal and maternal mortality. Nor is there evidence that current obstetric practices can reduce the risk. While obstetric intervention in the presence of signs of possible hypoxia may prevent fetal death, there is no evidence that such intervention will limit the prevalence or severity of cerebral palsy.[2]

Nevertheless, very distressed parents continue to search for causes and explanations through the courts. This chapter illustrates the issues that can arise when it is argued that neurological injury is the result of delay or misuse of forceps.

....

The first case highlights the difficulties that occur when there are protracted passages of time between a cerebral palsy birth and a court hearing. Statute of limitation legislation governs the time in which negligence cases must be commenced in Australian states and territories (there is a judicial discretion to extend these times),[3] and children have an extended period in which to claim. In practice, claims by children are usually brought much earlier through a 'next friend'. ('Next friend' is a person who conducts a legal action as plaintiff or defendant on behalf of a minor or on behalf of a person of unsound mind).[4]

The standard against which care is measured is that prevailing at the time of the alleged incident, not when the case is heard.

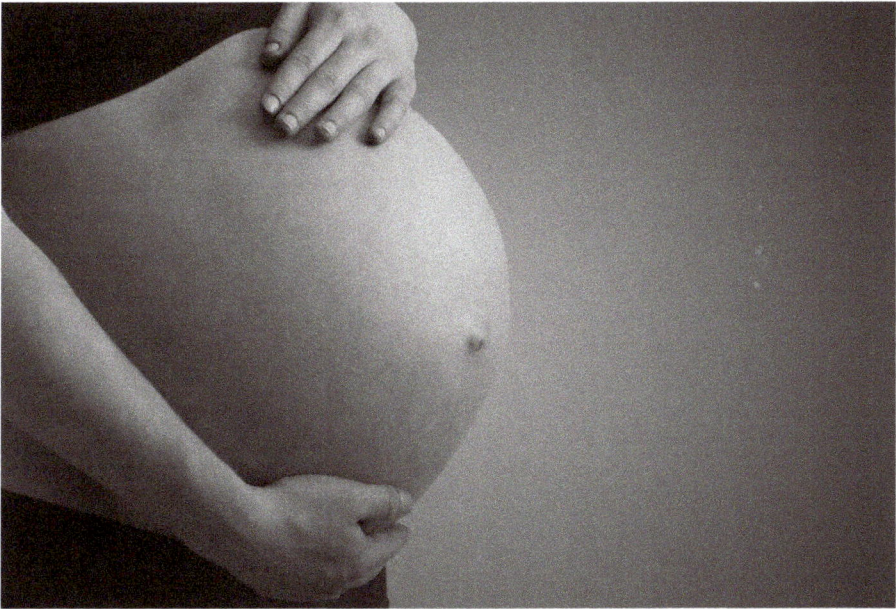

Dissidomino v Newnham & Anor [Aus, 1994]⁵

The facts

On 21 July 1963, Gina's membranes ruptured and she was admitted to hospital. When labour commenced the following morning, meconium- stained liquor was noted at 7 am. The GP, who had supervised the antenatal period, delivered the baby with the assistance of forceps at 3.00 pm. Baby Elena suffered from cerebral palsy.

The trial

It was alleged that both the GP and the hospital had been negligent and that this caused Elena's anoxia and brain damage. When her case first came to court in 1993, thirty years later, Elena had a chronological age of 30 and a mental age of 12 months. The court found in favour of the doctor and the hospital.

Elena appealed.

The appeal

It was argued that when meconium liquor was noted at 7.00 am on the day of Elena's birth it was likely that asphyxia or hypoxia had begun a few hours earlier. The GP should have attended and called a specialist. It was further argued that the hospital should have called another doctor when the GP failed to attend. The failure to induce her mother's labour or carry out a caesarean section had increased Elena's level of disability.

A GP in 1963. The appeal court heard evidence that a reasonably competent GP in 1963 should only have considered taking further steps if labour had not commenced by the middle of the day. There was no reason to perform a caesarean section if the heart rate was normal. Calling a specialist would have made no difference and there was no need to interfere with a labour that was proceeding normally.

Extraordinary lapse of time. The court (in 1994), noted the 'extraordinary lapse of time'[6] between events surrounding the birth and the hearings. The hospital records had been destroyed in 1978; the GP was now age 75 years and the attending midwife 78 years.

Perception and recollection distorted. In addition, the passage of time and the effects of drugs given during labour would have dimmed Gina's perception and recollection of the day of her daughter's birth. The fact that her family had had to care for Elena for 30 years could be expected to 'distort and obscure'[7] Gina's memory. She reported, for example, that the midwife had asked her to push before she was fully dilated early in labour. The judge did not accept this. The court heard that competent midwives would know that pushing before the patient is fully dilated could injure the fetus.

Gina contended that she had been in the lithotomy position for two hours. This also was not accepted. The court heard evidence that the lithotomy position is not used until delivery is imminent.

The decision

The appeal was unsuccessful. The court held that, apart from the meconium stained liquor (occurring in 10 per cent to 15 per cent of all births), there was no apparent abnormality of the fetus. Attendance by the GP or any other doctor was therefore not warranted. The birth itself would not have caused such devastating brain damage and it was likely that placental insufficiency had caused the baby to be anoxic even before labour commenced. This could have occurred days or even weeks before the birth. Unless placental insufficiency was severe, meconium would not be passed.

Gina had therefore failed to show that anything the GP or hospital had done, or failed to do, had had any adverse effect on her condition.

....

Time between the decision to deliver by caesarean section, getting the OR team together and delivering the baby is central to the next group of cases.

In the first of these cases a British judge heard evidence of the practical realities of meeting the 'decision to incision' 30-minute standard. Even so, the judge found this did not explain a 55-minute delay.

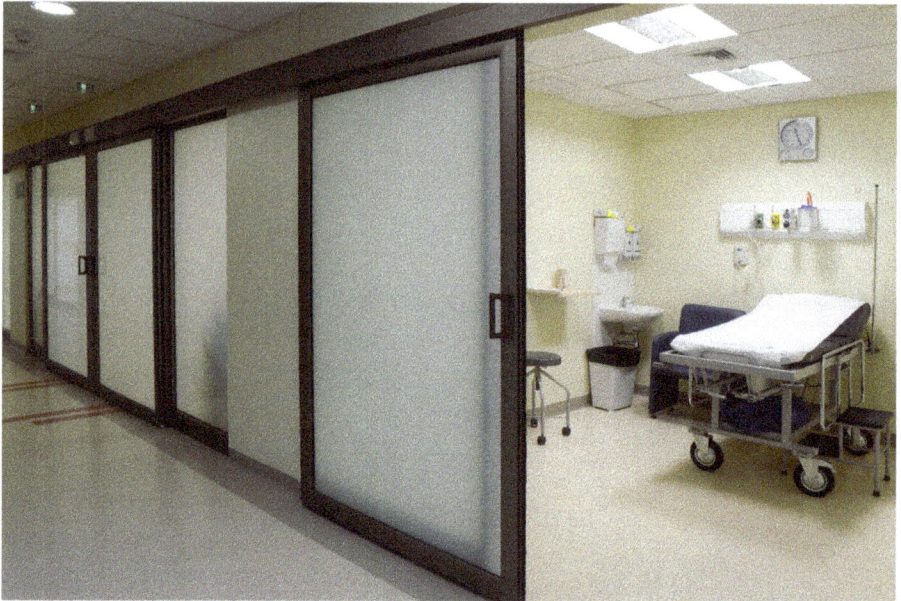

Richards (a child) v Swansea NHS Trust [UK, 2007][8]

The facts

Robyn became pregnant for the first time in 1996 following fertility treatment. The consultant obstetrician saw Robyn when she was 11 days post-term and arranged for her to be admitted to hospital for induction of labour. She was admitted to the labour ward at 8.30 am at term plus 13 days. At 9.10 am, monitoring commenced by CTG.

Four basic CTG features. The court was later to hear evidence that the CTG device records the fetal heart rate (FHR) and the mother's contractions by tracing a line on a moving roll of paper divided into 1 cm columns that represent 1 minute of time. The FHR is recorded in the top section, and the mother's contractions in the bottom section.

   [Note: Four basic features (and others) are defined in the Clinical Guideline (No. 8) published by the Royal College of Obstetricians and Gynaecologists in 2001—the NICE Guideline:[9]

1. Baseline: the mean level of the FHR expressed in beats per minute (bpm) over a period of 5 to 10 minutes.
2. Baseline or beat to beat variability (BTBV): the difference in bpm between the highest peak and the lowest trough of fluctuation in the FHR over one minute.
3. Accelerations: where FHR is at least 15 bpm above the baseline for 15 seconds or more.
4. Decelerations: where the FHR is at least 15 bpm below the baseline for 15 seconds or more.

Accelerations are generally seen as a sign of fetal wellbeing; decelerations as a sign of fetal distress- especially when the decelerations are 'late', that is, where they begin after the onset of a contraction—reach their nadir more than 20 seconds after the peak of the contraction, and end after the ending of the contraction.

9.30 am	At 9.30 am, midwife Tyson noted that the baseline was 140 bpm and 'flatish'[10] — lacking btbv; this continued after Robyn was moved onto her left side. The obstetrician saw Robyn at this point and directed that the FHR monitoring continue. Shortly afterwards, the registrar conducted a vaginal examination and was unhappy about inducing labour before the obstetrician had seen the trace. The registrar advised that the trace be continued for 30 minutes.
10.00 am	Midwife Tyson noted that the baseline continued to be flat with poor btbv despite changes in the maternal position.
10.45 am	Robyn was reviewed again by the obstetrician, then transferred to the central delivery suite either for induction of labour or for a caesarean section. Monitoring stopped.
11.25 am	By 11.25 am, the CTG trace had been recommenced. Robyn was now under the care of a new registrar whose note of a conversation with the obstetrician recorded that labour should be induced with Prostin and the patient closely monitored 'if any deceleration for LSCS'.[11]
11.30 am	A student midwife took over from midwife Tyson with midwife Rowan as her mentor.
12.30 pm	The student midwife made a note (referring to the earlier discussion between the obstetrician and the registrar):

'Prostaglandin 1 mg if any deterioration in ECTG then for emergency LCS'.[12]

The obstetrician (who had no independent memory of managing Robyn's labour and was dependent on the team's notes) later said that he would have said/or have been understood to say that there should be a caesarean section if there was a 'pathological' deceleration or decelerations that were late or deep, or suggested something was amiss. The judge later accepted that the obstetrician would have used the word 'deceleration' rather than 'deterioration', as noted by the student midwife.

Expert witnesses. Obstetricians giving expert evidence disagreed as to much of the interpretation of the trace, including the period between 9.10 am to 11.30 am. The obstetrician (for Robyn) believed that, notwithstanding a number of accelerations from about 9.38 am, this part of the trace was suspicious because of the flat baseline and a shallow deceleration at about 9.17 am. Although not falling within the NICE Guideline, this ought to have been of concern. The guideline says that it is only where btbv is less than 5 bpm over a period of 40 minutes that lack of btbv renders the trace 'non reassuring.'[13] The obstetrician pointed out that (a) no-one knew for how long the FHR had been flat before the CTG was commenced, and (b) where a mother is 38 years as well as being 13 days post-term, there would be concern about placental sufficiency and liquor depletion. Although the obstetrician (for the hospital) disagreed, both obstetricians did agree that a responsible body of professional opinion would support the management plan set by Robyn's obstetrician.

12.10 pm   At 12.10 pm, 12.20 pm and 12.40 pm, there were decelerations that were close to falling within the NICE Guidelines.

12.57 pm   A deceleration occurred from a baseline of about 135 bpm to a nadir of about 90 bpm that lasted between 1 ½ and 2 minutes (within the NICE definition). The student midwife noted the deceleration as 'late'.[14]

(At 12.50 pm, or immediately after the 12.57 deceleration, midwife Rowan contacted the registrar after the student midwife had drawn her attention to the trace.)

13.05 pm   The registrar noted: 'Asked to see due to further decelerations on CTG. Late deceleration noted. Plan for LSCS.'

13.10 pm   Midwife Rowan noted that registrar had attended and decision made for emergency LCS.

From these times, the judge concluded that the registrar was on the scene at
1.05 pm, had reviewed the situation for 5 minutes, then decided at 1.10 pm
that there should be an emergency caesarean section.

1.25 pm   Robyn was prepared and taken to theatre at 1.25 pm. She
recalled no sense of urgency. The CTG was discontinued and
never recommenced. Both obstetric experts agreed that had
it been continued, clinicians would have been alerted to the
fetal bradycardia induced by the acute hypoxic ischaemic insult beginning at 1.45 pm. 'EM LSCS' was handwritten at the
end of the trace (probably by the student midwife). The anaesthetist recorded the operation as an 'Emergency LSCS'.[15]

1.30 pm   From this record, the judge determined that Robyn arrived
in theatre at 1.30 pm; a spinal anaesthetic was administered
at 1.45 pm; the surgeon put knife to skin at 1.58-1.59 pm.
Baby Ned was born at 2. 05 pm with cerebral palsy.

It was alleged that negligent delay in performing the caesarean section was
the cause of the baby's injuries. At the time of the trial Ned was ten years old
and severely disabled.

Categories of urgency.   The judge heard evidence that the previous classification of caesarean sections as being elective or non-elective (and the latter as emergency or not) was unsatisfactory. The emergency category was
too broad, covering 'crash' sections where there are only minutes to save the
baby and, at the other end of the scale, situations where mother and baby are
well but an early delivery becomes advisable.

Following the 1995 National Confidential Enquiry into Perioperative
Deaths,[16] four grades of urgency had been recognized:

1. immediate threat to the woman or the fetus,
2. maternal or fetal compromise not immediately life threatening,
3. no maternal or fetal compromise but needs early delivery and
4. delivery timed to suit the woman and staff.

The judge treated Robyn's situation as a grade 2 case.

The National Sentinel Caesarean Section Audit report published by the RCOG in 2001[17] states that in cases of serious maternal or fetal compromise the decision-to-delivery time by caesarean section should be 30 minutes but noted that there was minimal research evidence to show this improved fetal outcomes. In these circumstances, delivery should be accomplished as fast as possible but without endangering the life of the mother. The 30-minute interval should remain the benchmark for service provision for caesarean sections of grade 1 and grade 2 urgency.

The same approach was taken in 2004 in the clinical guideline published by NICE and the RCOG.

Delivery at emergency CS for maternal or fetal compromise should be accomplished as quickly as possible, taking into account that rapid delivery has the potential to do harm. A decision-to-delivery interval of less than 30 minutes is not in itself critical in influencing baby outcome, but remains an audit standard for response to emergencies within maternity services.[18]

It was agreed that the '30-minute standard' was operating in 1996.

The obstetrician giving expert evidence for Ned said there was no greater risk in achieving his birth in 30 minutes than in 60 minutes. The obstetrician for the hospital, while not agreeing that the 12.57 pm deceleration meant a caesarean section was very urgent, accepted that it would have been technically possible for Ned to have been delivered within 30 minutes and that Robyn could have been prepared for theatre in ten minutes, rather than the 15 minutes it had taken.

The court was referred to two research papers. *(1)'Interval between decision and delivery by caesarean section — are current standards achievable?'* by Tufnell, et al.[19] *(2)'National cross sectional survey to determine whether the decision to deliver is critical in emergency caesarean section'* by Thomas, et al.)[20] Tufnell described the caesarean section as a complex, multidisciplinary procedure usually requiring a team of seven, including a surgeon, anaesthetist, OR assistant, a nurse, a midwife and a paediatrician. Tasks to be done between decision and delivery range from blood sent for analysis, shaving and catheterizing the mother, setting the theatre, moving the mother to theatre, instilling the anaesthetic, and skin and uterine incisions. Expert witnesses agreed that some tasks could be done concurrently.

The data analysed in the Thomas paper related to 17,780 singleton births (99 per cent of all births) delivered by caesarean section in England and Wales between 1 May 2000 and 31 July 2000. Results showed that 46.2 per cent of the grade 1 cases (total 4,622) were performed within 30 minutes, 73.1 per cent within 45 minutes, 83.8 per cent within 60 minutes and 88.4 per cent within 75 minutes. Corresponding figures for grade 2 cases (total 9,122) were 15.5 per cent (30 minutes), 36.44 per cent (45 minutes), 57.2 per cent (60 minutes) and 68.8 per cent (75 minutes).

The cases were also analysed in three grades of urgency in terms of primary indication for caesarean section as reported by the doctors involved. Fetal (as distinct from maternal) primary indications were: failure to progress; breech presentation; malpresentation or unstable lie; presumed fetal compromise (intrauterine growth, retardation, or abnormal cardiotocogram); cord prolapse; chorioamnionitis and other. The indication applicable to Ned's case was presumed fetal compromise. The percentage of presumed fetal compromise cases in grade 2 (total 9,122) was 33 per cent.

The decision

In the judge's opinion, once the decision had been taken to deliver Ned by emergency caesarean section, a duty was owed to deliver him as quickly as possible with the aim of trying to achieve delivery within 30 minutes. This meant that although there was no indication of immediate danger, there was a risk that the baby could deteriorate at any time and with disastrous consequences. To guard against this risk, the operation had to be performed as quickly as possible without subjecting Robyn to unnecessary risk. This was the approach in the NICE/ RCOG guideline and reflected the approach in 1996.

Practical difficulties. While the research papers showed the practical difficulties of meeting the 30-minute standard, this did not provide a justification for the 55 minutes taken to deliver Ned. The failure to achieve the 30-minute standard, or at the very least, delivery within 45 minutes, must have been due to one or more of the following:

  a. some exculpatory external constraint on the team, such as competing demands for the surgeon or anaesthetist's services,
  b. a misguided mindset or
  c. a failure to exercise the necessary skill or expertise.

As the hospital had not produced evidence from witnesses, records or notes that would explain that there were logistical constraints preventing Ned being delivered within 45 minutes of 1.10 pm, the judge found that it had been established, on a balance of probabilities, that those attending Robyn negligently failed to deliver her son as fast as possible; had they not been so negligent, Ned would have been born before 1.55 pm and intact.

Although Ned succeeded in his primary claim, two other scenarios had been considered during the trial as alternative claims. Because the issues had been argued during the trial, the judge made the following findings. Note how the inferences are drawn:

1. The student midwife

The student midwife accepted that she should have reported the 12.10 pm, 12.20 pm, and 12.40 pm decelerations to her mentor, midwife Rowan. Had she done so, the senior midwife (under the obstetrician's management plan) would have reported this to the registrar at about 12.46 pm. The judge believed there was no doubt that the registrar would have come and examined the trace — as any reasonably competent registrar would have done. On the basis that it had taken the registrar 6-8 minutes to arrive after he had been called to consider the 12.57 pm deceleration, the judge found that had he been called at 12.46 pm as he should have been, he would have arrived before the 12.57 pm deceleration began and would have seen this deceleration occur as he was examining the trace.

On the basis of this reasoning the registrar would have decided on a caesarean section by 1.00 pm. As the actual decision-to-delivery time was 55 minutes, the inference was compelling that Ned would have been delivered in no longer a period of time. It followed that if the student midwife had reported the earlier three decelerations as she ought to have done, Ned would have been born intact.

2. Continuation of monitoring

As an alternative to relying on the time actually taken to deliver Ned, it had been argued that monitoring of the FHR should have continued throughout the caesarean procedure. If the events that actually occurred from 1.10 pm had happened ten minutes earlier (as the judge found they would have done), spinal anaesthesia would have been instilled at 1.35 pm and taken sufficiently for delivery to have commenced as soon as the monitor showed the onset of bradycardia to which Ned's FHR would have slumped at 1.45 pm. On this hypothesis, it followed that Ned would have been born by 1.55 pm and without injury.

Ned therefore succeeded on his primary claim and would have succeeded on either of the two alternative claims.

Damages awarded.

....

In the next case, the fact that the hospital was required to respond to an emergency on a public holiday was a matter for comment by the court. The question also arose whether 'emergency' had the same meaning for both labour ward and OR staff. As this misunderstanding can cause delay, good risk management needs to ensure that verbal communication between the two areas is unambiguous.

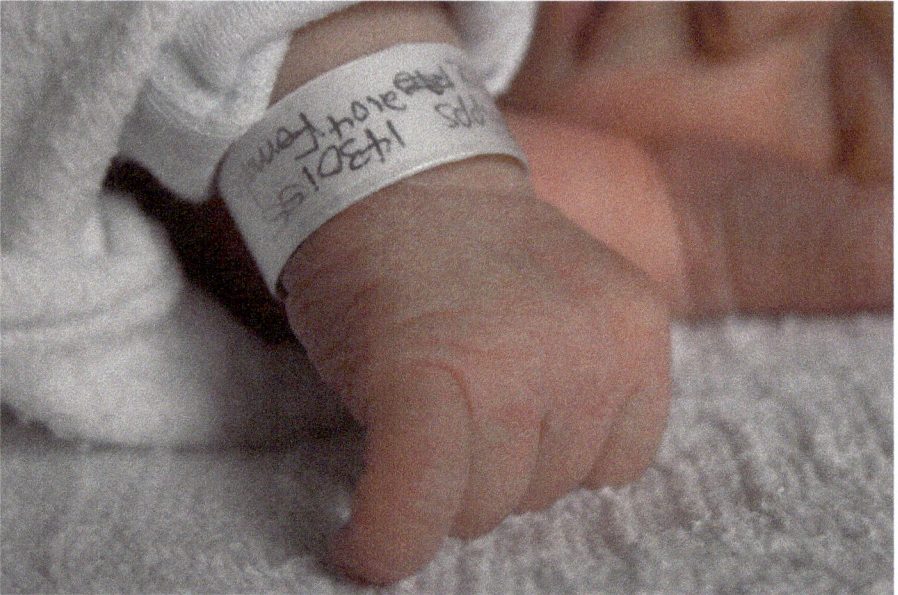

Ren v Mukerjee and Anor
[Aus, 1996][21]

The facts

Kate was admitted to hospital in labour on Easter Sunday. An obstetrician carried out a physical examination at 1.05 pm, a Syntocinon infusion was commenced the following day at 11.45 am and the obstetrician examined Kate again at 3 pm and 5.10 pm. The second stage of labour was reached at about 10.30 pm. The obstetrician performed an episiotomy at 11.40 pm and proceeded to apply forceps to rotate the fetal head towards the anterior position. That attempt was unsuccessful. At this time, the fetal heart was slow and difficult to count. After forceps were reapplied without success, the obstetrician decided to deliver by caesarean section. A delay then occurred while the on-call anaesthetist and nurse reached the hospital.

Negligence alleged. The baby was delivered by caesarean section at 1.16 am, suffering anoxia at birth. He was cyanosed, slow to take his first breaths, and began fitting after 20 minutes. Over the next 4–6 weeks it was

clear he had been born with cerebral palsy. The condition was predominant-
ly athetoid. Some repetitive involuntary movements were exhibited and also
some spastic movements. Negligence was alleged against both the obstetrician and the hospital.

The trial

The parents. It was argued that:

1. The insertion of the forceps precipitated fetal distress resulting in hypoxia and consequent damage.
2. The obstetrician should not have performed the forceps procedure but
   gone straight to caesarean section.
3. No reasonably competent obstetrician would have contemplated the
   forceps procedure with sufficient confidence to justify carrying out the
   procedure in the labour ward; there must have been sufficient doubt
   about the outcome to require the use of the operating room.
4. It was negligent to insert the forceps a second time.

The obstetrician. The obstetrician said that if he had any doubts that the
attempt at forceps delivery would fail, he would have performed the delivery
in the operating room.

The hospital. The hospital argued that even if a caesarean section had
been carried out immediately after the removal of the forceps, it would not
have made any difference. The damage done by the forceps was already irreversible. The obstetrician's duty was not one which could be delegated. He
had not taken adequate steps to make the hospital staff aware of the urgency
of the situation.

   The court had to decide exactly when the damage to the fetal brain had
occurred.

Fetal distress. The baby had begun to show signs of fetal distress from
11.43 pm, when the forceps were applied, to 12.05 am, when the fetal heartbeat was slow and difficult to hear. Fetal distress continued from about 12.07
am until 12.50 am, when a tachycardia was noted. There was a degree of
cardiovascular resuscitation between 12.30 am and the time of birth. The
question then arose as to whether all the damage had been done when the
forceps were used, or whether the delay in performing the caesarean section
was causally related to the baby's condition.

Expert medical evidence. On the basis of expert evidence, the court found that the forceps did not cause irreversible harm, but triggered asphyxial changes to the fetal heart rate. If birth had occurred within 30-60 minutes of the cessation of forceps, the baby's condition would not have been as severe. It was probable that if asphyxia had been terminated shortly after the birth by the administration of oxygen, then in all probability the baby would have been born without disability. Cerebral palsy with athetosis is widely accepted to be the result of acute short-lived asphyxia of less than 30 minutes in labour. Spastic quadriplegia is more likely to be caused by chronic asphyxia lasting more than an hour before birth.

Delay. The court found that damage initiated by the forceps was continued and aggravated by the delay in performing the caesarean section. Whether the labour ward or the operating theatre was the appropriate place to apply forceps depended on the circumstances. If the obstetrician was sufficiently confident about a successful delivery, the labour ward was considered to be an appropriate place for the procedure. To require the procedure to be carried out in the operating room would put unnecessary stress on the mother and make unnecessary demands on the hospital and staff.

Reasonable obstetric practice. The overwhelming view of expert witnesses was that the obstetrician, in attempting a forceps delivery, had acted in accordance with reasonable standards. The decision to attempt the delivery in the labour ward, instead of proceeding to a trial of forceps, was in accordance with reasonable obstetric practice. The court did not find that a greater degree of force or pressure had been used than was usual. Evidence from the obstetrician was accepted that failure to rotate the fetal head on the first attempt may have been because of a misapplication of the blades. The decision to proceed with a second attempt was neither grossly negligent nor reckless.

Labour ward. The decision to attempt the delivery in the labour ward precluded delivery within five to ten minutes of that failure. The decision to attempt a forceps delivery in the labour ward was a reasonable one. Therefore, failure to organise the operating theatre to carry out a caesarean section within five to ten minutes, after the attempt to rotate the head, involved no lack of reasonable care by either the obstetrician or the hospital.

Duty of hospital. The court accepted that the obstetrician's duty was not one which could be delegated as far as his obstetric functions were concerned. Nevertheless, it was the duty of the hospital to provide an operating theatre, equipped for a caesarean section, as soon as reasonably possible, having regard to the need for urgency. In the event of a failed forceps delivery, the caesarean section should have been carried out within 30 minutes. The hospital was therefore in breach of its duty to take proper care unless it had a procedure in place for the preparation of an operating room equipped for a caesarean section within 30-60 minutes of notification by the obstetrician.

OR to be ready. The obstetrician had done all that could reasonably be expected of a competent obstetrician in his position. He was entitled to expect the operating room to be ready within 30-40 minutes after staff were notified of the urgency.

The decision

Getting the message right. The court found there had clearly been a breakdown in communication among hospital staff. Had it been understood that the OR was needed for a caesarean section following a failed attempt at forceps delivery, and not for a trial by forceps, with possible caesarean section, it was likely that delay would have been avoided. This error was due to the negligence of the hospital. It was an error that could have been avoided by the simple exercise of getting the message right.

Damages awarded.

....

The following case is concerned with an allegation that the doctor failed to plan for the potential need of an OR and staff.

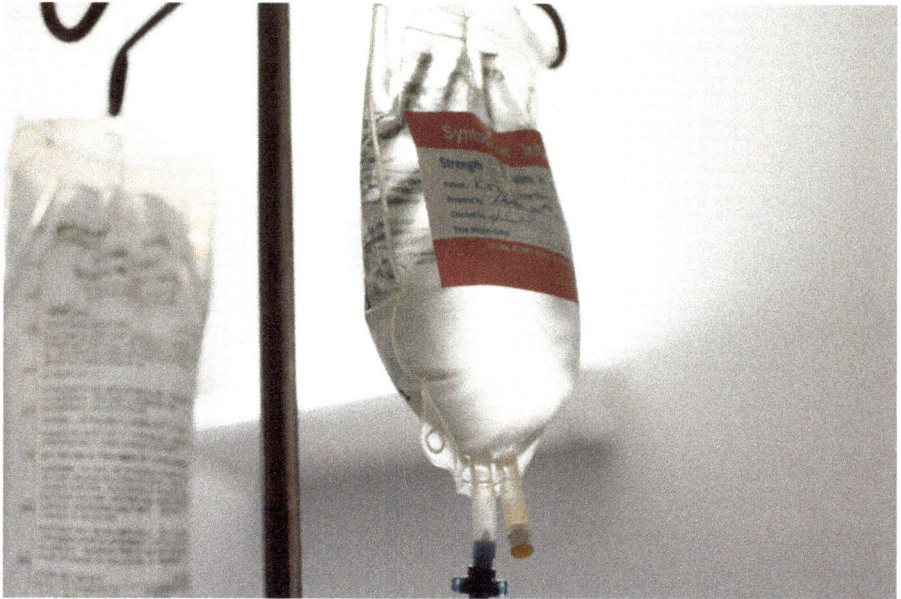

Allen (Next Friend of) v University Hospital's Board [Can, 2000][22]

The facts

Dr Hall and Dr Peters had a 'shared care' approach to obstetric patients. Both saw patients during their antenatal care, the doctor on-call handling the labour and delivery.

Possibility of caesarean. At 7.50 am, Dr Peters examined Sally and performed an artificial rupture of the membranes. At 9.20 am, Dr Hall saw the fetal heart strip, ordered an IV, then noted the possibility of a caesarean section. At 10.00 am, he consulted with the midwives. Morphine was ordered, but Dr Peters did not examine or speak to Sally. At this point, the fetal monitor was unhooked, then reattached by Sally at 10.30 am

Emergency delivery. At 11.00 a.m, Sally, concerned about the pattern on the monitor, called for a midwife. RMO Dr North examined her, found a compound presentation and did an ultrasound. At 11.20 am, Sally was told an emergency caesarean section was urgently needed. She was prepared and wheeled into the operating room at 11.40, where surgery commenced at

11.54 am. The baby, delivered at 12.01 pm, was resuscitated, intubated, and bagged with oxygen. The prevailing view was that the baby suffered from birth asphyxia.

The trial

In the negligence case that followed, Dr Hall explained that it had taken longer than anticipated to perform the caesarean section because of the unavailability of an operating room. This explanation was rejected.

Operating room availability. The judge found that while the hospital had no dedicated theatre for performing caesarean sections, there were in fact 14 operating theatres in use on the date of the incident. Dr Hall was himself alerted after his examination of Sally at 9.20 am that there was a distinct possibility that a caesarean section would be needed. He even took the precaution of ordering an IV at the time in anticipation of this. If, as Dr Hall contended, it was difficult to get operating rooms, he should have checked that possibility. The judge stated:

He did not do so and in my view this failure to communicate the potential need and to explore the potential need with the appropriate administrative personnel was substandard care afforded to (the patient) when in the end result it took from 11.10 till 12.01 to complete the C-section. In the circumstances, 45 to 50 minutes to do an urgent C-section in a tertiary care hospital is substandard care. The evidence indicates a 10 to 30 minute time frame is acceptable.[23]

The decision

The judge held that the negligence of the doctors had materially contributed to the neurological damage sustained by the baby, even if she was prone to be autistic, and even if autism is caused by faulty genes. The clinical symptoms displayed at birth were consistent with a 'mild to moderate intermittent hypoxic eschemia.'[24]

Although the RMO in the next case was found to be 'a little slow'[25] in getting an obstetrician involved, the negligence of midwives was found to be the major cause of the baby's neurological injuries.

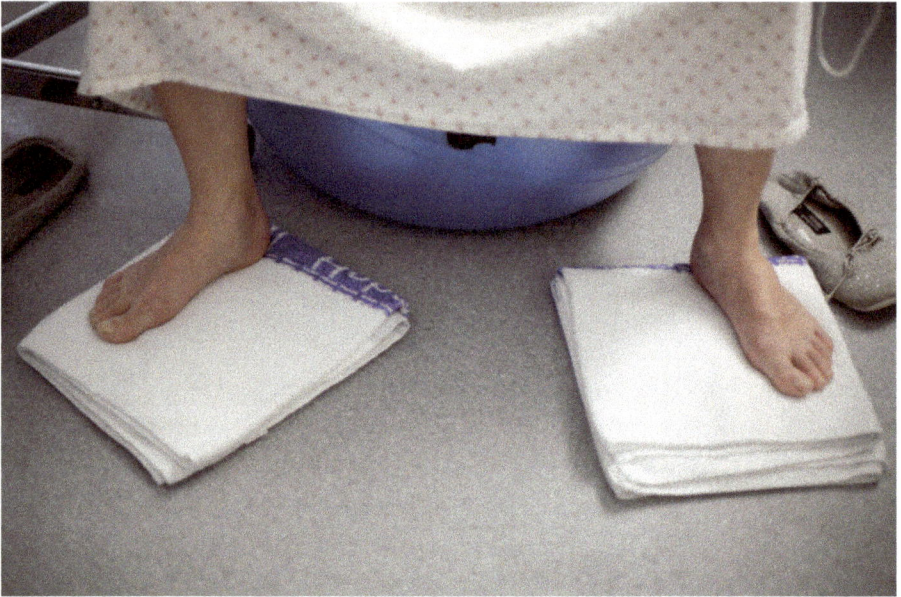

Bauer v Seager [Can, 2000][26]

The facts

As the baby was in breech position, midwives knew that the mother, Gwen, was high-risk. At 12.10 am, the midwife noted she was fully dilated and that the second stage of labour had started. At 12.25 am, the fetal heart monitor showed deep decelerations, with contractions. At 12.30 am, pushing commenced. At 12.40 am, the fetal heart strip showed deep variables, with contractions, and the fetal heart beat dropping to 75-80 bpm for 30-40 seconds. The midwife called the RMO and at 12.45 am applied oxygen. At 1.12 am, the buttocks and body were delivered.

Forceps delivery attempted. At 1.19 am, an obstetrician and the RMO attempted to use forceps to deliver the head, but were unable to properly attach the forceps and the baby's head was ultimately delivered manually. The baby was not breathing and suffered from cerebral palsy. She was, at the time of the trial, significantly mentally and physically impaired.

The trial

It was alleged that the doctors failed to consider or implement a caesarean section on a timely basis.

The decision

The judge was satisfied that the cause of the baby's injuries was asphyxia, which commenced prior to her birth, at approximately 12.10 am, and continued during the delivery and resuscitation process. If a caesarean section had been performed, the baby would probably have been born without injury.

Failure to notify doctor. The midwives' actions and inactions in failing to notify the doctors of the problems of the fetus in a timely fashion (from the commencement of the second stage of labour at 12.10 am until 12.40 am) was conduct which fell below a reasonable standard of care for each midwife. This negligence had caused or contributed to the hypoxia and resulting injuries.

Time is of the essence. A caesarean section could have, and probably should have, been performed at, or as shortly after 12.25 am or 12.30 am as reasonably possible (probably within 15-20 minutes if proper steps had been taken). Some brain damage probably occurred by 12.45 am or 12.50 am. A caesarean delivery then, or very quickly after, would in all probability have reduced the degree or extent of brain damage.

The judge :

Time is of the essence and it simply took too long for the midwives to alert the doctor as to the emergent status of this fetus.[27]

The court then considered whether the RMO was negligent in the management of the situation around 12.45 am.

Caesarean section not best option. It had taken the RMO more than 15 minutes to notify the obstetrician of the critical situation that was apparent at 12.45 am. The obstetrician had responded promptly, then decided that labour had progressed to the point where a caesarean section was not the best option.

The issue then became whether the option of performing a caesarean section was effectively taken away from the obstetrician because she was not notified until after 12.10 am.

Emergency situation. The judge found that the RMO had been put in a very difficult emergency situation by the delay of the midwives in calling her to the labour room after 12.10 am. Nevertheless, she should have responded differently and more quickly at or very shortly after 12.45 am. She should have immediately notified the obstetrician and got the mother to the double set-up room more quickly for immediate examination and decision by the obstetrician.

While the RMO was not negligent in her decision to defer to the obstetrician the decision as to the method of delivery, she was a little too slow in getting the obstetrician involved and getting the mother to the case room.

The judge:

In finding that the RMO did not meet the acceptable standard of care at or shortly after 12.45 am and before the obstetrician was finally notified, I remain strongly convinced that the negligence of the midwives was the chief contributing cause of the hypoxia and resulting brain damage.... More timely action by the RMO at or very shortly after 12.45 am, which would have permitted a caesarean section, would only have reduced the length of hypoxia and probably reduced the degree of brain damage. It would not likely have prevented the brain damage.[28]

The court found that the midwives were 80 per cent at fault and the RMO 20 per cent.

....

A number of cases in this chapter have involved intervention with forceps. The classic judicial statement on the difference between 'an error of judgment' and 'negligence' occurred in an English case concerned with a trial of forceps.

In *Whitehouse v Jordan* a trial of forceps is described as 'a tentative procedure, requiring delicate handling of the baby with forceps and a continuous review of the baby's progress down the birth canal. Traction should be stopped if it appears that the delivery cannot proceed without risk.'[29]

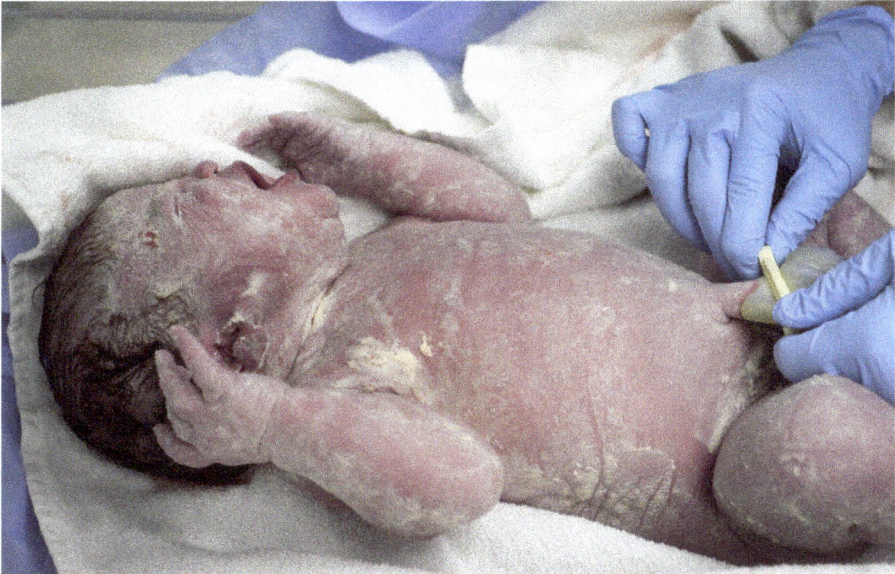

Whitehouse v Jordan
[UK, 1981][30]

The facts

Mrs Whitehouse, aged 30 years, was pregnant for the first time. She was 4 ft 10 in in height, and described as a 'difficult, nervous and at times aggressive patient.'[31] She refused a vaginal examination or a lateral X-ray during her pregnancy. The consultant obstetrician's notes identified a difficult pregnancy and stated that a 'trial of forceps' would have to be tried before proceeding to a caesarean section.

Mrs Whitehouse was admitted to hospital at 2.00 am shortly after her membranes had ruptured. The vertex was engaged at 2.30 am and this was confirmed by a consultant at 10.00 am who noted 'fair sized baby.'[32] At 11.30 am she was given an epidural and examined by a doctor who reported 'vertex engaged, fetal heart satisfactory... pelvis seems adequate.'[33]

At 11.30 pm, Dr Jordan, a senior registrar (quasi-consultant status) took charge after Mrs Whitehouse had been in labour for some time. He recorded 'small gynaecoid' against 'pelvis' and then 'Normal delivery out of the question.'[34]

'Too long and too hard'. Dr Jordan embarked on a trial of forceps. He pulled on the baby six times, with the forceps coincident with the mother's contractions. When there was no movement on the fifth and sixth pulls he decided, some 25 minutes after the trial commenced, to abandon the procedure. The baby was quickly and competently delivered by caesarean section but suffered severe brain damage due to asphyxia. It was alleged Dr Jordan had pulled too long and too hard on the baby's head.

The trial. Mrs Whitehouse gave evidence that she was 'lifted off'[35] the bed by the application of the forceps. The judge rejected this as being clinically impossible. An expert witness interpreted the mother's evidence to mean that the forceps were applied with such force that she was pulled towards the bottom of the bed in a manner inconsistent with a properly carried out trial.

No further progress. Dr Jordan said that when there was no progress on the fifth pull of the forceps, he pulled once more to see if he could ease the head past what might have been only a minimal obstruction. As there was no further progress, he decided to proceed to caesarean section and had easily pushed the head slightly upwards to effect this procedure. Dr Jordan said the head had not been wedged or stuck prior to the surgery. The judge interpreted this explanation to mean that the registrar had pulled too long and too hard, causing the head to become wedged or stuck.

Disimpaction. A consultant obstetrician who had examined the medical notes and spoken to Dr Jordan prepared a report for the hospital. This report found the mother had received correct and skilled treatment. However, the consultant had referred three times to 'disimpaction'[36] of the head prior to the caesarean section. At the trial, the consultant said that he had used that term as meaning no more than that a gentle push of the head up the birth canal was needed before the caesarean.

No agreement. There was no agreement among the medical experts as to the meaning of 'impacted',[37] or whether it had meant that there had been excessive or unprofessional traction with the forceps. The experts were clear that the amount of force to be properly used in a trial of forceps was a matter of clinical judgment. There should be no attempt to pull the fetus past a bony obstruction. If the head became so stuck as to cause asphyxia, excessive force had been used.

The decision

The judge inferred from the consultant's use of the term 'disimpacted'[38] that the baby's head had become firmly wedged or stuck and that in doing so, or in getting the head unwedged or unstuck, the registrar had caused the asphyxia. The registrar had therefore used the forceps below the required standard of skill expected from the ordinary competent specialist. Damages were awarded.

The appeal

Lord Denning in the Court of Appeal reversed this decision. The trial judge's ruling that Dr Jordan had pulled too hard or too long amounted only to an 'error of clinical judgment'[39] and was not negligent in law.

We must say, and say firmly, that in a professional man an error of judgment is not negligent.[40]

Appeal to the House of Lords

The House of Lords rejected the distinction drawn by Lord Denning. Lord Fraser said that what Lord Denning must have meant was that 'an error of judgment is not *necessarily* negligent:'

The true position is that an error of judgment may or may not be negligent; it depends on the nature of the error. If it is one that would not have been made by a reasonably competent professional man professing to have the same standard and type of skill that the defendant held himself out as having, and acting with ordinary care, then it is negligent. If, on the other hand, it is an error that a man, acting with ordinary care, might have made, then it is not negligent.[41]

Inference not justified. The House of Lords found the evidence did not justify the inference that Dr Jordan negligently pulled too long or too hard. In the final analysis, the registrar was considered to have done his best.

....

The concluding case in this chapter was reported in 1999 in the Spring issue of *A Quarterly Newsletter.*[42] The report (which does not identify the parties) concerns the settlement of a negligence action against (a) an obstetrician for an unwarranted and traumatic forceps delivery, and (b) against a paediatrician for failure to diagnose and treat polycythemia in the immediate newborn period. Note that the nurses brought the higher than normal hemacrit level to the attention of the paediatrician but he chose to disregard this.

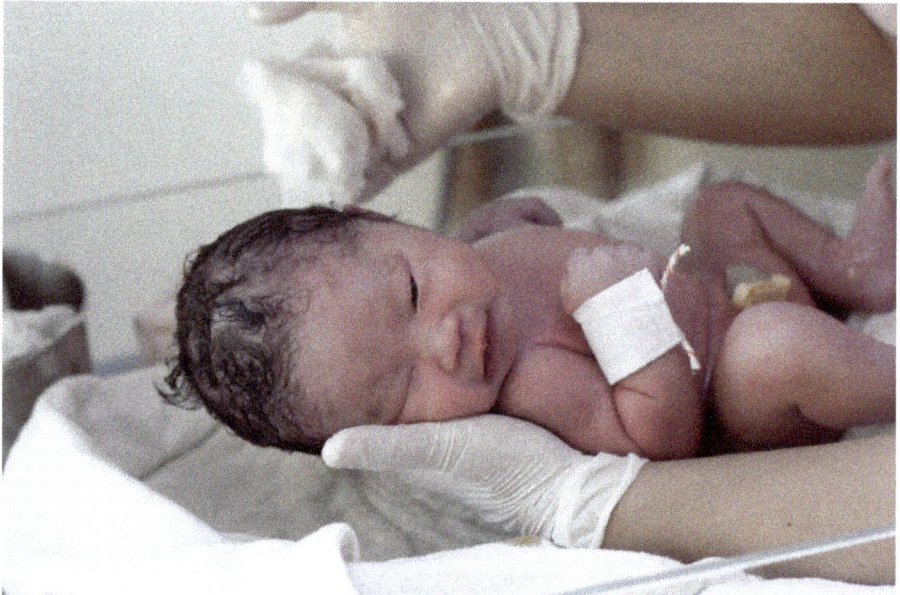

The facts

Pauline was admitted to hospital and labour progressed slowly throughout the night. The following day the obstetrician augmented the labour with pitocin, which resulted in a good labour pattern. Three hours later the cervix was completely dilated and the mother ready to push. After just a few pushes with contractions, the obstetrician decided to intervene with forceps (not described). The obstetrician then changed to Tucker-McLean forceps and, with the assistance of a traction bar, used a constant pull technique for eight minutes to effect delivery. The baby suffered neurologic injury. A negligence action was brought against both the obstetrician and the paediatrician.

Arguments and allegations

The obstetrician
Forceps. There was substantial evidence that the forceps were traumatic and caused the baby's brain injury. The record documented bruising on both sides of the temples, the cheeks, the left ear and the eyebrow. Bruising was still evident three days later. The CT scan showed evidence of swelling of the baby's brain in the first three days.

The obstetrician claimed that the intervention was due to fetal distress, dysfunctional labour, left occiput posterior position (LOP) and maternal exhaustion. With the exception of the LOP position, none of these conditions was noted in the mother's medical record or documented on the fetal heart monitor strip.

Contraindication. It was argued that the intervention by forceps was without medical justification. Pauline, though tired, had been willing and able to continue pushing toward delivery. Evidence was given that the LOP position is not an indication for the use of forceps and in the vast majority of cases the fetus will rotate spontaneously out of that position.

A medical expert conducted a survey which revealed that, on average, a forceps procedure takes about four minutes from insertion of the first blade of the forceps until the entire delivery of the fetus is completed.

The paediatrician
Failure to recognize polycythemia. Following delivery, the baby's care was transferred to a paediatrician, who, it was alleged, failed to recognize polycythemia[43] and to initiate treatment to decrease the risk of neurological injury

It was argued that the paediatrician failed to diagnose this condition despite laboratory evidence documenting its presence.

The nurses

Haematocrit level. The standing order at the hospital required that nurses determine the haematocrit level by heel stick within six hours of birth, and that they contact the doctor if the value is greater than 60 or less than 40. The haematocrit would then be re-checked from a central venous source. If polycythemia is confirmed, a partial exchange transfusion may be performed to dilute and reduce the hyperviscosity of the blood.

Polycythemia not contemplated. The paediatrician had been notified that the first heel stick haematocrit was 72.9, but decided to disregard this because in his experience the central venous haematocrit was always lower than the heel stick. He was not thinking in terms of polycythemia and did not alert nursing staff to watch for clinical signs and symptoms of polycythemia, which can be subtle.

It was argued that the combination of the bleeding and swelling from the trauma, and the viscosity from the polycythemia, combined to produce the baby's neurological injury. This was described as left-sided hemiparesis, borderline mental retardation, some moderate speech defects and an ongoing seizure disorder.

The case was settled, the majority of the damages being borne by the obstetrician.

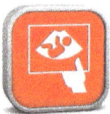

Discussion of key issues

When allegations are made that delay has caused or contributed to cerebral palsy, courts frequently hear evidence that 30 minutes is the 'gold' standard for transferring the patient to the operating room. This standard has also been described as an unrealistic expectation. Nevertheless, two questions arise in these cases. What was happening between the decision to perform the caesarean section and the actual procedure, and how long did it take to get the OR team together?

- What clinical implications would you draw from the times in each of the cases in this chapter?
- Do you agree that a hospital has 30 minutes in which to:
  a. explain the procedure and get the patient's written consent,

b. inform delivery suite, anaesthetist, theatre nurses and porters,

c. take blood sample in case transfusion is necessary;

d. remove jewellery,

e. disconnect patient from monitors and

f. transfer to theatre.

- Is there anything you would add or subtract from this list?

....

In *In Re MB* (Chapter 2) the judge found that 'the temporary factors of confusion, shock, fatigue, pain or drugs may completely erode capacity to refuse consent'.[44]

- How many of these factors could be present in the labouring woman asked to consent to an emergency caesarean?
- What is the alternative?
- Do you agree that the word 'emergency' can have different meanings for the obstetric/midwifery area and OR staff?
- How do you communicate to the OR at your hospital in relation to an emergency caesarean section? Staff may have worked in other hospitals where the term 'emergency' is interpreted differently. List and discuss the different ways 'emergency' is communicated.

....

Any emergency dash to the OR can be frightening to both patient and carers. For example, the patient's mother in *Allin* (Chapter 11) described it as 'all hell broke loose.'

- Does your unit provide adequate explanation and debriefing?

....

In *Richards* the primary claim was a) an unacceptable 55-minute delay between decision and incision. Alternatively it was argued b) the student midwife had delayed reporting three decelerations to midwife and (c) that CTG monitoring should have continued throughout the caesarean procedure.

- Discuss the merits of each claim

....

In *Ren* the judge found that the hospital had a duty to provide an operating theatre, equipped for a caesarean section, as soon as reasonably possible, having regard to the need for urgency.

The judge also found that breakdown in communication between hospital staff was at the heart of the problem. Had it been understood that the OR was needed for a caesarean section, following a failed attempt at forceps delivery, and not for a trial by forceps, with possible caesarean section, it was likely that delay would have been avoided.

- Do you agree?

The delay in this case happened on a public holiday.

- Identify the 'risk' days at your hospital.
- On average, how long does it take on-call staff to reach the OR for an emergency caesarean section at your hospital?

....

Allen. This case raises the issue of ORs not being booked or not being available.

- Can there be difficulty in finding an operating room for an emergency caesarean section in your hospital?
- Have you known an emergency theatre to be mis-used?

Telephone communication between midwives and doctors was a factor in most of these cases. Calls needs to be clearly documented as to time and content.

- Will your documentation demonstrate that you have recognised a problem and responded accordingly?
- Is there a process in place to resolve the issue where a midwife telephones with a concern about a patient, but the doctor refuses to alter treatment or come to the hospital?
- If not, what would you suggest?

NOTES

1. MJA 162: 85-90 The Australian and New Zealand Perinatal Societies, *The Origins of Cerebral Palsy — Consensus- Statement*. Alastair H MacLennan, Assoc. Prof. Ob/Gyn, University of Adelaide, Consensus Conference Chair, p.7 (1997).
2. Ibid., p.1.
3. CCH Australian Health and Medical Law Reporter, *Time Limitations*, 16-740.
4. *Concise Australian Legal Dictionary*, Butterworths, Australia (2004).
5. *Dissidomino v Newnham & Anor*, Supreme Court of Western Australia, No. 84, CCH Australian Health & Medical Law Reporter 77084 (12 April 1994).
6. Ibid.
7. Ibid.
8. *Richards (a child) v Swansea NHS Trust*, 96 MLR 180 (2007).
9. Ibid., p.182.
10. Ibid., p.183.
11. Ibid.
12. Ibid.
13. Ibid., p.184.
14. Ibid.
15. Ibid.
16. Ibid, p.185.
17. Ibid.
18. Ibid., p.186.
19. BMJ 2001:322:1300-3. *'Interval between Decision and Delivery by Caesarean Section — Are Current Standards Achievable?'* Tufnell, et al.
20. BMJ 2004, *'National Cross Sectional Survey To Determine Whether the Decision to Delivery Interval Is Critical in Emergency Caesarean Section'*, Thomas, et al., BMJ, doi.10.1136/bmj.38031.775845.7C.
21. *Ren v Mukerjee and Anor*, ACT Supreme Court, No. SC 440, 12 (Dec. 1996).
22. *Allen (next friend of) v University Hospital's Board*, A.J. No.880 (QB) (QL) Alberta Court of Queens Bench (2000). Case note based on Bogoroch, R.M. and Levine, S.A. (Bogoroch & Associates), *Forceps and Caesarean Deliveries and Informed Consent: New Issues And Dangers in Child Delivery Methods.* 26 (Mar. 2002). www.bogoroch.com/articles/index.php.
23. Ibid., p.11.
24. Ibid.
25. *Bauer (litigation guardian of) v Seager*, MJ., No.356 (QB) (QL) (Canada, 2000). Case note based on Bogoroch & Associates article. (as above), pp. 12–16.
26. Ibid.

27. Ibid.
28. Ibid.
29. B. Dimond, *Legal Aspects of Midwifery*, 2d ed. BFM, commenting on *Whitehouse v Jordan*, at p. 226.
30. *Whitehouse v Jordan*, 1 All ER 267 (1981).
31. Ibid., p.271.
32. Ibid., p.271.
33. Ibid.
34. Ibid.
35. Ibid., p.278.
36. Ibid., p.282-3.
37. Ibid., p.283.
38. Ibid.
39. Ibid., p.281.
40. Ibid.
41. Ibid.
42. *A Quarterly Newsletter*, pp. 2–3 (Spring 1999). http/www.sjblaw.com/news/
43. (Polycythemia is an abnormally high number of red blood cells which have the effect of thickening or 'sludging' the blood, thereby increasing the risk of clotting due to the hyperviscosity.)
44. *In Re MB:* See Chapter 2.

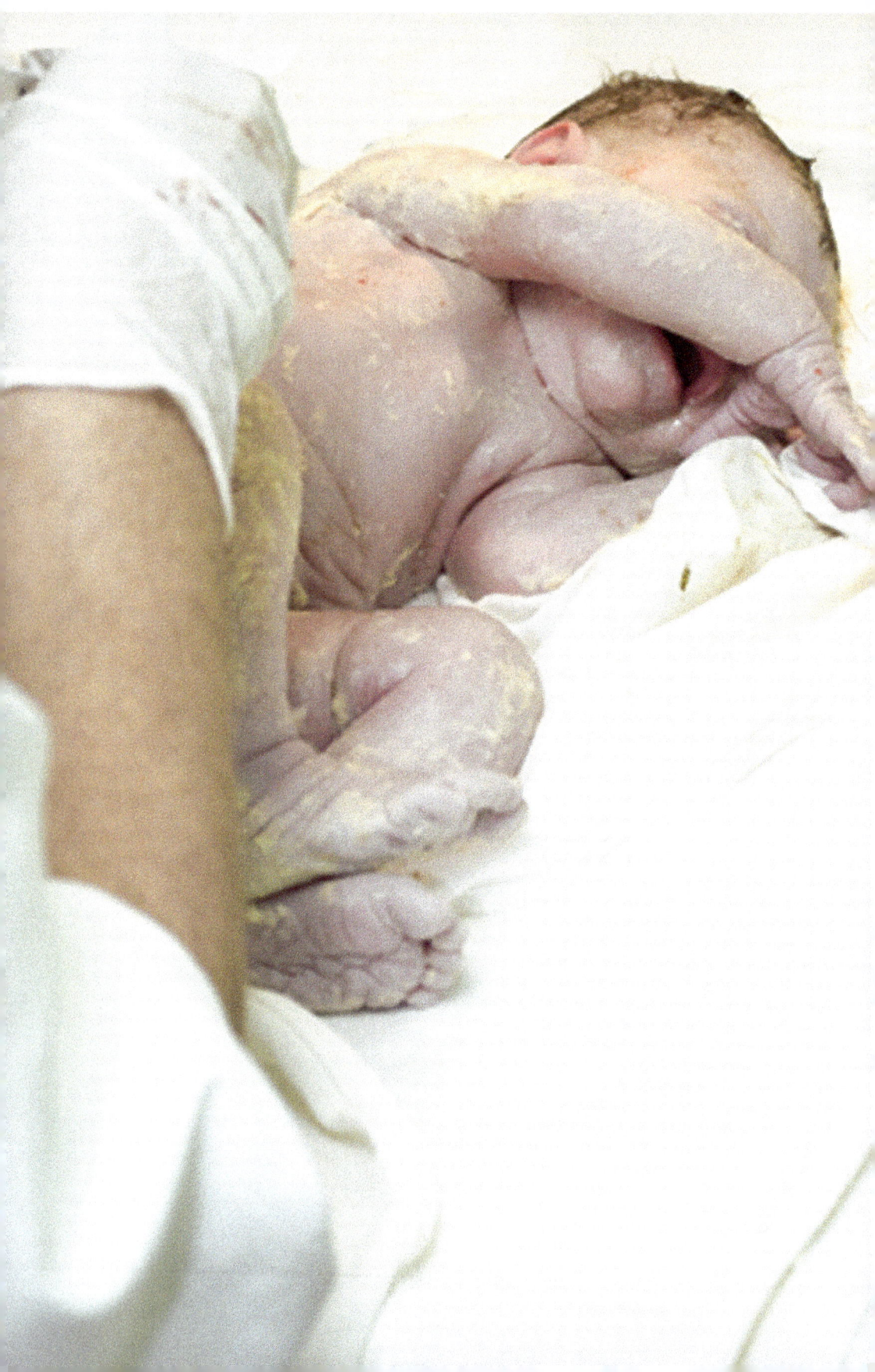

CHAPTER 6

Shoulder dystocia

'The assumption that the presence of an injury is evidence that traction must have been applied is no longer valid. Injury may occur regardless of the best efforts of the midwife.'

—Justice Hickinbottom.

Introduction

English obstetrician Dr Roger Clements describes shoulder dystocia as 'the most frightening of all obstetric emergencies.'[1] It may follow spontaneous delivery of the head, but is more commonly seen after forceps or ventouse delivery when the chin fails to clear the perineum. Shoulder dystocia is disastrous for the baby unless its shoulders can be released within a few minutes. Excessive traction with lateral flexion of the neck may leave the baby with a paralysed arm (Erb's or Klumpke's paralysis), or the baby may suffer asphyxia because the chest cannot be expanded.

Clements notes that textbooks can present a 'multiplicity of confusing and often inappropriate advice'[2] and considers that the combination of the McRobert's manoeuvre, extreme hip flexion, generous episiotomy and suprapubic pressure will often free the impacted anterior shoulder. If not, 'the shoulders must be rotated within the pelvis (Wood's screw) to bring the posterior shoulder under the symphysis pubis and into the pelvis.'[3]

The problem 'can and should'[4] be anticipated if the baby is known to be large (over four kilos), the mother has gained excessive weight, the pregnancy is postdates or the labour dysfunctional and operative delivery necessary from the midpelvis. Where possible, a senior doctor should be present at delivery.

....

The first of the following three cases focuses not so much on the management of the obstruction but on the failure of the obstetric team to abandon vaginal delivery at an appropriate time. The second case questions whether shoulder dystocia should have been anticipated, and if so, how the delivery should have been handled. The third case illustrates how medical thinking and case law have changed.

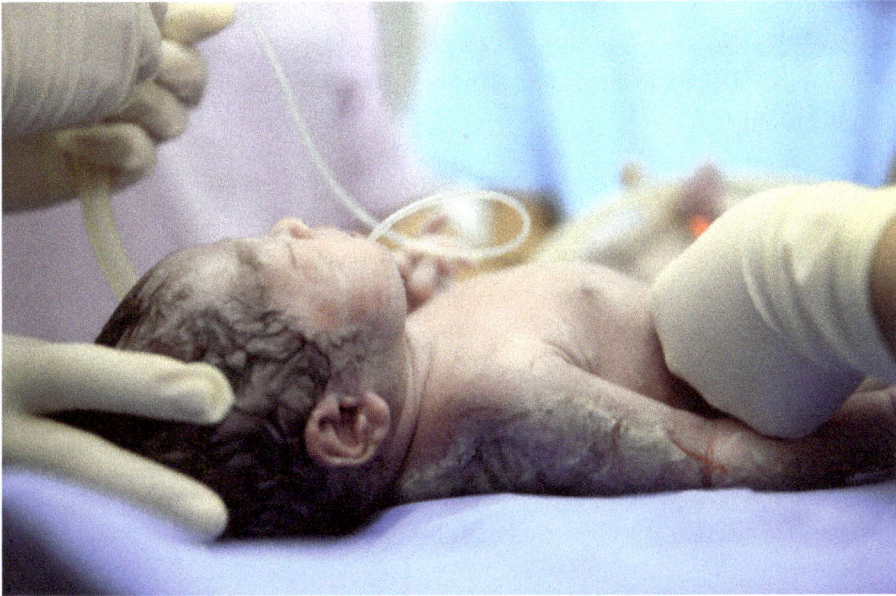

Dowdie v Camberwell Health Authority [UK, 1997][5]

The facts

Susan's estimated date of delivery for her second child (the first born 13 years earlier) was 28 December 1991. On 6 December, the symphysial fundal height was assessed at the hospital as 40 cm. This being large for the stage of gestation, Susan was referred to the Fetal Assessment Unit. On 10 December, an ultrasound scan showed the fetal abdominal circumference at 33.4 cm (placing it on the 50th centile) and the fetal weight at 3.181 kg.

Discrepancy in weight. On 20 December, the symphysial fundal height was again recorded at 40 cm. On 27 December, the fetal weight, based on clinical examination by a doctor, was assessed at 4.2 kg. Where there was a significant discrepancy between weight assessed on ultrasound and on clinical examination, it was the doctor's practice to manage a patient on the scan assessment. However, even on the basis of 4.2 kg he did not consider further action was appropriate or that cephalopelvic disproportion (CPD) or shoulder dystocia was indicated.

Admission to hospital. Early on 31 December, Susan showed signs of bleeding and contractions, and was admitted to hospital at 4.30 am. Records showed she was having weak and irregular contractions, but 'not in established labour.'[6]

First vaginal examination. A midwife examined Susan at 7.30 am. Symphysial fundal height was 42 cm. Fifteen minutes later a senior house officer carried out the first vaginal examination. The cervix was noted to be 2 cm long, 1 cm dilated. A senior registrar, accompanied by registrar Dr Walsh, saw Susan on a ward round at 8.50 am. The senior registrar's note suggested labour should be induced.

Second vaginal examination. At 10.00 am, Dr Walsh carried out the second vaginal examination. The cervix was found to be soft, 75 per cent effaced and 2 cm dilated. The notes recorded artificial rupture of the membranes and the direction that staff 'wait one hour for contractions then start Syntocinon.'[7] A partogram was commenced. A midwife clinically estimated the fetal weight at 4 kg. A CTG, which had been used intermittently since 4.30 am, was recommenced.

Syntocinon. The administration of Syntocinon began at 11.15 am at a rate of 10 drops per minute (dpm), increased to 20 dpm at 11.30 am. Two minutes later a midwife recorded the fetal heart as having a baseline of 130 beats per minute (bpm) with early deceleration of 109 bpm and 'fairly good recovery to baseline.'[8]

Syntocinon was increased to 30 dpm at 11.45 am. Ten minutes later the same midwife recorded a fetal heart baseline of 138 bpm and 'shallow deceleration (early) to 120 with good recovery to baseline.'[9] At noon, Syntocinon was increased to 40 dpm. At 12.13 pm the midwife noted 'further early deceleration to 100 bpm with fair recovery to 138 bpm. Trace is reactive.'[10]

Third vaginal examination. The attending midwife carried out the third vaginal examination at 12.20 pm when applying a scalp electrode, noting: 'Os 3 cms dilated. Cephalic 2 cms above ischial spines.'[11] Syntocinon was then increased to 50 dpm. The senior house officer was informed of progress. A note by SHO Dr Talbot at 12.40 pm referred to shallow decelerations and to 'mild–moderate contractions only 1 in 5 comfortable.'[12]

At 12.50 pm, the midwife noted continuing early decelerations with each contraction, a fetal heart baseline of 126, no accelerations and 'contracting 4:10 moderate.'[13] Syntocinon was increased to 60 dpm at 1.00 pm. Susan was experiencing some distress with contractions. Five minutes later the midwife noted a baseline of 129 and early decelerations to 105-110, with slow recovery to baseline. Soon afterwards, Dr Talbot recorded 'Trace much improved.'[14]

Fourth vaginal examination. At 1.30 pm, Susan was transferred to another room. The fetal heart was beating at 90 bpm when the CTG was reconnected, recovering to 117 and then 124 bpm. At 1.45 pm, the midwife carried out the fourth vaginal examination, noting 'cervix effaced, thick, loosely applied to presenting part. Os 4 cm dilated. Cephalic 2 cm above ischial spines.'[15] The fetal heart was at 124 bpm following the examination.

A second midwife, accompanied by a student midwife, then took over Susan's care. She immediately noted early deceleration down to 85 bpm, recovering to a baseline of 120 bpm. Dr Talbot was called, confirming 'some deep decelerations to 80, this in the context of CTG reactive with accelerations.'[16] Five minutes later the fetal heart was recorded at 135 bpm. The CTG tracing continued to show deep decelerations.

Fifth vaginal examination. Dr Walsh saw Susan at 2.25 pm. The Syntocinon was reduced to 40 dpm. At 2.50 pm, Dr Walsh performed the fifth vaginal examination and found the cervix 5-6 cm dilated. A fetal blood sample was within normal limits (and therefore contra-indicative of fetal distress). At 3.15 pm, early decelerations were noted to 80 bpm with reasonable recovery to a baseline of 132. Sytocinon continued at 40 dpm. Contractions were strong, remaining so at 3.30 pm.

Sixth vaginal examination. At 3.45 pm, when a prolonged bradycardia was observed, the midwife stopped the Syntocinon. Dr Walsh was satisfied that the fetal heart had picked up rapidly and the tracing was normal. Because the contractions were beginning to decrease, the Syntocinon was started again gradually. Dr Walsh carried out the sixth vaginal examination, finding the cervix to be 8 cm dilated. He believed Susan was making progress. On Dr Walsh's instructions the Syntocinon was recommenced at 10 dpm at 4.05 pm, and increased to 20 dpm at 4.20 pm. The fetal heart was about 122 bpm.

Seventh vaginal examination. At 4.20 or 4.33 pm, the midwife found the cervix still eight centimeters dilated. There was moulding and caput. The head was one centimeter above the ischial spines and not palpable on abdominal examination. The Syntocinon was increased to 30 dpm shortly afterwards.

At 4.46 pm, Dr Talbot attended and was pleased with the CTG trace. Within four minutes it was showing early decelerations. Syntocinon was reduced to 20 dpm, but increased to 25 dpm at 5.05 pm. Fifteen minutes later the senior registrar came on a ward round noting 'CTG satisfactory … all well.'[17] Syntocinon was increased to 30 dpm at 5.30 pm and to 35 dpm at 5.40, with the note 'baseline reactive.'[18]

Eighth vaginal examination. At 5.48 pm, the midwife was concerned about early decelerations and reduced the Syntocinon to 15 dpm. Dr Talbot carried out the eighth vaginal examination. The cervix was now nine centimeters dilated. There was caput and moulding. The leading part of the head was at the level of the ischial spines. Syntocinon was increased to 25 dpm but almost immediately reduced by the midwife to 20 dpm. The notes recorded 'early deceleration with slow pick up to baseline.'[19] It was then reduced to 10 dpm.

Dr Talbot came and ordered that Syntocinon be increased to 15 dpm, whereupon the CTG improved. It was now 6.05 pm. During the next hour, the midwife twice increased the Syntocinon and then decreased it to 20 dpm, so that at 6.55 pm the CTG was noted as recording 'deceleration deep with fairish pick up to baseline.'[20]

Ninth vaginal examination. Dr Talbot saw Susan at 7.00pm and interpreted the CTG as some 'further decelerations with fair recovery to a reactive baseline.'[21] On the ninth vaginal examination she found the cervix to be nine centimeters dilated. The head was at the level of the ischial spines in the right occipito-anterior position. At 7.08pm, the midwife observed a period of bradycardia at 90-95 bpm; she turned the Syntocinon off.

Tenth vaginal examination. Dr Talbot came back. The baseline returned to an acceptable level. Dr Talbot ordered the Syntocinon to be recommenced. It was 10 dpm at 7.15 pm, increasing to 20 dpm five minutes later. At 7.30 pm, the notes recorded 'CTG very much improved,'[22] with the baseline at 120 bpm. However, at 7.50pm there was another episode of bradycardia at 80-90 bpm. The Syntocinon was stopped and Dr Talbot was asked to return. She ordered the Syntocinon to be resumed at 20 dpm. A tenth vaginal examination showed the cervix to be nine centimeters dilated. Dr Talbot considered the CTG 'suboptimal'[23] and decided to bring in registrar, Dr Walsh, with a view to a possible instrumental delivery.

Increased risks. Dr Walsh considered, then rejected, performing a caesarean section, believing that there were increased risks at that stage of labour:

---

*At 8.00 pm I saw 'Susan'... I performed an abdominal examina-
tion and was unable to feel any of the fetal head. A vaginal examination was performed. The cervix was fully dilated, the fetal head
was at the spines and the position of the occiput was directly anterior. There was no evidence of cephalo-pelvic disproportion as
there was only +1 of caput and the head passed into the maternal
pelvis. I decided that a ventouse delivery was indicated. A puden-
dal block was inserted of 10 ml 1 per cent lignocaine to each of the
ischial spine. Susan was catheterised and Dr Talbot performed the
ventouse delivery under my direct supervision. The ventouse cup
was applied to the fetal head and carefully checked to ensure no
vaginal skin was caught. The suction was gradually increased to
a level of 0.8 PSI. The fetal head was delivered easily with three
contractions and an episiotomy.[24]*

The emergency. The doctors then realised that the baby was stuck and
that the reason was a shoulder dystocia. As not all shoulder dystocias are
equally severe, the lesser ones sometimes responding to relatively straightforward manoeuvres, Dr Walsh was initially content to let Dr Talbot continue to attempt to deliver. Dr Walsh applied supra-pubic pressure, while Dr
Talbot applied traction. Dr Walsh then took over. By this time, the obstetric
emergency was becoming more intense. It was obvious that if the baby was
not successfully delivered within a little more than five minutes, he would
die or suffer serious brain damage. Although what happened next was the
subject of debate, the judge found the probable sequence of events was as
described below:

Intra-vaginal manipulation. Dr Walsh took over from Dr Talbot, applying some (but not very much) traction as part of his assessment. The
midwife applied supra-pubic pressure. Dr Walsh then commenced a vaginal
examination and attempted an intra-vaginal manipulation of the baby. In

doing so, he twice extended the episiotomy, which Dr Talbot had performed earlier.

Humerus fractured. Dr Walsh tried intra-vaginal manipulation twice, attempting to rotate the posterior shoulder. The baby's head was becoming blue on the perineum. In the course of the second attempt, he caused a fracture of the left humerus. This resulted in a reduction in the resistance to rotation and he was able to rotate the shoulders marginally to an oblique position.

Injury. Baby Thomas was delivered by traction, weighing 4.28 kg. He suffered serious brachial plexus injury involving the avulsion of three of the nerve roots from the spinal cord. Negligence was alleged.

The trial

Pre-delivery
It was argued that:

1. The obstetric team ought to have predicted, or suspected, that Thomas was going to be a macrosomic baby, with the possibility of cephalopelvic disproportion. They should therefore have concluded that it was unsafe to seek a vaginal delivery in circumstances which called for a caesarean section.
2. A caesarean section became all the more necessary after secondary arrest of labour and signs of fetal distress.
3. The management of the labour was characterised by over stimulation with Syntocinon.
4. CTG abnormalities ought to have diverted the doctors from proceeding with a vaginal delivery.

Delivery

5. The use of traction by Dr Talbot, and/or Dr Walsh, prior to Dr Walsh undertaking intravaginal manipulation was excessive.

The defence. It was argued in defence that it was obvious traction had been applied; otherwise, the baby would not have been delivered. Dr Walsh agreed that he had used considerable force when the humerus cracked:

I was in a situation of either having a dead baby or a baby with palsy and I felt that a baby that survived is better than one who did not survive and, secondly, I was also worried that as time went on there was an increasing chance that this baby would end up with cerebral palsy as well as an Erb palsy due to anoxia.[25]

The decision

The judge held that Thomas's claim succeeded because:

1. It was highly probable that when traction was applied between the time of the fracture and delivery, Dr Walsh went through a process of having to apply increasing force in order to achieve the delivery of a baby who might otherwise have been born dead or seriously brain damaged. It was more probable than not that the brachial plexus injury was caused at that stage rather than at the earlier stages by either Dr Talbot or Dr Walsh.

2. There was clear evidence of secondary arrest from 6.00 pm onwards and a very high probability that this was mainly caused by mechanical difficulty arising from macrosomia size and position.

3. As at 7.00 pm, the safe and proper conclusion was that the CTG trace was suspicious rather than abnormal, indicating periods of fetal stress rather than distress. Neither doctor had secondary arrest or macrosomia in mind at that stage, as they should have.

4. Dr Talbot should not have persisted towards a vaginal delivery at 7.00 pm.

5. At 7.55 pm, when Dr Talbot found that the cervix remained at 9 cm dilated, her decision to proceed by way of an assisted vaginal delivery rather than by caesarean section was not negligent.

6. In the hour before Thomas was born, there were unequivocal abnormalities shown on the CTG trace from about 7.40 pm. In the light of his clinical findings at 8.05 pm as to station and full cervical dilatation, Dr Walsh's decision to proceed by way of a ventouse delivery rather than by caesarean section was a decision within the range of acceptable practice. Thereafter, neither he nor Dr Talbot acted negligently as they attempted, in increasingly fraught circumstances, to deliver a live and uninjured baby.

7. If there had been a decision to proceed by way of caesarean section at 7.00 pm, it was highly probable that Thomas would have been born uninjured.

The judge:

I recognise that, in this area, even more than in many other areas of medical litigation, a great deal revolves around matters of judgment, that more than one view can coexist within the range of the acceptable and that one must be careful before categorising something as negligent if it was simply an alternative but acceptable judgment which has only become unfortunate with the benefit of hindsight. I am also conscious of the need to make allowances for the pressures within which decisions have to be taken by clinicians. However, I am satisfied that the management of the mother at 7.00 pm was negligent.[26]

Damages awarded.

Commenting on this case, English barrister, Margaret Puxon QC, makes the following key points:

1. The *Dowdie* case is complicated and in some aspects confused by the conflicting antenatal findings and the advent of secondary arrest in labour. While a prenatal diagnosis of macrosomia would probably have made all the difference to the outcome, the definition of macrosomia is itself uncertain. In the United Kingdom, a diagnostic factor is a child of 4 kg or more, or above the 97 percentile; in the United States, it is 4.5 kg (as at 1997). While it was understandable that the registrar took the earlier ultrasound figure of 3.181 kg rather than trust his own clinical assessment of 4.2 kg, a repeat scan might have come nearer his clinical figure and forewarned of possible shoulder dystocia.[27]
2. The secondary arrest of labour from 6.00 pm onwards was crucial to the baby. The team's failure to recognise the arrest, or bear in mind the size of the baby, meant they were not alerted to the chance of CPD. In the judge's view it had been negligent to continue 'down the Syntocinon road rather than deliver straight away.'[28]

3. As there was no evidence of fetal distress (and the mother was reacting to the Syntocinon), there was some sympathy with the defence argument. It had not been proved that any doctor using reasonable skill and care would have performed a caesarean section at 7.00 pm, unless they had an accurate diagnosis of macrosomia, rather than the 'impression'[29] of the midwife confirming the clinical assessment as against the scan. While it should be remembered that the majority of shoulder dystocia cases are unrelated to macrosomia, *Dowdie* is a warning of the importance of awareness of the risks of shoulder dystocia when the baby is large.

4. The finding of no negligence in delivery emphasizes the 'immense difficulty and urgency'[30] of the situation. The decision recognizes the dilemma of an obstetrician faced with the need to save the baby by a swift delivery yet avoid the risk of brachial plexus injury by heroic manipulation. According to the judge in *Dowdie*, 'The danger of a baby suffocating in the birth canal while half delivered from compression of the chest and umbilical cord makes shoulder dystocia the ultimate horror in obstetrics.'[31]

....

In the next case, the court is concerned with whether shoulder dystocia should have been anticipated and, if so, how the delivery should have been managed. Daniel was born with injury to the right brachial plexus and with Erb's palsy of the right arm.

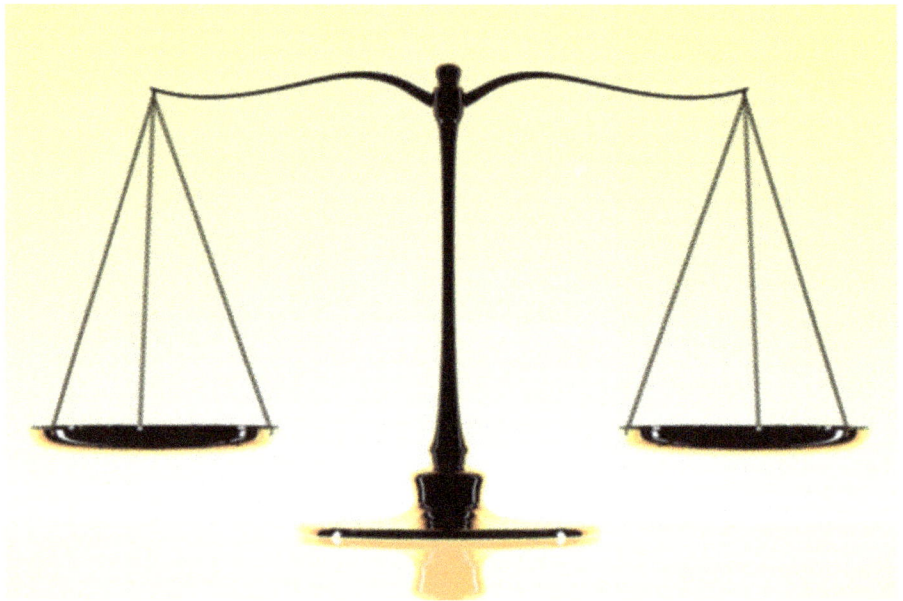

Gaughan v Bedfordshire Health Authority [UK, 1997][32]

The facts

Mary, aged 32, was due to give birth to her third child on 8 February 1991. Her first son weighed 3.9 kg at birth in 1982; a second son 4 kg in 1987. Both were spontaneous deliveries. At 20 weeks into the third pregnancy, Mary was 'significantly overweight at 98.6 kg,'[33] having gained an above average weight of 5.8 kg at 30 weeks. At 33 weeks, the baby's estimated weight was 2.9 kg. Mary was told the baby was in good condition and would be big.

By 30 January, Mary weighed 110.3 kg. A doctor examining her on 13 February did not consider the baby would be larger than 4 kg, nor did he anticipate any particular problems. But he noted Mary's obesity might make the baby's position difficult to define. Arrangements were made to induce labour on 15 February, but contractions began on 14 February and Mary was admitted to hospital at 9.15 pm.

'Big baby.' Documentation noted a cephalic presentation, the baby estimated to be 3/5 palpable above the pelvic brim. The partogram and labour notes noted 'Big Baby.'[34] From 10.30 pm to 10.35 pm the baby remained 3/5 palpable; the cervix had dilated from 3 cm to 4 cm. At 10.40 pm, the midwife ruptured the membranes. At 4.15 am, the cervix was fully dilated and the baby fully descended.

Labour notes made between 4.10 and 4.23 am read:

04.10   CTG variability improved — feels like pushing.

04.15   VE. no cvx felt, pp celp in m/c (mid cavity) pushing well with contractions. FSE fell off, pp advancing very well so FH not recorded.

04.23   Big Baby Boy delivered.

Shoulder dystocia, poor condition and cord loosely round neck x 1. Immediately transferred to NNU.[35]

The labour summary noted Daniel's birth weight as 4.945 kg and an Agpar of 3:1 at one minute, rising to 9:10 at ten minutes.

Allegations. It was alleged that the injuries to Daniel's arm were the result of the midwife's negligence.

The trial

The midwife, described to the court as 'extremely experienced,'[36] had been in practice for 20 years and delivered between 4,000 and 5,000 babies. She had encountered shoulder dystocia, or some degree of obstruction, on eight to ten occasions. Each baby had been delivered by traction without injury. The midwife was first asked for a written statement four years after Daniel's birth. At the trial, she was dependent on her notes for recalling the delivery. The judge found some gaps in the notes, as well as disputes about what had occurred. Despite this, the judge determined that Daniel's head was delivered quickly by the midwife at 4.20 am, within five minutes of a vaginal examination at 4.15 am. It was also established that two contractions had occurred between delivery of the head at 4.20 am and the body at 4.23 am.

Shoulder dystocia suspected. The midwife said that after delivery of Daniel's head on the first contraction his head had restituted and retracted against the perineum. She checked the umbilical cord was loose, and then cleared the airway by suction. Suspecting shoulder dystocia, she asked Mary, prior to the second contraction, to push out. When nothing happened, she asked the student midwife to call for assistance and removed one section of the mattress to give herself more room. She said she rejected the idea of getting Mary on her side, this having failed earlier because of Mary's obesity.

Trouble. The parents said the midwife had told Mary, now in a squatting position on the edge of the mattress and supported by her husband, that the baby was in trouble. She must give as hard a push as she could on the next contraction.

Traction. The midwife then held Daniel's head with both hands, giving continuous steady traction downwards at an angle of 25 to 30 degrees. She had done so while Mary was pushing, so that she could deliver the anterior shoulder. These pushes probably lasted between 15 to 20 seconds or longer. The midwife said the idea was to deliver the baby. If he had been left longer, the outcome could have included stillbirth. However, she had managed such life-threatening situations before and was very confident she could do so again. She believed she had dealt with the delivery to the best of her ability in the three minutes between delivery of the head and of the shoulders and body. Daniel was delivered on the third contraction, as other midwives arrived in the room.

The time factor. A midwife, giving expert evidence for Daniel, said that the standard estimate of time available to achieve delivery and save a baby's life was eight minutes. A consultant obstetrician for the defence agreed that, if a baby had not yet turned puce, a midwife or obstetrician still had time to try different methods of dislodging the obstructed shoulder. At one stage in her evidence the midwife who had delivered Daniel said there was nothing more she could have done between contractions. The judge noted that she had earlier explained to the court that alternatives were to improve the position of the mother, and to use supra-pubic and fundal pressure.

The judge identified four significant issues:

1. Should a reasonably competent midwife have predicted or anticipated shoulder dystocia?

The judge was not satisfied that a reasonably competent midwife would have done more than the midwife had done. She was aware of the risk factors,

in particular of Daniel being a large baby. This had been noted on the partogram and progress notes. She had borne in mind possible complications,
including shoulder dystocia.

2. Should the medical team have been notified?

An obstetrician giving expert evidence for Daniel said that, given the assessment of a large baby, the medical team should have been put on standby
when Mary was approaching full dilatation. He agreed the midwife's note of
'Big Baby' would serve to 'heighten awareness'[37] of possible problems, but
believed this was not sufficient and that the team should have been alerted.

An obstetrician for the defence, while agreeing it would be good practice to inform the registrar of a potential problem, considered it would be a
'counsel of perfection'[38] to expect the midwife to let the registrar know when
stage two of the labour had been reached. He was firmly of the view that experienced midwives were perfectly capable of running a labour room on their
own. There was no need to call for assistance unless a problem arose. (About
50 per cent of shoulder dystocia cases occur in babies who are not macrosomic.) The obstetrician believed the labour ward coverage by the midwives
was adequate, provided the midwives had a clear idea of what to do if shoulder dystocia did occur. In the obstetrician's words, 'In reality, they are more
skilled than doctors in delivery, unless more manipulative or invasive procedures become necessary.'[39]

The judge concluded that the midwife had not fallen below a reasonable
standard by not alerting the team, putting the team on standby or securing
the attendance of a doctor before a problem occurred. The midwife had considerable experience and her action in documenting 'Big Baby' was sufficient.

3. Position.

The midwife had Mary, supported by her husband, squatting at an angle
of 45 degrees and perched on the edge of the mattress. Thighs were flexed
against the abdomen. The McRobert's position, i.e., the mother being nearly
prone on her back, head supported by a low pillow and weight off her sa-
crum, had been introduced in Canada in the 1980s. It was not widely known
in the United Kingdom or favoured by some experts until 1992.

The judge found that the midwife's choice of position in the circumstances,
and by 1991 standards, was appropriate.

4. Traction.

After hearing expert midwifery and obstetric opinion for both parties, the
judge accepted that traction for very short periods of time (four to six sec-

onds) was a recognised and acceptable method of dealing with the problem of an impeded shoulder. But this was with the proviso that the shoulder showed signs of coming free during its application. It was not a recognised or acceptable method if a modest increase in force beyond what was normally required to deliver the body was required, and if there was no feeling that the shoulder was coming free.

Asked how she judged how little traction to use, the midwife answered :

A: *You try traction and obviously eventually the shoulders will come ... The anterior shoulder will be delivered but, if it doesn't, then you try a little bit more. But you are not just giving it all the time.*

Q: *And if the shoulder did not come free?*

A: *Obviously, you have to use a little bit more traction then ... try again, and that is with the mum pushing at the same time.*[40]

The judge found the midwife negligent in this regard. She should not have continued to use traction after realizing she was dealing with shoulder dystocia, unless she was sure the shoulder was becoming free. There was no evidence that she thought this was occurring, or even that she was concerned to ascertain if the shoulder was becoming free. Instead of ceasing traction after the second contraction, and trying either suprapubic pressure or rotation of the shoulders, she had increased the amount of traction in accordance with her general practice until the baby was delivered.

On a balance of probabilities, the midwife had used more force for longer than was acceptable. Daniel's severe brachial plexus injury was entirely consistent with application of excessive traction. Acknowledging that even with 'best practice' no technique is without risk of injury, the judge found either alternative, on a balance of probabilities, would have resulted in no injuries or less severe injuries.

The midwife, otherwise described as having a 'highly professional approach,'[41] had fallen below the standard of a reasonably competent midwife. In the judge's opinion, this was possibly due to over-confidence (engendered by her previous successful deliveries in shoulder dystocia cases) that traction would solve the problem.

Damages awarded.

Change

By 2009, however, established medical thinking and case law had changed. One judge explained:[42]

.

> It had been generally thought that natural uterine propulsive forces on the baby's neck during delivery were not sufficient, or in the right directional plane, to cause damage to the brachial plexus. The accepted medical view of causation of such injuries during delivery was that in all cases the nerve damage was caused by the application of lateral and downward traction to the fetal head while the anterior shoulder was impacted against the symphesis pubis. So, in the majority of cases where a baby was born with such injuries, there would be an assumption that the cause was excessive traction.

> This change was prompted by a recognition that the single mechanism of lateral and downwards traction of the baby's head against resistance cannot readily explain all of the available data, such as reports of significant numbers of injuries being suffered to the posterior shoulder and/or of obstetric brachial plexus injury without any evidence of shoulder dystocia.

In *Bennion v North East Wales NHS Trust* (24 February 2009, unreported) the judge reviewed over 80 pieces of literature and heard evidence from biomedical engineers and orthopaedic surgeons as well as obstetric experts, concluding:

> Causation of obstetric brachial plexus injury is multifactorial; evidence suggests that while some cases are traction mediated, others

may not be. There is growing acceptance in both medical literature and case law that the propulsive forces of uterine contraction may play a part.

The assumption that the presence of an injury is evidence that traction must have been applied is no longer valid. Injury may occur regardless of the best efforts of the midwife. Diagnostic traction is acceptable and claimants now need to demonstrate factual evidence of the use of excessive force or other inappropriate management to succeed in arguing negligent management.

Negligence must therefore be proved not only on the basis of all available evidence but, in particular, on the evidence of eye-witnesses to the delivery.

....

This was the approach taken by the court in the final case in this chapter, *Croft v Heart of England NHS Foundation Trust 2012 WL 1933467.*[43]

During his birth in 1997, Mark suffered an injury to the nerves of his neck which resulted in a permanent loss of function in his right arm. Nine years later it was alleged that the midwife had encountered shoulder dystocia and over a period of 5-10 minutes had negligently pulled his head, 'repeatedly and with force', before summoning assistance.

The midwife could not remember Mark's birth, but, relying on her notes and usual practice in 1997, denied that she had been negligent. The case came to court in 2012.

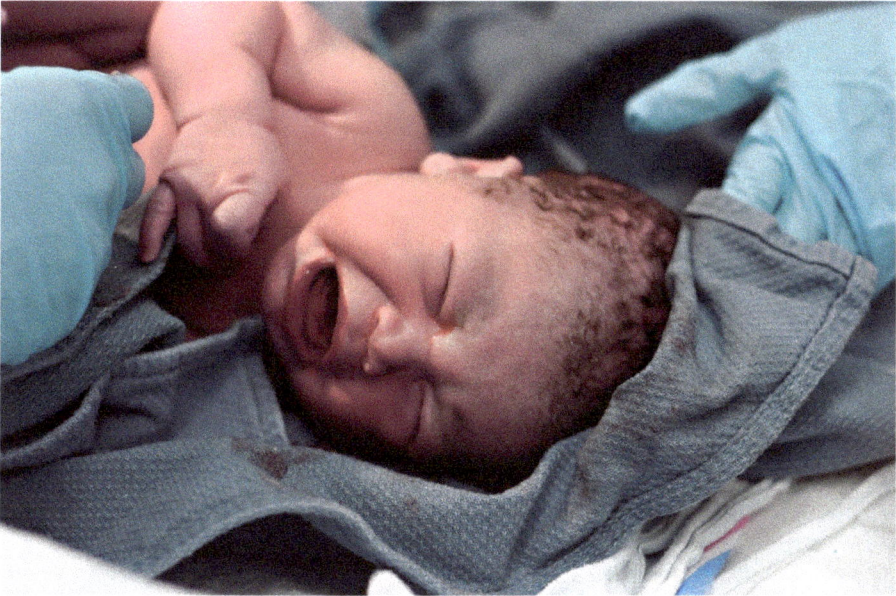

Croft v Heart of England NHS Foundation Trust 2012 WL 1933467

The facts

Joanne's first pregnancy was uncomplicated, with a successful forceps delivery and her second pregnancy was essentially normal. The due date was 19 April and Joanne was admitted to the delivery suite at 12.10 am on 14 April. The progress of labour was described as 'perhaps slightly slower than usual for a second birth'[44] but otherwise normal. The midwife came on duty just before midnight and Joanne was given an epidural anaesthetic around midnight.

The midwife then noted:[45]

1.45 am	Contractions 4: 10 mild (every two and a half minutes).
08.00	Cervix dilated, with baby's head in the left occipito–posterior position (this was the only noted position of the baby's head).

03.00	Cervix fully dilated — with no urge to push.
04.00	Complaining of rectal pressure.
04.15	Commenced pushing– Presenting part visible.
04.31	Normal delivery of live male.

Moderate shoulder dystocia.

Apgar 8 & 9.

3rd stage complete — Blood loss 100 ml.

2nd degree tear sutured.

[Birth weight] 4.390 kg.

Epidural catheter removed intact.

IVI discontinued.

Baby to be seen by paediatrician — Re Shoulder dystocia.

(What happened in the sixteen minutes between 04.15 and 04.31 became critical to the negligence claim.)

The trial

The mother. Joanne said it had taken some time to come to terms with her son's disability and its possible causes. However, despite the fifteen-year interval, she had a clear memory of what happened in the sixteen minutes between starting to push and the baby's delivery; it had been a frightening experience.

Forceful pulls. She was asked to push which she found difficult. The midwife had taken what seemed a long time trying to get the baby's head out, then said she needed help. Then it seemed that a lot of people came into the room. Joanne put the time between the midwife getting the head out and pressing the emergency buzzer at between 4-5 minutes — certainly more than 1-2 minutes and less than ten minutes. Though she could not see the midwife's hands, Joanne said she seemed to be struggling and gave the baby's head 'two or three forceful pulls.'[46]

The father. Evan said he had been standing beside his wife, near her head, so could not see the midwife's hands but could see her body making pulling motions. The midwife had suddenly hit a buzzer and panic followed.

The 'mystery' midwife. Joanne also had a vivid memory of a woman getting up on the bed, straddling her (with her back towards Joanne's face) and pushing down on 'the bump.'[47] No one had said anything about this. At the same time, other midwives were pushing her legs back towards her abdomen. The woman had removed herself before the baby was born.

Evan could not recollect seeing anyone get onto the bed but did recall a woman of Asian appearance, with a ponytail, on his wife in the position she remembered. He had been 'alarmed at the procedure' but had not said anything.

Other claims.
It was also claimed that :

- the hospital did not have a shoulder dystocia protocol and
- the midwife's notes were sparse and substandard.

The defence

The midwife was experienced, had held a senior position for seven years, was involved in the informal training of other midwives and had encountered a few cases of shoulder dystocia per year. She could not recall Mark's birth but relied on her notes and her usual practice in 1997.

The midwife said it was clear from the record that Joanne had begun to push at 04.15 and would probably have required urging to push because of the epidural anaesthetic. She could not say when the baby's head was delivered but it would only have been after delivery of the head that a problem with the shoulders would have been apparent.

Signs of shoulder dystocia. The midwife said 'turtling' (the retreat of the head back into the vagina) was a sign of shoulder dystocia as was encountering resistance to delivery during the uterine contraction following delivery of the head.

Usual practice. Her usual practice, immediately upon recognising this emergency (she could not say whether 'turtling' or resistance had occurred in Mark's case), would have been to push the emergency buzzer and shout 'shoulder dystocia' to alert other midwives. The on-call obstetrician, senior house officer and paediatrician would be summoned by bleep and be expected to attend within 2-3 minutes of the alarm being sounded; sooner, if they were nearby.

McRobert's manoeuvre. Meanwhile, she and other midwives would have continued to try to deliver the baby by performing the McRobert's manoeuvre and possibly the application of supra-pubic pressure.

Times. As Mark had been delivered before the doctors arrived and intervened, she thought Mark had been delivered within about 3 minutes of her pressing the emergency buzzer.

Putting Joanne into the McRobert's position, with knees flexed towards her chest, would have taken no more than one and a half to two minutes. On the basis that contractions continued at the rate of one every two and one half minutes and that the doctors were not involved in the delivery, the midwife said it was likely that Mark had been delivered on the first contraction after the buzzer was sounded.

Episiotomy. As her notes referred to a second-degree tear (and not to an episiotomy), the midwife did not think an episiotomy was performed.

'An incredible allegation.' The midwife found the allegation that a midwife had straddled Joanne, in the way Joanne and her husband had described, was 'incredible.' Not only would it have been physically difficult given the height and narrowness of the bed, but she would have told the midwife to desist 'in no uncertain terms';[48] she would have remembered the incident.

The decision

The judge examined each allegation:

1. Baby's head pulled repeatedly and with force.
The judge acknowledged that the parents were honestly trying to recollect what happened but that these events had occurred in an unfamiliar, stressful and frightening context. Joanne had been in labour for sixteen hours and neither she nor Evan had had any significant sleep when they suddenly found themselves facing a potential emergency. Their evidence differed significantly and their recollection was patchy.

The judge accepted the midwife's evidence that she would pull with modest and steady force, stop at any suggestion of an obstruction and would never pull a baby's head more than once during a contraction.

The judge also accepted that the midwife, in accordance with her usual practice, would have summoned assistance after the first contraction after that which delivered the baby's head, as the recognised steps to overcome the problem require more than one clinician.

2. The 'mystery midwife'.

Considerable time was spent examining the allegation that a midwife had sat astride Joanne, the judge concluding that it was false. This, in turn, undermined the parent's credibility as to what else had occurred.

3. Sub-standard records.

One expert witness described the midwife's delivery notes as 'dreadful,'[49] others found them 'sufficient', and the judge accepted they may have fallen below the standard reasonably expected in 1997. However, this did not show the midwife was incompetent. She had recorded the problems encountered with shoulder dystocia as 'moderate'[50] suggesting that the problems were reasonably, straightforwardly, and routinely overcome.

While the midwife accepted that her notes would have been inadequate if the outcome had not been good and while she recognised that there was some injury to the baby's arm, no one then knew the extent of that injury or its permanence.

4. Lack of a protocol.

The judge heard evidence that in 1997 some hospitals had a protocol on shoulder dystocia and others didn't. It was not in dispute that any protocol would set out a number of sets of manoeuvres that included (i) a call for help, (ii) the McRobert's manoeuvre, and (iii) the application of supra-pubic pressure.

The judge found that even if the hospital had a shoulder dystocia protocol in 1997, it would have done no more than set out the steps which the midwife had taken. Immediately upon diagnosing the condition she had called for assistance and put the mother in the Mc Robert's position.

Clear evidence. In the judge's view, the evidence was clear. The midwife had summoned assistance because she had diagnosed a shoulder dystocia and required assistance with that emergency. The timings were consistent with her story and she had shown she was aware of the correct procedures.

The Draycott paper. The judge also referred to the Draycott paper.[51] This paper contained a checklist containing criteria for reviewing the strength of a brachial plexus injury claim. The authors suggest that 'although each criterion by itself does not establish causation ... the more positives there are in the iatrogenic injury group the more likely the injury is to have been caused by the midwife/clinician.'[52]

Checklist:

PROPULSION INJURY	IATROGENIC INJURY
Posterior arm injured	Anterior arm injured
No shoulder dystocia	Shoulder dystocia
Up-to-date training	No recent training
Appropriate protocol followed manoeuvres	Incorrect manoeuvres
Performed manoeuvre	Ineffective manoeuvre
No evidence of excess traction	Evidence of excess traction
Correct number of birth attendants	Insufficient birth attendants
Precipitous second stage	Fundal pressure
Temporary injury	Permanent injury

The judge found that in Mark's case, the anterior arm was injured; there was shoulder dystocia and the injury was permanent. However, neither 'precipitous second stage' or 'fundal pressure' applied and there were sufficient birth attendants present. The issue of training had been dealt with by direct evidence of the midwife's experience and seniority.

While the judge found the checklist useful, he noted that the authors also stressed that whether a particular brachial plexus injury is caused by excessive traction will depend largely upon evidence of what occurred in the delivery room in the crucial time between delivery of the head, and the delivery of the shoulders and the body.

No negligence. On all the evidence, the midwife had not pulled Mark's head repeatedly or at any time with excessive force. She had diagnosed shoulder dystocia, stopped all traction and called for immediate assistance. There was no causative negligence in the assistance that was then given.

The negligence claim failed.

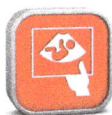

Discussion of Key Issues

In all three cases a child was left damaged, but alive. Parents claimed damages (on behalf of the child) for these injuries, as many parents will when confronted with a child's permanent injury.

In *Dowdie* the judge gives six reasons why a caesarean section should have been performed, concluding that it was 'highly probable'[53] that if one had been, Thomas would have then been born uninjured.

- Discuss the merits of each reason.

Margaret Puxon QC comments that the negligence in *Dowdie* was not in the management of the obstruction, but in the failure of the obstetric team to abandon vaginal delivery at the appropriate time.

- Have you experienced a situation where there were differences of opinion in the obstetric team about whether a vaginal delivery should be abandoned in similar circumstances? How was the matter resolved?

Puxon also observes that the *Dowdie* case is complicated, and in some aspects confused, by the conflicting findings and advent of secondary labour.

- Discuss whether Puxon is justified in her reasoning in points 2-6 (see preceding text).

....

In *Gaughan* the issues were:

1. Should a reasonably competent midwife have anticipated shoulder dystocia?
2. Should the medical team have been notified?
3. Was the patient positioned correctly?
4. Was traction used appropriately?
   - Discuss the judge's conclusions.

....

In *Croft* the issues included:

1. Had the midwife pulled the baby's head repeatedly and with force?
2. Had a 'mystery midwife' sat on the mother and applied force?
3. Did the hospital have a shoulder dystocia protocol?
4. Were the midwife's notes sparse/substandard?
   - Discuss the judge's conclusions.

....

The judge in *Croft* stressed that eye-witness accounts of what happens between delivery of the head and delivery of the shoulders and the rest of the body will be particularly important evidence.

In both *Gaughan* and *Croft,* midwives cannot recall what happened six and fifteen years before. Both relied on their documentation and evidence of usual practice.

- Would your documentation support you in similar circumstances?
- What policies/protocols/other evidence would be available to support your evidence of 'usual practice' six or more years later?

Note in all three cases in this chapter how times become critical to the narrative.

....

The judge in *Croft* described the recall of events by the parents as inconsistent, patchy and in one case, false.

- Do you agree that stress, lack of sleep and fear can alter the perception of events by mothers/parents/others during labour and delivery?
- Could these factors have contributed to the parent's evidence about the 'mystery midwife?'
- Have you known mothers to report similar/bizarre happenings?
- Do mothers have a chance to 'de-brief' after stressful experiences?
- Is this process documented?

NOTES

1. Powers & Harris, *Medical Negligence,* 2d ed., Butterworths, London, p.943 (1994).
2. Ibid.
3. Ibid.
4. Ibid.
5. *Dowdie.*
6. Ibid., p.370.
7. Ibid.
8. Ibid.
9. Ibid.
10. Ibid.
11. Ibid.
12. Ibid.
13. Ibid.
14. Ibid.
15. Ibid.
16. Ibid.
17. Ibid., p.371.
18. Ibid., p.371.
19. Ibid.
20. Ibid.
21. Ibid
22. Ibid.
23. Ibid.
24. Ibid.
25. Ibid., p.372.
26. Ibid.
27. Ibid. p.376.
28. Ibid.
29. Ibid.
30. Ibid.
31. Ibid.
32. *Gaughan v Bedfordshire Health Authority,* 8 Med.L.R 182 (1997).
33. Ibid., p.183.
34. Ibid., p.184.
35. Ibid.
36. Ibid.

37. Ibid., p.187.
38. Ibid.
39. Ibid.
40. Ibid., p.188.
41. Ibid., p.190.
42. *Croft v Heart of England NHS Foundation Trust,* WL 1933467 per Mr. Justice Hickinbotham, p. 2 (2012).
43. Ibid.
44 Ibid. p.2.
45. Ibid.p.4.
46. Ibid. p.6.
47. Ibid.p.7.
48. Ibid. p.5.
49. Ibid. p7.
50. Ibid.p.11
51. Draycott, T., et al., *A Template for Reviewing the Strength of Evidence for Obstetric Brachial Plexus Injury in Colinical Negligence Claims* ('The Draycott Paper'), Clinical Risk; 14:96–100 (2008).
52. Croft at p.11 (Draycott).
53. Ibid.

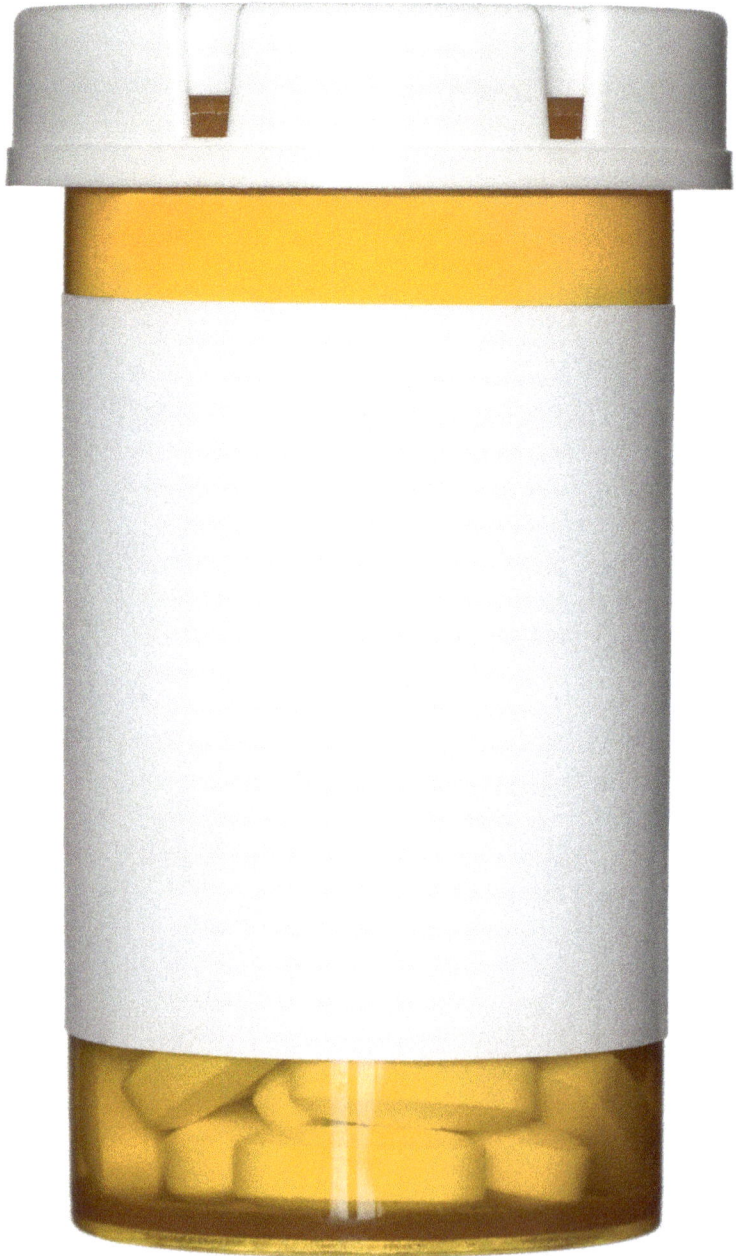

CHAPTER 7

Medication

'Drug errors are usually caused by failure to monitor a highly routine action.'

—Dr Currie.

Introduction

Safe management of medication starts with the trial, manufacture and packaging of a drug and continues through the prescribing, dispensing, storage and administration of that drug.

Prevention of adverse outcomes with medication includes the duty of a hospital to employ adequate numbers of competent staff. Competence includes ensuring that the right drug is administered in the right amount to the right patient by the right route at the right time. Competence includes knowledge of the cause and effect of a drug, together with the ability to recognise and respond to an adverse reaction or emergency.

Coroners investigating fatal drug errors hear evidence of hospital policies and protocols to determine whether they accord with accepted standards, how they are disseminated to staff and how new staff are orientated to their use.

As you might imagine, there is no shortage of litigation and coronial inquests dealing with drug errors. This chapter contains six cases. They focus on drugs given during pregnancy, at induction, during epidural anaesthesia and just prior to birth. Doctors, midwives and risk managers will all find guidance on effective risk management and policy development in this chapter.

....

In the first case a drug ingested by the mother during pregnancy caused injury to the fetus. The court had to determine whether the injury was caused before or after the doctor's negligent delay in organising tests and specialist examination.

The causation issue in this case is probably the most complex in this book, but it will show you how an appeal court insisted on keeping the issue a practical one. Note the court's caution that standard practice (against which a particular incident is measured in a negligence action) may *itself* be negligent when fraught with obvious risk.

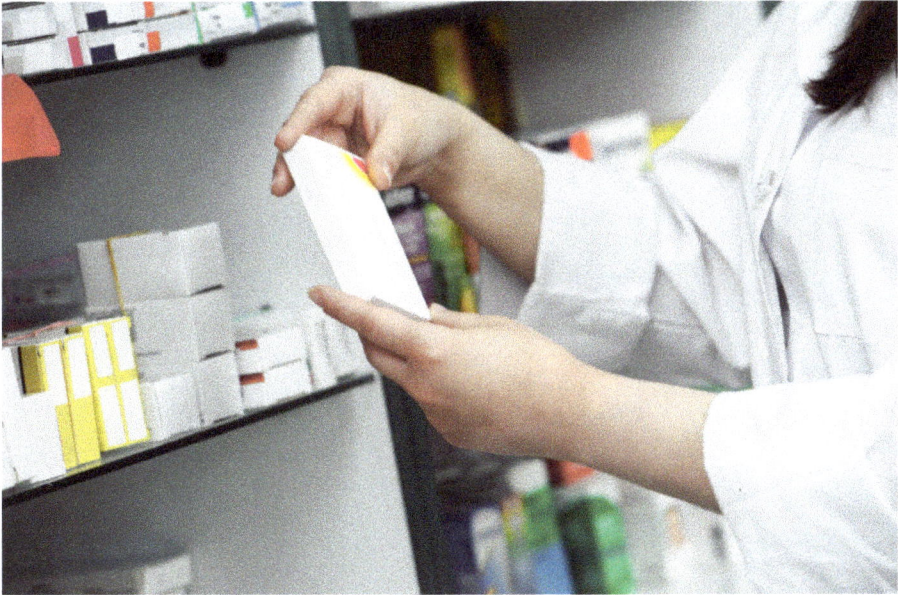

Webster v Chapman
[Can, 1998][1]

The facts

Grace, who suffered from pelvic thrombosis, was prescribed the blood thinner, warfarin (Coumadin) by a specialist. Her GP, Dr Hill, continued to monitor Grace's blood, warning her against becoming pregnant while on the medication. He did not specifically warn of the potential harm to a future child if she took warfarin when pregnant.

Warning against pregnancy. Dr Hill inserted an intrauterine device, but removed it two weeks later after Grace complained of discomfort and said that her husband objected. The doctor did so reluctantly, reiterating his advice against a further pregnancy. Grace reacted with some hostility, saying she and her husband 'would take care of it'.[2] Grace then transferred to Dr Casey, another doctor at the clinic.

Further warfarin. Dr Casey took over the blood monitoring and prescribed further quantities of warfarin. He said nothing about avoiding pregnancy, but was aware of Dr Hill's previous advice to Grace.

Pregnancy. In early February, Grace thought she might be pregnant. She did not consult a doctor, but arranged for a pregnancy test. The results were sent to Dr Casey, who saw them three days later (after the weekend) on 20 February. Dr Casey immediately arranged to see Grace on 22 February. He assessed her as 11 weeks pregnant. Dr Casey expressed concern about the pregnancy because of the warfarin, and then wrote a further prescription for the drug, advising Grace to keep taking it.

Ultrasound. Dr Casey arranged for Grace to have an ultrasound and to see an obstetrician. The appointment for the ultrasound was made for 9 March, the appointment with the obstetrician for 16 March. After reviewing the ultrasound result and examining Grace, the obstetrician assessed her to be 11 and 1/2 weeks pregnant, not the 14 weeks she would have been on the basis of Dr Casey's assessment. Dr Casey spoke to a haematologist by telephone, then advised Grace to stop taking warfarin, which she did.

Birth injuries. The baby was born prematurely on 3 August with congenital abnormalities, some of which were morphological and the rest of which were anomalies of the central nervous system (CNS). Consequently, the baby was severely and permanently disabled, both physically and mentally.

The trial
Arguments and allegations

Dr Hill. It was alleged Dr Hill failed to advise Grace of the known risks to a fetus if warfarin was taken during pregnancy. The trial judge held there was no breach of duty. Dr Hill had been insistent the mother avoid pregnancy while on warfarin and was assured she and her husband would take care of birth control.

Highly speculative. Although not required to consider the question of causation (because no negligence had been found), the trial judge nevertheless found it 'highly speculative and unlikely'[3] that the mother would have taken better precautions against a pregnancy if she had been warned about a fetal risk.

An appeal court upheld the trial judge's decision, finding it 'difficult to imagine that even the most careful of doctors would have seen a need to add a warning that a child conceived while the mother was on the drug would be at risk.'[4]

Dr. Casey. The trial judge found Dr Casey negligent. He should have consulted a specialist more quickly to obtain advice about continuing the patient on warfarin once he knew she was pregnant and had failed to advise her of the risk to her unborn baby if she remained on the medication.

The appeal

Dr Casey appealed, arguing that it had not been demonstrated that 'a prudent and diligent doctor'[5] would have sought advice earlier. Two medical experts at the trial had approved his care of Grace after he had learned of the pregnancy.

Was the standard of care negligent? The appeal judge held that the standard of care of doctors is to conduct their practice in accordance with the conduct of prudent and diligent doctors in similar circumstances. But, while conformity to a practice will generally exonerate doctors, there are certain situations where the standard practice itself may be negligent:

This will only be the case where the standard practice is so 'fraught with obvious risk' that anyone is capable of finding it negligent without the necessity of having diagnostic or clinical expertise. Thus it is sometimes open to a judge to find negligence without proof of a general standard and despite expert evidence that exonerates the defending doctor. This was such a case.[6]

Need for consultation and disclosure. Dr Casey had been justifiably uncertain as to fetal age. He was aware of the risk of fetal abnormality if a mother took warfarin during the first trimester. He was also aware of the risk to her of sudden withdrawal of the drug, as well as the need for specialised consultation. These factors would have alerted any prudent family doctor to the need for immediate consultation and for disclosure to the mother of both the risks involved and the treatment options. In the appeal judge's opinion, the trial judge had been entirely justified in finding Dr Casey negligent.

Causation. The critical question was whether the damage occurred before Dr Casey's negligence or resulted, at least in part, from the continued ingestion of warfarin between 22 February and 16 March.

Two facts had been established:

1. The baby's anomalies were caused by her mother's ingestion of warfarin during pregnancy.
2. Her morphological anomalies were caused by ingestion of warfarin in the early weeks before Dr Casey knew of it.

But it was not known as a scientific fact when, or in what manner, warfarin affects the development of the CNS. All that was known is that ingestion during the first trimester can result in the kind of CNS anomalies which afflicted Grace's baby.

No proper scientific basis. As neither party would accept the impossibility of proving the point at which the CNS damage occurred, the trial judge was asked to make a decision and had done so. The appeal court found the trial judge had not been entitled to make such a decision on the evidence:

(The judge) had gone down a road previously untravelled by any medical person, finding, without a proper scientific basis, that a mother's ingestion of warfarin prior to the ninth week of pregnancy could by itself – could and did – cause the damage to the CNS of the fetus.[7]

In order to link Dr Casey's negligence to the damage to the CNS, it was sufficient for Grace to have proved on the balance of probability that her ingestion of warfarin between 22 February, when Dr Casey renewed her prescription, and 16 March, when the obstetrician advised her to stop, materially contributed to the damage.

'A practical question of fact'. The appeal judge held that causation need not be determined by scientific precision, but is essentially a practical question of fact which is best answered by ordinary common sense rather than abstract metaphysical theory. The judge referred to Lord Salmon's comments on this point in *McGhee v National Coal Board*:

In the circumstance of the present case, the possibility of a distinction existing between (a) having materially increased the risk of contracting the disease, and (b) having materially contributed to causing the disease, may no doubt be a fruitful source of interesting discussion between students of philosophy. Such a distinction is, however, too unreal to be recognised by the common law.[8]

The decision

Material increase of risk.
The appeal judge held :

- The baby's injuries were caused by warfarin being taken over a period which began before, and continued after, the act of negligence.
- It could readily be said that the continued use of the drug materially increased the risk of the damage which resulted. This was the case, notwithstanding that the drug remains in the system and continues to affect it to a reduced extent for a short while after it was last taken.
- No distinction should therefore be made between materially increasing the risk of damage and materially contributing to the damage. If taking warfarin during the critical period was a cause of the damage, then negligent administration during part of that period, must, at a practical level, be seen as a materially contributing factor.

Damages awarded.

....

The causation issue in the next case, though not as complex as in *Webster,* is again decisive. The failure of the midwives to monitor a patient who had received Prostin was found to be negligent.

But was this the cause of the baby's brain damage? Courts hear that Prostin can be used to induce labour in women who have a normal pregnancy; it works by softening and dilating the neck of the womb and stimulating contractions. The active ingredient in Prostin E2 (gel) is dinoprostone.[9]

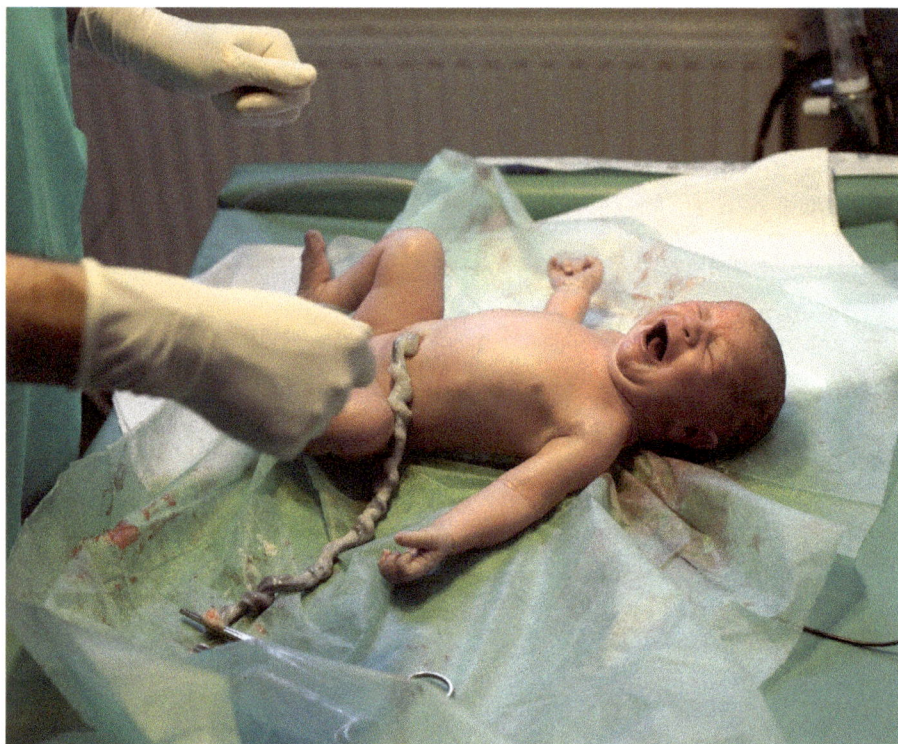

Look, et al. v Himel [Can, 1991][10]

The facts

Gayle was two weeks overdue when she was admitted to hospital and Prostin administered to induce labour. Gayle then experienced sudden and intense labour. The baby was born severely brain damaged.

The trial

Fetal distress unrecognised. Gayle alleged that the immediate, 'strong and unremitting'[11] contractions caused by the Prostin had compromised oxygen delivery to the fetus. She argued that the fetal distress should have been anticipated and diagnosed, with resultant monitoring of fetal status and uterine activity. As there had not been continuous monitoring, the fetal distress had gone unrecognized.

Extent of expertise. The court found the midwives were experienced in monitoring and assessing patients during labour. This expertise extended to their determining the intensity of the contractions, the location of the fetus, the significance of any movement of the fetus in the birth canal, as well as any change in the contractions. They were also experienced in the significance of cervical dilatation.

The decision

Failure to monitor. With the exception of a one-hour period, the court found the midwives' care had been satisfactory. But it was significant that for one hour, just after the contractions began, the midwives had failed to monitor Gayle. The risks associated with Prostin and post-maturity were common knowledge. Given the circumstances, a one-hour period without monitoring was negligent.

Causation. But had this failure caused the brain damage? As the cause of the baby's brain damage was unclear, harm could not be attributed, on the balance of probabilities, to the midwives' actions or inactions. Gayle's case therefore failed.

....

In the next case, a coroner investigates whether it is 'standard practice' to discharge a woman home after the administration of Prostin.

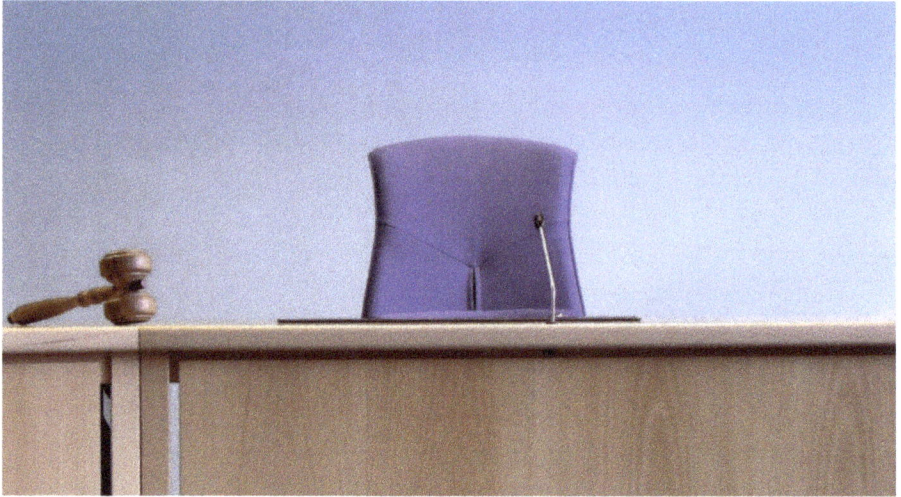

Coronial Inquest [Aus, 2006][12]

The facts

Lauren, aged 33, had an uncomplicated second pregnancy and underwent antenatal care as part of a hospital's birth centre programme. Pathology testing and ultrasounds were normal, except small uterine haemorrhage noted in the ultrasound at 12 and 1/2 weeks. When Lauren was approximately two weeks post-term, induction was discussed with the birth centre midwife and GP/obstetrician, Dr Craig.

At 42 weeks and two days, Lauren was admitted to hospital, where Dr Hayward saw her for the first time in the delivery suite. Midwife Silva explained that she would be assisting the doctors in the administration of the Prostin intra-vaginally. At 4.24 pm, midwife Silva commenced monitoring by CTG. On her return at approximately 4.50 pm, she noted a marked deceleration in the fetal heart rate, from a baseline of 130 beats per minute (bpm) to 90 bpm. The 20-minute trace contained no other worrying features.

At approximately 5.20 pm, midwife Silva reviewed the CTG with Dr Hayward At 5.30 pm, Dr Hayward found Lauren to be clinically stable:

> *The CTG trace had returned to normal baseline, variability and reactivity and had remained as such for 35 minutes following the initial dip.*[13]

Insertion of Prostin. After Dr Hayward and the midwife agreed the isolated dip was not a cause for concern, Dr Hayward proceeded to insert the Prostin gel. CTG sensors were applied. Dr Hayward understood that Dr Craig would be reviewing Lauren within the next one to two hours and asked midwife Silva to inform him of the dip.

Three further decelerations. Following the insertion of the Prostin, three further heart rate decelerations were noted by the midwife. She telephoned Dr Craig, who came to the hospital and ordered the CTG to continue for a further 60 minutes. No further decelerations were noted and the trace became reactive, with good variability. Dr Craig asked Lauren to remain at the hospital for a further period of observation and for the CTG to be repeated after a further lapse of 60 minutes.

Caesarean section not indicated. No further decelerations occurred during the 25 minutes following the reapplication of the sensors at 8.30 pm. Dr Craig was reassured that an immediate caesarean section was not indicated. He said that Lauren could be discharged home and return to hospital the next morning for induction, or sooner if labour ensued. Midwife Silva was present during this discussion, as was the midwife coming onto the night shift as well as the consultant obstetrician.

Midwife Silva:

> *They were offered a choice of staying in the hospital, or going home and returning if labour started or if they had any concerns. They elected to go home.*[14]

Discharge and re-admission. Lauren was discharged at approximately 9.00 pm. At 4.00 am, she awoke with lower abdominal pain and began to experience more regular pain at 4.30 am. At approximately 5.20 am, the membranes ruptured. Lauren re-presented to the labour ward at 6.20 am, where she was found to be in early labour, with the cervix 2 cm dilated.

CTG was commenced at approximately 6.42 am and fetal heart rate decelerations (more sustained than the previous day) noted.

Transfer to OR. Dr Craig arrived at 7.15 am and consulted the obstetrician. As it was still within the after-hours period, OR staff were called in. Lauren was transferred to the OR at 8.05 am, surgery commenced at 8.27 am and the baby was born at 8.33 am.

Apgar scores. The baby's Apgar scores were 1 at one minute and 3 at five minutes. There was no heart beat at birth and no respiratory effort. Following intubation and resuscitation, the baby (whose first gasp occurred at 22 minutes) was transferred to a neonatal intensive care unit at another hospital. Critically ill, he died there eight days later.

At autopsy, cause of death was given as perinatal asphyxia.

Expert medical opinion. During the investigation which followed, an independent obstetrician and gynaecologist was asked to review the management of Lauren and her baby.

The obstetrician was of the opinion that the interpretation of the CTGs and the subsequent action was correct. Lauren's decision to go home (following the administration of the Prostin) was an appropriately informed one and the time taken to perform the caesarean section was reasonable:

I think that had they remained it may have been possible to perform the caesarean sooner, but this would have made little difference to the outcome.[15]

The obstetrician expressed some concern that an amniotic fluid index (AFI) was not performed before the Prostin induction but subsequently conceded that AFIs were not so prevalent in 2003.

Comment

The coroner noted that while many hospitals allow a patient to be discharged after the administration of Prostin if there are no signs of labour, another medical witness was of the opinion that optimal obstetric care requires the patient to stay in hospital. This was now standard practice at the hospital in question.

Unexplained loss. The obstetrician explained that the reason for induction of labour as a routine at about 42 weeks is the rate of unexplained loss of babies, which increases slowly from about 36 weeks when it is very low. At 42 weeks, the rate of risk starts to rise more rapidly; thus the need to induce.

Critical stage. Lauren had been at the critical stage of 42 weeks and two day's gestation. In the coroner's opinion, remaining in hospital after the administration of an induction agent should be a consequence of the aim to reduce risk of loss.

Recommendation

The coroner recommended a universal practice of continued admission after the administration of Prostin for induction of labour.

....

In the next case the wrong drug was injected during epidural anaesthesia, with consequent injuries to the mother. What the drug was, or how it came to be on the anaesthetist's trolley, remained a mystery. The judge was left to draw inferences from all the circumstances. This case illustrates the risks of departing from hospital protocol on checking, queries how a drug cupboard is stocked, and demonstrates how an article by Australian anaesthetists persuaded an English judge that fatigue can contribute to drug error.

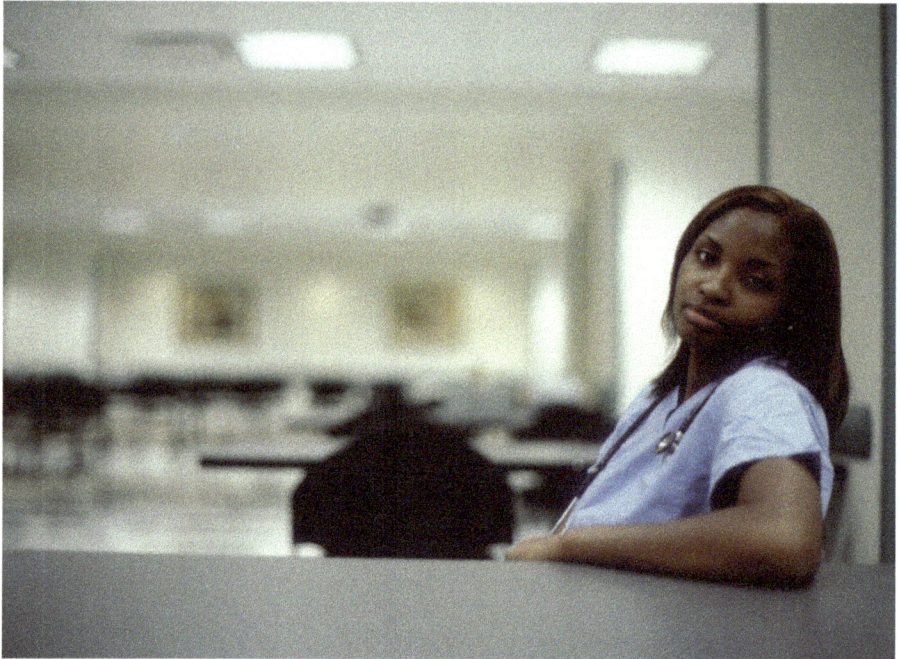

Ritchie v Chichester
Health Authority [UK, 1994][16]

The facts

Admission. Joanna was in her early thirties when she miscarried during her first pregnancy in November 1988. Her previous medical history indicated a potential for her to suffer from high blood pressure at times of stress and anxiety, but there was no indication of hypertension. Two months after the miscarriage Joanna became pregnant again, this time with twins. On 16 September (at 36 weeks), she was admitted to hospital with stomach pain and a small loss of blood. She was discharged the same day after routine monitoring indicated that she had settled down. On 26 September 1989, Joanna, now 38 weeks into her 'largely uneventful' pregnancy, had a small loss of blood. She was admitted to hospital and when a scan indicated the size of the babies an unsuccessful attempt was made to induce labour on 28 September. A further, and this time successful, induction was made on the afternoon of 29 September.

Labour. By evening, labour had begun in earnest. Notes at 10.45 pm described Joanna as 'rather tense to examine',[18] and dilation was noted at 4-5 cm. Midwife Cullen performed an artificial rupture of the membranes. At 11.00 pm, Joanna was transferred to the labour ward, where she came under the care of student midwife Stone (an RN who passed her midwifery exams two months after this event).

Student midwife. Stone described Joanna as 'crying and cursing', 'not coping well' and with 'ferocious contractions'.[19] Joanna had not attended antenatal classes, so had not received any advice on coping with labour pains.

The epidural. Dr Baez, who had been on duty since 9.00 am, was called to the labour ward late in the evening and set up an epidural around midnight. 1000 ml of Hartmann's solution IV was administered prior to giving the epidural. Dr Baez was an overseas-trained doctor who had considerable experience performing obstetric anaesthesia, but had not progressed beyond the trainee post of registrar in England. He was described by staff as kind and caring, but with some language difficulty and a tendency to sweat a lot. (The judge later found this could have caused people to think the doctor was flustered when he was not.) Also present were midwife Stone and Joanna's husband. Dr Baez asked Joanna to lie on her left side, with her knees up as far as they would go.

'Unbearable pain'. Joanna said she felt an injection, then a dreadful pain immediately shoot down into her legs, principally down her left leg. She had screamed and asked the anaesthetist to stop. Dr Baez told her to keep still. Midwive Stone told her to 'take deep breaths to try to breathe the pain away.'[20] Joanna said she continued to scream about the awful pain in her legs and pleaded with the doctor to stop. Eventually, Dr Baez said he was going to take the needle out but would put it back after she had a rest. Joanna said she had some difficulty understanding what he was saying. After the needle came out, the pain eased a little, but 'an awful ache'[21] persisted in her legs.

Less intense pain. Shortly after the needle was reinserted, Joanna again felt the pain shoot down her leg, though less intensely this time. She was again told to 'lie still and to breathe the pain away'.[22] Joanna described the pain as 'ten times worse'[23] than the contractions, running down from the site of the injection, through her buttocks and into her legs. The third injection was uneventful. She was left with just an ache in her legs.

The obstetric epidural record. The record showed an initial dose of 3 ml of 0.5 per cent bupivacaine was inserted at 12. 25 am, another 3 ml at 12. 35; the remainder at 12. 45. Blood pressure was taken at five minute intervals over an hour and recorded by the midwife. At 1.00 am, student midwife Stone noted on the labour record that the epidural was working quite well. At 1.15 am, she recorded the cervix was 8 cm dilated.

Top-up. It seemed there was a top-up of the epidural by Dr Baez at 1.45 am when the student midwife was absent from the room. No record of this was made on the obstetric epidural record, but it was recorded by student midwife Stone on the labour record. This was a clear breach of procedure. The ampoule used was clearly not checked by her before being passed to Dr Baez. No record was made by Dr Baez of the patient's blood pressure at the time of this top-up, nor during the subsequent half-hour.

After 30 minutes, Dr Baez was satisfied that the top-up was giving good results. As delivery did not appear imminent, he left, remaining on-call.

Dilation. From the labour record, it seemed that the epidural was working reasonably well. At 2.00 am it was recorded that Joanna was 'relaxing well' and at 2.30 pm that she was 'coping well'. Blood pressure and a further top-up was recorded at 2.55 am. The cervix was recorded as being 8 cm dilated.

At 3.45 am Joanna was described as 'relaxed and pain free'.[25] At 4.30 am student midwife Stone took a meal break and was replaced by midwife Hogg, a more experienced midwife. Midwife Hogg recorded that Joanna was pain free but that there was no external sign of full dilation. At 5.00 am, she recorded dilation at 5-6 cm which surprised her, given the earlier recording of 8 cm. She recorded an epidural top-up and also noted blood pressure at the appropriate times.

Passing of urine. Midwife Hogg later said that Joanna had not complained to her of an inordinate degree of pain at the commencement of the epidural. She recorded that 100 ml of urine was passed at 5.00 am. The record showed that Joanna did not pass urine at 6.45 am and was unable to do so. A top-up was recorded at this time together with blood pressure readings, but the degree of cervical dilation was not recorded. By 7.00 am Joanna was resting between contractions and at 7.30 am a catheter was fitted, which resulted in reasonably good drainage.

New team. About 8 am, there was a change of staff and a student midwife recorded at 7.50 am that Joanna was feeling pain all over. Further top-ups were given and the cervix recorded as 8 cm dilated. A doctor performed top-ups at increased levels at 9.15 am and 11.15 am.

Delivery. At 11.45 am, when cervical dilation was arrested at 8 cm, twins were delivered by caesarean section, the first at 12.45 am, the second two minutes later. There had been no indication of fetal distress prior to the delivery.

Post-delivery. The following day, Joanna complained of numbness from the top of the buttocks downwards through part of her thighs into her feet. The midwifery staff (who Joanna described as 'fairly dismissive'[26]) assured her that this was normal; various doctors examined her over the next two days. A myelogram showed no compressive abnormality, but did show an abnormal CFS with quite a high protein level.

Injury. Joanna left hospital 19 days after the twins' birth with permanent paralysis in the saddle area, double incontinence and loss of vaginal sensation. These conditions were permanent. A negligence case was brought against the hospital, alleging that a neurotoxic substance was injected at the induction of the epidural process.

The trial

Defence. The hospital contended that any injury sustained was due to ischaemia, the cause of which was either a fibrocartilaginous embolus (FCE), which occluded the anterior spinal artery and blocked the blood supply to the conus medullaris, or a sudden and spontaneous interruption of the blood supply to the lower end of the spinal cord or the cauda equina.

Dr Baez (giving evidence by written statement because of ill health) explained that he would have warned Joanna that she would have to put up with an uncomfortable procedure and not move during the insertion.

Preparation. Dr Baez said that he had prepared her back with an antiseptic solution, identified the site of the injection, then administered a local anaesthetic of lignocaine into the skin and deeper tissues. He used an orange needle, followed by a blue needle. As the local injections seemed to cause more pain than usual, he had waited three minutes for the anaesthetic to take effect before inserting the 18-gauge epidural needle in the midline between the third and fourth lumbar vertebrae, using loss of resistance to air to detect the epidural space. The needle insertion was uneventful, with no blood or fluid seen to issue from the needle.

Catheter threaded. However, when he threaded the catheter through the needle Joanna had complained of a very sharp pain shooting down her left leg. When he had withdrawn the needle and catheter completely, the pain had stopped.

Reinsertion of needle. When contraction pains were reduced and when Joanna was happy for him to continue, Dr Baez said he reinserted the needle after further local anaesthetic infiltration in the same space. This time the catheter was inserted without difficulty. He had no recollection of Joanna screaming at any time during the procedure.

No recollection by student midwife. Student midwife Stone had no recollection of how many injections were given, but said the epidural had gone in easily, with good effect. She insisted the only pain Joanna suffered was from contractions and that she had at no time complained of pain or aching in her legs.

Wife's pain possibly normal. Joanna's husband, who had been standing near her, confirmed that Joanna had complained about the tremendous pain in her legs. He described Dr Baez as 'obviously very ruffled, not explaining anything',[27] with quite bad English. He thought his wife's pain was possibly normal, and believed that 'you leave it to the professionals'.[28]

The decision

The judge preferred the evidence of Joanna and her husband, (supported as it was by Dr Baez's account) to that of the student midwife, who he did not find a very satisfactory witness:

In the first place she seems to have remembered the trivia and forgotten the essentials. She said she remembered talking to (the patient) about her previous employment with the county council, discussing the decoration of the nursery and the nursery curtains, and the fitted bedroom in the patient's sister's house. Conversely, she seemed to have no recollection of the set up of the epidural. She had no recollection of how many injections (the anaesthetist) gave

.... she said the epidural was fine. She said there was no complaint
at all...when the epidural went in. That is a flat contradiction not
only of what the patient and her husband say about it, but also of
what (Dr Baez) said.[29]

The judge commented that Joanna had not been prepared to cope with the
pains of labour by attending antenatal classes:

Antenatal classes might have reduced her anxiety and increased
her ability to cope with the pain. On the other side of the coin, I
think nurses, and especially midwives, are liable to develop a certain immunity to cries of pain in a labour ward as they must occur
very frequently.[30]

The judge also rejected criticism of Joanna's husband for not calling the anaesthetist to stop once he saw had badly his wife was suffering.

While theoretically a patient in a dentist's chair might be able to
stand up and say 'enough is enough' and call a halt to the treatment, preferring to suffer the toothache, such an option is not open
to women in labour. Childbirth is an irreversible process from
which one is unable to contract out because one finds the contractions too painful. Most husbands present at a confinement (and I
would put Mr R in that category) probably feel that they are there
under sufferance, that their role is purely that of comforter to their
wives, and that they have no right to interfere or to question or to
tell the professionals how their job should be done.[31]

Epidural procedure

Ward protocols. Evidence was given that the insertion of the catheter
should be painless, but may on occasion touch a nerve root, resulting in a
sudden shooting pain either in the back or down one leg. If this occurs, the
catheter and needle should be removed and the procedure started again.

This procedure was also to be followed if the catheter and needle penetrated a blood vessel. If the procedure was correctly followed, the catheter could not touch the spinal cord or the delicate nerve roots of the cauda equina, which are protected by the relatively strong dura mater.

Test dose. A small test dose, usually 3 ml of bupivacaine, is then injected through a filter and cap fitted to the end of the catheter. If there has been inadvertent penetration of the dura, the result is likely to be a widespread spinal block. Provided the catheter is in the epidural space, numbness will begin around the L1/2 level and spread up and down. If all is well, further local anaesthetic is inserted after about five minutes. Evidence was accepted that the raised protein level and presence of xanthochromia indicated that there had been a penetration of the dura.[32]

The checking process. Protocols had been developed by the consultant anaesthetist to avoid the risk of mistake. Only the appropriate drugs, and no other, should be placed on the anaesthetic trolley. The ampoules (in this instance bipuvacaine) should be picked up by the midwife, who reads the name on the ampoule to make sure it is the correct one, then hands the ampoule to the anaesthetist, who checks that he has been given the correct drug.

Were the protocols observed?

Documentation. There had been considerable criticism of Dr Baez's documentation during the trial, including his failure to note in the epidural record the need to withdraw the Touhy needle and catheter, as well as re-inserting it.

Checking. The top-up at 1.45 am had been given in the student midwife's absence but Dr Baez had not recorded this on the epidural chart. Nor was blood pressure documented. Dr Baez's explanation that he always checked that he was drawing the correct drug in the correct strength into the syringe before administering it was described as 'totally unsatisfactory.'[33] There was no emergency. The first line of safety checks had therefore been eliminated.

Fatigue. Dr Baez, who was in his late forties, had been on duty about 15 hours by the time he was called to see Joanna. The judge was referred to an article by Australian anaesthetists[34] cautioning that errors are usually caused by failure to monitor a highly routine action, and that this failure is much more likely when limited cognitive resources are compromised by haste, inattention, distraction or fatigue.

Protocols not observed. The judge found that although the protocols were not being observed, this in itself did not necessarily mean that a neurotoxic drug was injected into the patient. If there was none on the trolley, no harm could befall the patient, no matter how inattentive the anaesthetist or the midwife had been.

Could there have been a neurotoxic drug on the trolley? Had Joanna received a toxic substance by mistake?

The consultant anaesthetist who had developed the protocols said that their observance would preclude the presence of neurotoxic drugs on the trolley. The judge found this had to be viewed in the light of evidence given by an operating room assistant.

The drug cupboard. The OR assistant said the drug cupboard in the operating room (next door to the delivery room where Joanna had her epidural) contained a list of available drugs on the door of the cupboard. This list was not 100 per cent accurate in that some anaesthetists would put additional drugs in the cupboard.

Potential for wrong drug. The judge concluded that there was the same potential for the wrong drug to find its way onto the anaesthetic trolley as there was for the wrong drug to be picked up in the adjoining operating theatre. This had to be inferred as all the ampoules had been destroyed.

The decision

The judge accepted the consensus of expert opinion that a neurotoxic substance had been inadvertently injected at the commencement of, but not during, the epidural process. As one consultant neurologist had explained to the court:

I think the lesion occurred at the time of induction of the epidural. The basis of my opinion is the history. In neurology you must be attentive to the history. What was so important was the severe instant bilateral pain involving both buttocks, both thighs and perineum. Its uniqueness has implications: it must be a unique cause. The plaintiff's complaints are entirely consistent with the subsequent physical signs elicited. I cannot conceive of any patient, not a neurologist, able to describe these symptoms then develop the signs the plaintiff had.[35]

Damages awarded.

English barrister Margaret Puxon QC comments:

The risk of introducing a toxic substance into the spinal canal is so well recognised that it is the rule in many, if not most, (English) hospitals that no drugs be allowed in the anaesthetic room which could conceivably be dangerous if mistakenly injected in the course of a spinal or epidural anaesthetic ... This precaution is in addition to the adaptation of a rigid protocol of checking by medical and nursing staff.[36]

....

Finally, a case where Syntometrine instead of Pethidine was administered prior to a birth. Courts hear that Syntometrine (a combination of ergometrine and syntocinon) is used to cause an immediate and sustained contraction of the uterine muscle following the birth of the baby. This is to aid in the delivery of the placenta and to reduce the risk of significant bleeding following delivery. Single checking, the preparation and placement of Sytometrine, and the difficulty in locating a reversing agent were central to the following investigation.

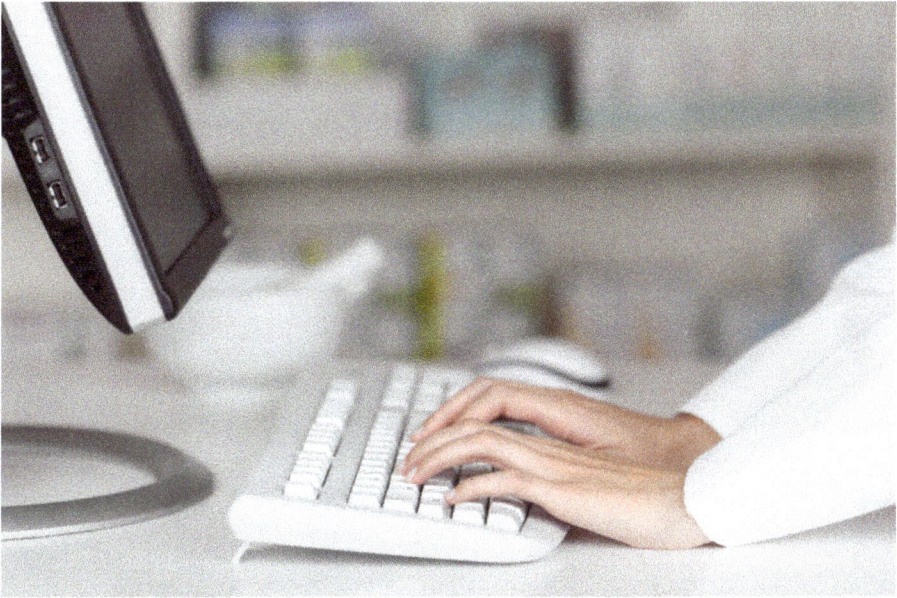

Coronial Investigation
[Aus, 2004][37]

The facts

Margaret's first child was expected on 10 August 2002. On 18 August, she presented at hospital after experiencing quite painful contractions for several hours. At approximately 10.00 am, a doctor confirmed cervical dilation of 2-3 cm, performed an amniotomy and prescribed 100 mg Pethidine prn. Maternal and fetal observations between 10.00 am and 12.30 pm were normal. During this period, Margaret used nitrous oxide. At 12.30 pm, the doctor prescribed Maxolon to be given concurrently with the Pethidine. At 3.30 pm, a further 100 mg of Pethidine was prescribed, as Margaret was complaining of considerable pain.

Signing the drug book. After the doctor ordered further pain relief at 3.30 pm, a midwife checked and signed the drug book, with a nurse, for 100 mg Pethidine.

Placement of Pethidine and Syntometrine. The midwife said she put the Pethidine syringe (2 ml clear liquid) in a green kidney dish, and placed this adjacent to a blue kidney dish, which contained a similar syringe with Syntometrine (1 mL clear liquid), a medication she had previously drawn up.

The error. After administering what she thought was Pethidine at 3.55 pm, the midwife then realized she had injected Syntometrine (1 mL). She contacted the doctor, who came immediately. He found the cervix was 8 cm dilated. Initially, the CTG was unchanged, but after approximately five minutes the fetal heart rate precipitously declined to 60 bpm, then failed to record.

Search for tocolytic. The medical record noted increased uterine tone at this time. This was not well represented on the CTG. The doctor asked for theatre to be prepared for a caesarean section and looked for tocolytics that might reverse the Syntometrine. He was unable to find any Ventolin or similar medication and instructed Pethidine (100 mg) to be given. This was administered by the midwife at 4.15 pm. The doctor contacted his partner to come and assist, but was unable to locate a surgeon. The midwife was asked to insert a urinary catheter.

Delivery. At 4.35 pm, the doctor re-examined Margaret, finding she was fully dilated and a vaginal delivery feasible. A spinal anaesthetic was administered at 4.42 pm. After an unsuccessful application of the ventouse, a live but floppy baby, weighing 3275 g, was delivered by Neville Barnes forceps. The baby responded to resuscitation, the heart rate rapidly increasing from 60 bpm to 100 bpm. But, while a good colour, the baby remained flaccid, with no spontaneous respiratory effort, until approximately 60 minutes after birth. The severe and sustained acute hypoxic ischaemic encephalopathy was found to be the primary cause of the baby's eventual death.

The inquest

Six issues emerged:

1.The intra-muscular administration of dangerous drugs
The midwife said she had gone to the general ward and asked a nurse to come and check the Pethidine. The nurse had accompanied her to the drug cupboard:

The midwife:

> *I had the keys to the drug cupboard and I removed one ampoule from the drug cupboard. We both signed the drug book and I took the Pethidine with me. We also checked the date. As I knew the general ward was busy, I indicated to (the nurse) that there was no need to check the patient as I had only one patient in the Birthing Suite/Labour Ward.*

Single checking. The nurse confirmed that she had asked the midwife if she wanted her to come to the labour ward to check the Pethidine with the patient and that the midwife replied: 'No, I am right.' The nurse explained that it was common practice at the hospital for RNs not to follow the established protocol (i.e., for two RNs to go to the bedside to check the dangerous drug with the patient). The nurse suggested two unit managers would have been aware of this practice. One unit manager confirmed this was the case.

Standard practice. The coroner found it was standard nursing practice for two nurses to double-check the checking out and intra-muscular administration of dangerous drugs such as Pethidine. That protocol was not contained in the Nurse Manual in the Delivery Suite due to an oversight at the time the manual was compiled. The coroner found this was not a 'telling circumstance', as staff were aware of the protocol and the rationale underlying it.

While not agreeing this was common practice, the doctor conceded that he was aware unsupervised intramuscular injections of drugs such as Pethidine occurred from time to time. In the obstetrician's opinion, the mistake would have been avoided had standard hospital operating procedures for the administration of controlled drugs (opiates) been adhered to by nursing (and midwifery) staff.

Systems failure. Were procedures followed at the hospital? Was this an aberration, an isolated case? Or was it common practice that one midwife/nurse, unsupervised, administered intra-muscularly? If so, it was a significant 'systems failure.'

The director of nursing conceded she had been aware of the administration of drugs intramuscularly without supervision because various nurses had told her of this. She had endeavoured to stop the practice and believed it had stopped before August 2002. The coroner did not find this evidence 'particularly compelling', finding the practice had clearly not stopped and that if the director of nursing had seriously inquired she would have learnt this.

'A blinkered eye.' The coroner found this 'alarming situation' was a common practice and probably known to the director of nursing, with an attendant risk to patients:

Permitting the situation to continue demonstrates a deficiency in training and supervision. It would appear a 'blind-eye' (or at least a blinkered eye) had been turned to this practice for years.

In the coroner's view, if the situation was not known to senior management, it should have been:

Either way the situation, which I accept altered after this tragedy, represents a significant deficiency in management and was a contributing causal factor in (the baby's) death.

---

2. Preparation and placement of Syntometrine
The midwife explained:

It was my normal practice to have the drug ready for delivery as (the doctor) normally likes the drug administered after the head and shoulders have been delivered.

Best practice. A director of delivery services at a tertiary hospital gave expert medical evidence of best practice for the administration of Syntometrine.

In order to minimise the inadvertent administration of this drug it is recommended that the individual conducting or assisting with the delivery does not draw the drug up until the woman has commenced the active phase of the second stage of labour. Having checked the contents and expiry date of the vial, the contents should be drawn up into a 2 ml syringe. The syringe and vial are kept in separate kidney dishes and removed from the patient and the neo-natal resuscitator to minimise inadvertent premature administration to the neonate. Prior to administration as an intramuscular/intravenous injection, the vial should be again checked by the administrator and counter checked by an independent practitioner.

The coroner found that the early preparation of Syntometrine, which was then placed adjacent to the syringe containing Pethidine, fell far short of best practice. It represented a causal link in the chain of causation of the baby's death.

3. Difficulty in locating a reversing agent (tocolytic)
*A **serious deficiency**.* The doctor had been unable to find a tocolytic in the delivery suite. In fact, the reversing agent Ventolin Obstetric was kept in the labour ward. The coroner found it was not in a conspicuous location and that staff should have known precisely where it was kept.

The obstetrician believed that the administration of a tocolytic:

. . . had one been available, may have sufficiently mitigated the effects of the Syntometrine, so as to have significantly altered the eventual neonatal outcome. That he was unable to find such an agent on the delivery unit is, in my opinion, a serious deficiency in the provision of obstetric services. Such drugs should be standard in any delivery unit drug cupboard.

The obstetrician, while maintaining the appropriateness of the administration of a tocolytic to reverse the uterine tonicity, conceded that he had no experience in trying to reverse Syntometrine. He could not say whether it would have worked. The coroner noted that the Royal Australian and New Zealand College of Obstetricians and Gynaecologists recommended a tocolytic. This suggested that there would be a good prospect of reversal.

A 'background circumstance'. Ultimately, the coroner was uncomfortable in making a firm finding on whether the inability to locate a tocolytic was a contributing factor, concluding it was a 'background circumstance.'

4. Delay in calling NETS

In spite of the baby's precarious condition, and despite urging by several senior nurses (including the director of nursing), the doctor did not call the NETS team until four hours after the birth. By the time the team arrived, the baby had no gag or suck reflexes; pupils were fixed and not responsive to light. The coroner accepted the doctor's assurance that there had not been a 'cover up', but found the delay could not be justified. Nevertheless, as the baby had already suffered irreversible brain damage, medical management following his birth did not further contribute to that damage. The delay was therefore another background circumstance rather than one of several causes of the baby's death.

5. Complaints

Three previous drug errors had been attributed to the midwife and there had been a number of complaints to middle management about her competence. The coroner found these should have sent 'alarm bells ringing.'

6. Incident reports

The coroner also heard evidence of deficiencies in the system of incident reporting: 'The incident reports (if indeed they were made) lacked precision and detail to the extent that meaningful action to remedy any deficiency in performance was nigh on impossible.'

Conclusion

Individual and systems problems. The coroner found that the baby died as a result of a terrible but preventable mistake by the midwife. This occurred in the setting of several systems failures, inadequate checks and balances, omissions in recognised duties and deficiencies in management – which in combination were the cause of his death.

Recommendations

The coroner adopted the recommendations of the director of delivery services at a tertiary hospital in relation to the preparation and administration of Syntometrine:

1. The individual conducting or assisting with the delivery should not draw up the drug (Syntometrine) until the woman has commenced the active phase of the second stage of labour.
2. Having checked the contents and expiry date of the vial, the contents should be drawn up into a 2 ml syringe.
3. The syringe and vial should be kept in separate kidney dishes and should be removed from the patient and the neonatal resuscitator to minimise inadvertent administration to the neonate.
4. Prior to administration as an intramuscular/intravenous injection, the vial should again be checked by the administrator and counter checked by an independent practitioner.

The coroner also recommended that the health service should review/revise its incident reporting procedures to facilitate ease of identification of an individual who has made an error, either by act or omission, which has the potential to adversely impact a patient's wellbeing.

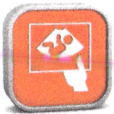

Discussion of key issues

Cause and effect

Webster clearly states that doctors have a duty of care to know the cause and effect of drugs they prescribe for pregnant women. But women also have a duty to take reasonable care for their own safety when giving a medical history about medications.

- Given the above reasoning, a court may hear evidence that foreseeable risks to the baby could have been minimized/ avoided if, during the taking of an antenatal history, the mother had been made aware that the taking of particular drugs, for example, non-prescription substances, will make a drug such as Narcan contraindicated if the baby requires resuscitation.
- Would your documentation demonstrate such a discussion took place?

- Knowing the cause and effect of a drug, as well as the condition of the patient, will dictate the appropriate level of monitoring. This was the central point in *Look* where the court found the risks of Prostin and post-maturity were common knowledge. Even though the patient's case failed on causation, an hour-long gap, during which the patient was not monitored by midwives, was considered negligent.
- What do the manufacturer's instructions say about monitoring following the administration of a drug to induce labour?
- Can appropriate monitoring of the patient during induction be compromised by staff/patient ratios and workload?

....

Coronial investigation. *(1)* The coroner noted that, while many hospitals allow a patient to be discharged after the administration of Prostin if there are no signs of labour, another medical witness was of the opinion that optimal obstetric care requires the patient to stay in hospital.

- What is 'standard practice' at your hospital?
- How would you justify this practice to a court?

....

The *Ritchie* case illustrates how a court will draw inferences from all the circumstances (circumstantial evidence) when there is an absence of direct evidence.

In this case there was evidence that the patient sustained a permanent injury consistent with the injection of a toxic substance. By the time she displayed symptoms of neurological damage, the ampoules had been cleaned away, so there was no direct evidence of what had been injected. But there was evidence of the anaesthetist's probable fatigue and failure to follow proper checking procedures, together with evidence that drug cupboards in the hospital could contain drugs not listed on the door of the drug cupboard. The inference drawn from all these circumstances was that a 'rogue ampoule' had found its way into the anaesthetic area and been injected by mistake.

- How many, if any, of the above risks (fatigue, failure to follow checking protocols, mismanagement of drug cupboard) could happen where you work?

- In your hospital, could a 'rogue ampoule' find its way into an area, such as a birthing suite, where epidural procedures are taking place? Could the contents then be injected? Either way, give reasons.
- If fatigue can contribute to a drug error, discuss the merits of doing the drug round at the end of a shift when on night duty.

Barrister Margaret Puxon comments that it is common practice in English hospitals that no drugs are allowed in the anaesthetic room which could conceivably be dangerous if mistakenly injected in the course of a spinal or epidural anaesthetic.

- Is this the case where you work?

....

There was evidence in *Ritchie* that the patient experienced painful contractions, that the anaesthetist warned her the epidural would be an uncomfortable procedure, and that the husband believed the management of pain relief should be left 'to the professionals'. The judge queried whether staff could become 'somewhat immune to cries of pain.'[54]

- Is it difficult to judge when 'normal' pain progresses to 'abnormal'?

....

In the *Coronial investigation. (2)* Syntometrine was administered instead of Pethidine, with fatal results to the baby.

- Discuss the reasons why this specific error could, or could not, happen where you work.

The coroner made a number of recommendations in relation to the safe preparation and placement of Syntometrine.

- What is the procedure at your hospital ?
- Give reasons for or against adopting the coroner's recommendations.

The doctor was unable to find a tocolytic in the delivery suite. In fact, the reversing agent Ventolin Obstetric was kept in the labour ward. The coroner found it was not in a conspicuous location and that staff should have known precisely where it was kept.

- Could either of these issues pose a risk at your hospital?

Numerous concerns relating to the management of medication were contributed by midwives at workshops I have facililitated. For example:

- An irritable uterus is a side effect of Prostin induction. This can endanger the baby and result in an LSCS. The worry I have is the reason for using Prostin – mainly for post-dates and greater than 40 weeks. The clinical tool of a BISHOP score is not enough to decide if Prostin induction is suitable. Doctors and midwives are put under a lot of pressure from women demanding inductions, but I wonder if these women are informed of the potential dangers?
- Two midwives were checking the Syntocinon infusion for a woman who had an epidural in situ. They checked the flask, correct dose and correct patient. I waited in the room to watch – which was just as well as one midwife began to connect the flask of IV fluid with Syntocinon into the epidural infusion.
- The patient had pre-eclampsia and was in the delivery suite for two - three days for control of her blood pressure post delivery. During this time, she was on antihypertensive drugs and magnesium sulphate sulphate. The anti-hypertensive drug was changed, but the new prescription was not sent to pharmacy. The patient was transferred to the postnatal ward and the nurses were told that she was self-medicating her hypertensive medication. Her BP remained high and she was then referred to a physician who queried the drug she was taking because that particular drug did not come in that dosage. When staff checked the medication in the patient's drawer, the discrepancy was discovered. It was later found that a new drug chart had 'run out of space' and the drugs were discontinued. The anti-hypertensive that the patient was self-medicating was on the first drug chart.
- Analgesic, such as morphine, is ordered in the delivery suite. The patient then has an emergency caesarean section and the same drug is re-written on the drug sheet. The first order should be cancelled by the doctor writing up the second order.

Discuss each incident with the view to minimizing or avoiding the same risk where you work. For example, in the last scenario:

- How are you informed about the medication a caesarean patient has received in the operating room or the post anaesthetic care unit?
- Grade the risk of not having time to read the patient's notes.
- Is the reason you do not have time to read due to a systems problem of heavy workload or inadequate staffing, or both?

Check whether protocols for standing orders in obstetric delivery wards are legal under the current drugs and poisons legislation in your State or Territory.

NOTES

1. *Webster v Chapman,* 155 D.L.R (4th) 83 (1998).
2. Ibid., p.85.
3. Ibid., p.87.
4. Ibid.
5. Ibid.
6. Ibid., p.92.
7. Ibid.
8. *McGhee v National Coal Board,* 1 W.L.R 1 (1973) per Lord Reid at pp.12–13.
9. Dinoprostone is a prostoglandin drug used mainly to induce labour. It is usually administered in a pessary or as a vaginal tablet or gel.
10. *Look, et al. v Himel,* Ont. Ct. (Gen. Div) (1991). Case note based on article by Louise Sanchez-Sweatman RN, BScN, LLB: Canadian Nurse, *'Legal Matters'* (Feb. 1996) p.47.
11. *Record of Investigation into Death,* No. 1765/03, State Coroner's Office, (Victoria, 2006), p.1.
12. No. 1765.
13. Ibid., p.2.
14. Ibid.
15. Ibid., p.3.
16. *Ritchie v Chichester Health Authority,* 187 (1994).
17 Ibid., p.188.
18. Ibid.

19. Ibid., p.189.
20. Ibid., p.190.
21. Ibid.
22. Ibid.
23. Ibid.
24. Ibid., p.192.
25. Ibid.
26. Ibid., p.193.
27. Ibid., p. 189.
28. Ibid., p.190.
29. Ibid., p.209.
30. Ibid., p.191.
31. Ibid., p.90.
32. Ibid., p.211.
33. Ibid., p.210.
34. Currie, et al., Anaesthetic Intensive Care 1993:21 'The- Wrong Drug Problem in Anaesthesia: an Analysis of 2,000 Incident Reports'.
35. Ritchie, p.210.
36. Ibid., at p.213.
37. Record of Investigation into Death, No. 2477/02, Victoria (Nov. 2004). Page references unavailable at time of writing: for access to findings www.coroners court.vic.gov.au/

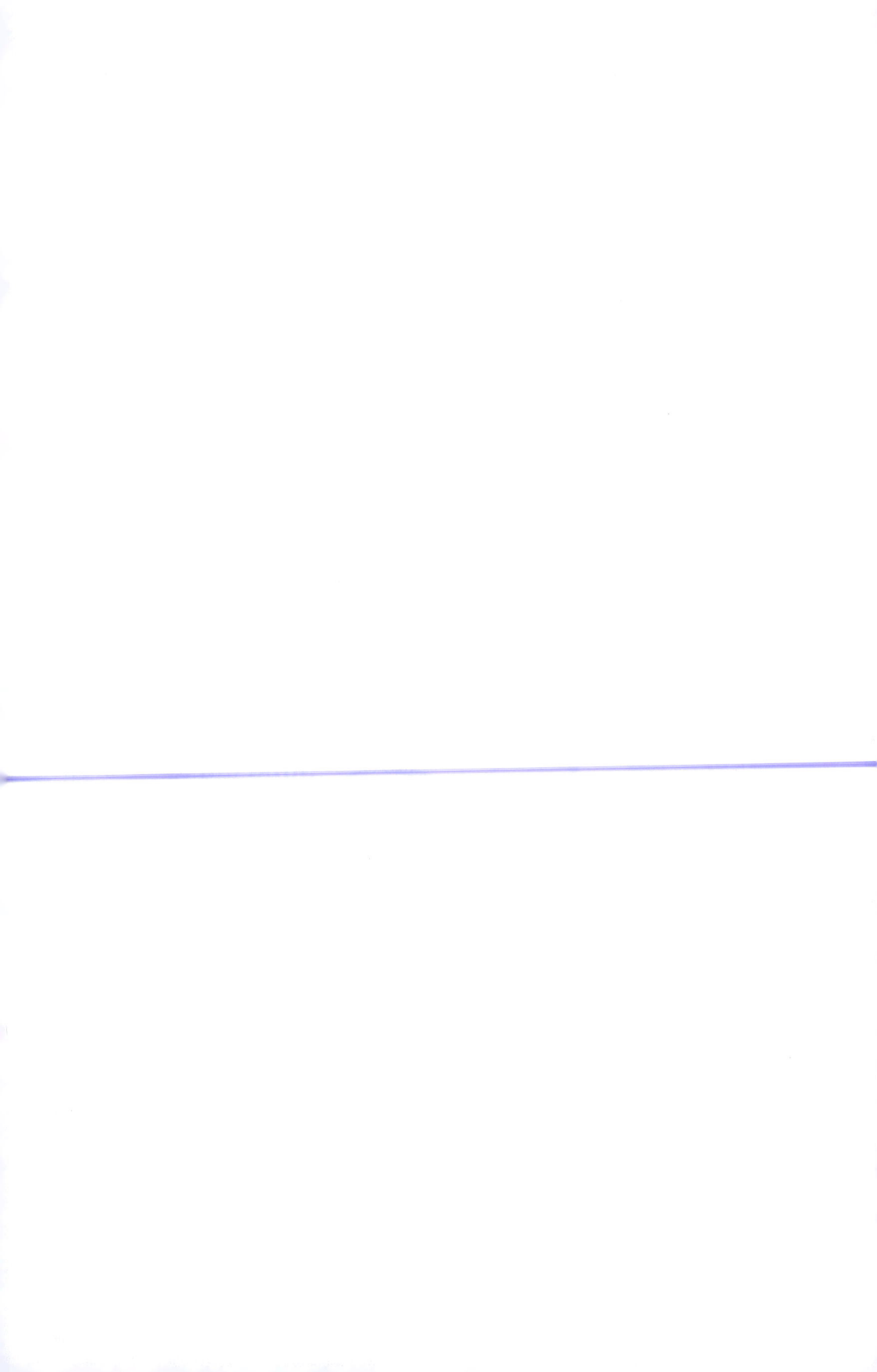

Introduction

General anaesthesia does not always produce unconsciousness and relief from pain. Patients have occasionally remained aware, recalling incidents during the operation. But, as English anaesthetists Professor M Rosen and Dr JN Horton have pointed out, 'awareness is not necessarily accompanied by pain, and the degree of recall can vary from brief episodes, when a single remark or sensation is experienced, to 'serious disaster', when the patient lies awake in extreme pain during the procedure.' Further, regional anaesthesia occasionally provides inadequate pain relief.[1]

While adverse outcomes can occur without negligence, medical defence organizations consider that it is almost impossible to defend a case where an anaesthetist has failed to adhere to generally accepted clinical practice in the choice of anaesthetic technique, failed to keep an adequate anaesthetic record, or faulty equipment was involved. If new means of detecting awareness become part of standard monitoring equipment, failure to use such a resource will become an issue.

Where awareness has apparently occurred, a full explanation should be given to the patient. Careful and sympathetic listening to the complaint (whether about pain, pressure, noise), together with an explanation, may reduce the likelihood of litigation. Some patients will need treatment to address post-traumatic stress.

As you will read in this chapter, flow-on damage from awareness and pain can include psychiatric illness, avoidance of surgery, difficulty bonding with the baby, and breakdown in relationships. Good risk management therefore requires that postoperative complaints are documented and followed up promptly.

....

The four cases in this chapter concern women who complained of extreme and unnecessary pain during the birth process. Two complain of awareness under general anesthetic, one of pain during an epidural, and one that no anaesthetic was given during the manual removal of the placenta.

The defence counsel's hopes must have faded in the first case when the judge described the patient's plight as 'the most horrifying experience it has ever been my misfortune to listen to recounted in these courts.'[2]

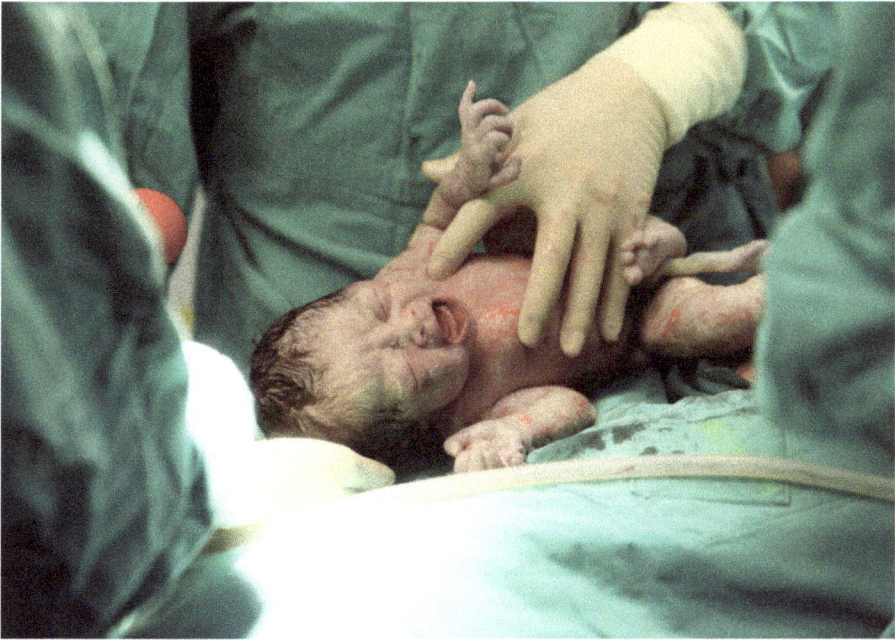

Ackers v Wigan Health Authority [UK, 1991][3]

The facts

Simone, with her first baby presenting in the breech position, was taken to the OR for a caesarean section. She said that she had lain paralysed in the operating room, unable to communicate and felt the insertion of the surgeon's knife 'like a red hot poker'.[4] Further 'excruciating'[5] pain followed as the uterus was cleaned and the incision sutured. Simone later told ward staff that she had felt everything.

Postnatal. Within 28 days of the birth, Simone experienced vaginal bleeding and returned to hospital. She was told she could have to undergo a general anaesthetic, so that she could be 'scraped'. Now terrified, Simone hid sanitary towels from the doctors in case they thought the blood loss warranted an operation. When a second pregnancy became a breech presentation, a caesarean section was again necessary. Sexual relations with her husband were affected because of her fear of a previously planned third pregnancy.

She experienced difficulties bonding with the child born after the original trauma, refused to undergo operations for the removal of a cyst and painful varicose veins, and suffered proximal insomnia, as well as periods of depression. Simone became withdrawn and fearful of the future.

Negligence was alleged.

The trial

Three levels of consciousness. An expert medical witness, who closely questioned Simone, explained to the court that when initially anaesthetized a patient can experience three levels of consciousness. The patient can be half conscious or dreaming; can drift in and out of consciousness; or remain awake, remembering everything clearly and without confusion. Simone had fallen into the last category.

Liability admitted. As the health authority admitted negligence, no details of what went amiss with the anaesthetic were disclosed. The case proceeded only on the amount of damages. The judge, hearing evidence that Simone planned to undergo therapy to deal with her experience, believed she was determined to get well.

Damages awarded.

....

In the next case, the hospital agreed that the patient might have experienced the sensations she described, but argued they occurred after the reversal of anaesthetic. This case is a good example of the importance of an accurate and contemporary anaesthetic record in the defence of a claim.

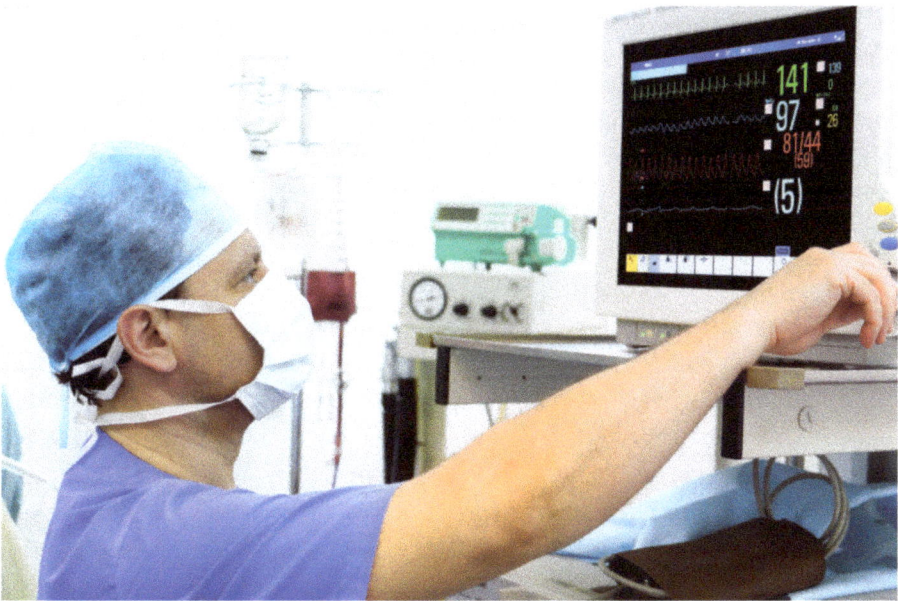

Taylor v Worcester & District Health Authority [UK, 1991][6]

The facts

Judith was admitted to hospital for a caesarean section. She recalled that she was crying as she was being taken to the operating theatre, given a mask to breathe through and that somebody started to count. She became unconscious after a few seconds, then remembered an increasingly acute pain, 'like a burning sensation,'[7] across her abdomen. This was followed by a strong sensation of something pressing down inside. She could not open her eyes nor move, and could hear a hissing sound. She felt as if the whole of her body was moving with a tugging sensation. There was also a constant pressure, followed by a release of pressure, on her chest. Judith said she was terrified. She felt she was going to die. She lost consciousness again, and then gradually heard voices. She still felt paralysed after the operation.

Nightmares. Judith said the only person she told of her experience was her mother, and that she started having nightmares when she returned home.

The trial

Judith contended that her episode of awareness was due to the negligence of the anaesthetist in failing to use the proper procedure, failing to exercise skill and judgment in the selection of drugs, and failing to monitor levels of the anaesthetic agent. The health authority contended that the patient's awareness occurred *after* the reversal of anaesthetic.

The anaesthetic record. The anaesthetist told the court she would have followed normal procedure. When she examined Judith at 7 am, just before anaesthesia, blood pressure was 140/100, heart normal. Induction, beginning with administration of 250 mg thiopentone and followed by 100 mg suxamethonium, began at 7.15 am. Judith was then intubated and given 50:50 nitrous oxide: oxygen and 0.5 per cent halothane at six-litre minute volume. Alcuronium in a 15 mg dose was given five minutes after induction.

As soon as the widest part of the baby was delivered, Judith received five units Syntocinon, plus a further five units after 14 mg of omnopon was administered when the cord was clamped.

Delivery. On delivery of the baby by fundal pressure at 7.30 am, nitrous oxide was increased to 70 per cent, oxygen decreased to 30 per cent, then the halothane turned off about four to five minutes after the omnopon. Blood pressure was 130, pulse normal. At 7.45 am, an extra dose of alcuronium was given and at 7.50 am to 7.55 am an extra dose of 2 mg omnopon. At 8.10 am, reversal commenced by administering atropine and neostigmine.

The anaesthetist said she saw no signs of awareness during the operation.

Expert medical evidence. A consultant anaesthetist giving expert evidence for the health authority (and whose opinions the judge found persuasive) gave the following explanations for Judith's experiences:[8]

1. Patients who experienced pain during a caesarean section would relate word for word any conversation they heard and would invariably hear the baby cry. They would feel touch and could usually tell on which side the person handed the baby was standing. They would remember the pressure of the intra-tracheal tube and be aware of the ventilator breathing for them. None of these descriptions had been given by Judith. The expert witness said he would have expected her to be aware of touch and auditory stimuli. The baby's Apgar score of 9 at 1 minute indicated it would have cried, and gone on crying.

2. The pain the patient had felt across her abdomen 'like a distant pain which had become acute'[9] was most likely explained by the swabbing of the wound after the stitches were put in, but before the wound was dressed. This was what would have been expected after the halothane was turned off; its full effect reducing gradually, as described.

3. The hissing noise was probably the noise of suction apparatus used to suck out the pharynx and mouth. This was usually switched on before the atropine and neostigmine were given and usually put under the patient's pillow. Sucking was only carried out at the very beginning and end of an operation.

4. The most likely explanation of the tugging sensation 'as if my whole body was moving',[10] was a prolonged period of coughing involving all abdominal muscles. This produced in patients who were awake a feeling as if the wound was being pulled apart at the stitches. The whole body would often be moving with such coughing movements. In addition, moving the patient onto her side before the tube was removed would stimulate the coughing or make it worse. The end of a caesarean section was a particularly difficult time. It was important to ensure the return of the airway reflexes and often patients experienced pain at this time. An adequate dose of omnopon would reduce, but not eliminate, pain.

5. There was nothing in the operation to explain Judith's description of constant pressure 'as if on the chest and released again.'[11] One explanation could be coughing. Another reason was that, after the operation, midwives often palpate the fundus of the uterus to find out if it had contracted satisfactorily, because of the risk of haemorrhage. If not, they might massage it with intermittent squeezing or pressure.

6. The expert witness agreed that the patient's pain had been excruciating. While not disbelieving her experiences, he believed they were a subjective interpretation of what was going on. Large numbers of women had similar experiences and anaesthetists were trying to address this problem.

7. In this case, the anaesthetic record did not contain evidence of pain or distress. There was no rise in blood pressure or pulse during the operation, and no record of any sweating or lacrimation. These were all signs the anaesthetist would have observed. In the consultant anaesthetist's opinion, a patient's blood pressure would have risen to a range of 160 to 200, and pulse to 120 to 140, if awareness had occurred with pain.

8. Although there had been disagreements over the anaesthetic process, if the anaesthetist's anaesthetic technique had been carried out as described, there would have been sufficient anaesthetic cover.

The decision

The judge found there had been an episode in which Judith suffered pain and discomfort, felt pressure and heard hissing. But her description of awareness was entirely consistent with events taking place at reversal, both individually and sequentially. There was nothing in her description exclusively referable to a time of the birth.

I am entirely clear in my mind ... that (the anaesthetist) was not negligent in any of the respects contended ... Even if the plaintiff's episode of awareness was during the operation, I entirely acquit the anaesthetist of negligence. I find she adopted a widely used technique of administering anaesthetics, a technique she carried out in a careful and competent manner. The technique carried with it a small statistical risk of awareness during the operation; a risk which arose from respectable and responsible medical opinion that halothane affected the contraction of the uterus after delivery.[12]

....

The following two cases focus on patients' claims that they received inadequate pain relief - in these instances from regional anaesthesia.

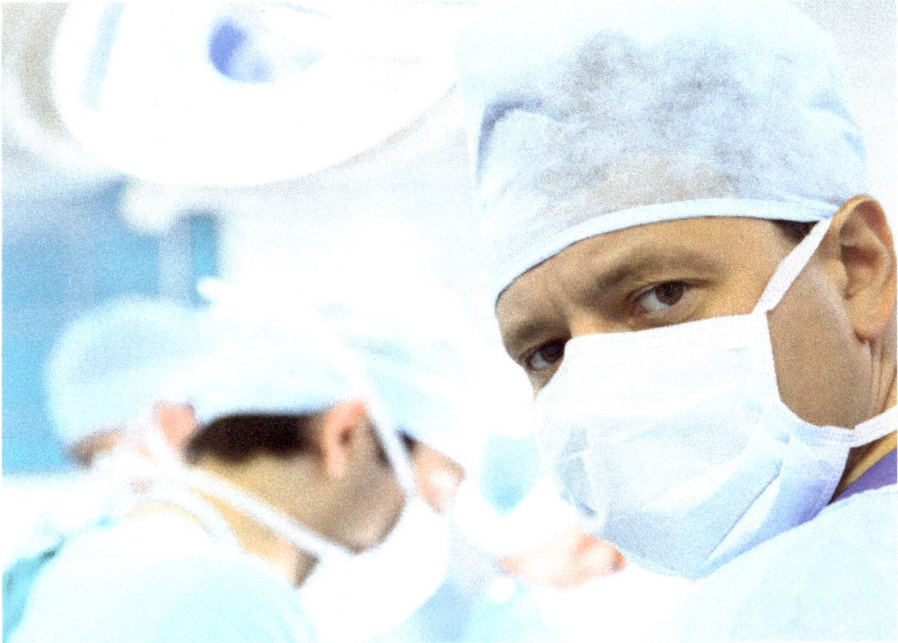

Tucker v Hospital Corporation Australia Pty Ltd & Ors [Aus, 1998][13]

The facts

Maxine was admitted to a private hospital for delivery of her child by cae-sarean section. A tubal ligation was performed immediately afterwards. The operation commenced at 9.35 pm and finished by 11. 05 pm.

The epidural. As Maxine had eaten on the night she went into labour, it was decided to use an epidural block. A mixture of lignocaine and adrenaline was inserted by epidural catheter and further amounts given when Maxine complained of pain. The anaesthetist administered Marcaine into the sub-arachnoid space and into the incision to provide further local anaesthesia; a mixture of Droperidol and Fentanyl was given intravenously for sedation. Despite Maxine's continuing complaints of pain, the doctors said they would have to proceed because the baby was in distress and at risk.

Traumatic. Maxine said she found the operation so traumatic that she did not want to look at the baby. She had asked that her daughter be taken away. Negligence was alleged.

The trial

Maxine said the doctors had not communicated with her during the procedure or appreciated the extent of her pain. She had felt a sharp piercing pain when the initial incision was made, and had shouted out as the pain was severe and shocking. She believed she was going to die. Her husband, who was present, corroborated this account, saying his wife was 'tense, apprehensive and upset.....her face was red and contorted.'[14] He had felt upset and sick.

Excruciating pain. Maxine said the continued cutting to deliver the baby had been 'excruciating, horrific pain.'[15] Her screaming only exacerbated this. She had breathed through the oxygen mask, but the pain got worse. The obstetrician had pushed down to deliver the baby and to deliver the placenta. She had groaned each time he pushed. Maxine said that during the tubal ligation she felt groggy, was still in pain, but had ceased complaining. At some stage, she had become unconscious and woke while she was being sutured.

Distorted memory. The doctors said it would have been professionally irresponsible and callous to have proceeded with the operation if a patient was experiencing such pain. They argued that her memory had become distorted about the severity of the pain over the years and that sedating drugs, given at the time of delivery, could have affected her memory. The obstetrician said he could not remember any specific complaints of pain, although he acknowledged Maxine could have experienced some discomfort. He said it was not unusual for patients to complain during delivery, as the fundus of the uterus is pushed hard at that time.

A stressful night. The anaesthetist said there had only been an initial complaint of pain and that Maxine had slept at some stage but was easily rousable. Both doctors denied she had screamed; both had an independent recollection of what went on, not relying on hospital records to give their evidence. The obstetrician described the procedure as 'unique',[16] saying it had been a 'stressful night'[17] for everyone concerned. The anaesthetist described it as 'something quite out of the ordinary'.[18]

The decision

The judge found the doctors negligent. The obstetrician and the anaesthetist had both failed to maintain the standard of care the law demands of medical practitioners. The judge referred to expert evidence that on occasions an epidural block and, less frequently, a subarachoid block may not be effective. In Maxine's case, the failure could have been the result of adhesions formed following her previous caesarean sections.

Greater level of distress. Despite arguments to the contrary, the judge was satisfied that the obstetrician and anaesthetist had observed a greater level of distress in Maxine than described in their evidence. Maxine's evidence that the anaesthetist had told her to 'hold on,'[19] or words to that effect, indicated that the doctors knew she was in a great deal of pain.

Fall in BP. In addition, recordings of blood pressure revealed a fall in pressure that could have been attributed to the subarachoid block. The rise in systolic pressure to just above 110 mm Hg could have been the initial pain Maxine felt when the incision was made. Her recall of the sequence of events was found to accord with that of the medical team.

Unacceptable level of pain. The judge was satisfied that Maxine suffered an unacceptable level of pain, not only at the outset of the operation but throughout the procedure. A general anaesthetic should have been administered. It was noted that the obstetrician had apologised to Maxine in the ward. Damages were awarded for distress, emotional problems and personality changes.

....

In the final case the patient alleges the patient's GP was negligent in attempting manual removal of the placenta without anaesthesia.

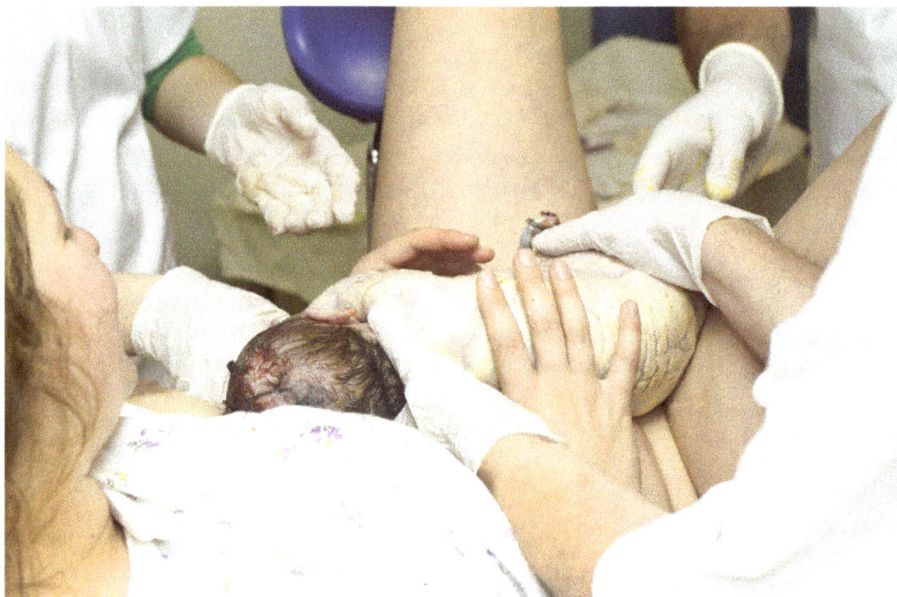

Lunn v Giblin (Aus, 1998)[20]

The facts

Leanne, aged 35 and pregnant, was worried that problems could arise at the birth. The GP reassured her that a specialist would be called in if necessary. When Leanne was admitted to hospital for an induced labour, a midwife, discovering the baby's head was not engaged, believed the induction should be postponed. Despite the midwife's concerns, the GP decided to proceed. The baby was delivered by forceps after a long and strenuous labour. When the placenta did not discharge spontaneously, the GP told Leanne he would remove it manually.

Removal of placenta. The GP inserted his hand through the cervix and into the uterus, scraping the uterus wall. Leanne said she was distressed, crying, shouting and writhing around as the doctor attempted the removal several times. He had left after removing the placenta and repairing the episiotomy.

Midwifery staff concerned. For eight hours afterwards Leanne experienced fainting episodes and had difficulty passing urine. For the next few days she passed blood clots, had a racing pulse and could not exert herself. Midwives were concerned at the first postnatal visit by the GP three days later, when the GP said that Leanne could go home. There was no discussion of retained products in the uterus, nor any referral for an ultrasound.

Ultrasound. When Leanne continued to suffer, she insisted on an ultrasound. This revealed 'echogenic foci consistent with presence of retained products.'[21]

Curette. Leanne was referred to a gynaecologist, who immediately admitted her to hospital for a curette. She was transfused after heavy blood loss and returned to surgery. An emergency developed which nearly required a hysterectomy, but surgeons were able to pack the uterus, leaving two packs in situ.

Asherman's syndrome. Leanne suffered postpartum haemorrhage and septicaemia; two days later surgery was required to remove the packs. She then experienced a long and drawn out process of symptoms and diagnoses—the final diagnosis being Asherman's syndrome. The court heard this syndrome is a rare condition in which the front and back wall of the uterine cavity adhere to each other in a way which may obliterate the cervical canal. Leanne said that by the time the condition was diagnosed the frustration, endless rounds of appointments and loss of libido were imposing a severe strain on her relationship with her partner. She was told surgery was possible but with no guarantee of success; a further pregnancy would be difficult.

Aftermath. Two unsuccessful hysteroscopies and a complicated laparotomy followed. When Leanne became pregnant about six months later, complications developed requiring hospitalization for four months until her second child was born. All these circumstances had an adverse effect on her relationship and studies. She was advised not to have any more children. Negligence was alleged.

The trial

The GP told the court that after delivering the baby he placed long forceps on the cord. These moved away from the vulva, which indicated that the placenta was separating. He then commenced the Brandt-Andrews technique of continuous cord traction, applying pressure to the cord to help ease the placenta off the wall of the uterus and deliver it through the cervix.

Manual removal. When this was unsuccessful, he undertook manual removal of the placenta. He had not waited 30 minutes, as was his usual practice, because Leanne was distressed. He was concerned about her bleeding. He had inserted his hand into the placental surface to begin peeling it off, noting that there was no distinction between the edge of the placenta and the wall of the uterus. The placenta appeared to be part of the uterus. He finally found an edge of the placenta that enabled him to start manually removing it. This process required firm strokes to dislodge it.

Abnormal situation. The GP noted that when the placenta did not come away easily, what had initially started out as a normal routine procedure had now become an abnormal situation. Despite this, he had continued the removal of the placenta for about ten minutes. This meant continually introducing his hand into the cervix and uterus. He had diagnosed placenta accreta, repaired the episiotomy, then left.

Implied term. Leanne said she had an express term in her contract with the doctor that he would bring a specialist in if complications arose. The doctor denied this, but conceded that the obligation to engage a specialist was an implied term of the contract.

Expert medical opinion

The following key points were made at the trial:

1. Expert witnesses were critical of the manual removal of the placenta. This procedure was considered to have been undertaken prematurely when there was ample opportunity to arrange for anaesthetic or specialist assistance. Hospital notes revealed that bleeding had been within normal range.
2. Standard procedure was to allow one hour from delivery before attempting removal of the placenta manually, unless life-threatening bleeding was an issue. The placenta will often separate and expel itself spontaneously.
3. Experts supported Leanne's allegation that the procedure would be extremely painful without anaesthesia.
4. One expert considered placenta accreta unlikely in a woman who had no surgery to the uterus.

The decision

The judge stated that the doctor owed his patient a duty of care and that the standard was that of an ordinarily careful and competent GP with considerable experience in obstetrics.

Failure to wait. The judge was satisfied that the manual delivery of the placenta was undertaken within a few minutes after the baby's birth and found the doctor's reasons for proceeding immediately were inadequate. Hospital notes described the blood loss as 'normal'.[22] The doctor's argument that an anaesthetic block may have run out was groundless. The doctor had been forced to agree that such a block was, in any event, completely ineffective in anaesthetising the uterine area. His normal practice was to wait 30 minutes. Failure to do so was 'largely inexplicable'.[23] The judge commented:

> *I consider that the defendant, having unreasonably entered upon the procedure, decided to continue with it but was unable to complete it. The defendant, recognising that his removal of the placenta was probably incomplete, thereafter merely hoped for the best.*[24]

Placenta accreta rejected. Neither placenta accreta, nor an abnormally adherent placenta, was recorded in the contemporary hospital notes.

Pain and suffering. Parts of the placenta were retained, causing subsequent complications, further surgery and severe trauma. Although Leanne had continued with her life 'remarkably well'.[25] the pain and suffering had continued over four years.

Damages awarded.

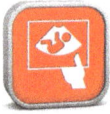

Discussion of Key Issues

Anaesthetists have a duty of care to act in accordance with good medical practice when providing pain relief. Note how decisive the anaesthetic record was in the defence of the anaesthetist in *Taylor*. The judge found that 'even if the plaintiff's episode of awareness was during the operation, I entirely acquit the anaesthetist of negligence. I find she adopted a widely used technique of administering anaesthetics, a technique she carried out in a careful and competent manner'.[26]

In *Ackers* and *Taylor*, the patients (both undergoing caesarean sections) complained of awareness under anaesthesia, with consequent mental trauma. *Taylor* provides detailed medical explanations of how awareness during anaesthetic can be consistent with reversal from the anaesthetic.

- Discuss the merits of each explanation.

Both cases identify the need for midwives/nurses to alert anesthetists to any complaints made in the postpartum period in order that an explanation can be given to the patient or the complaint further investigated. In *Ackers* the patient was clearly terrified of further surgery and made no complaints to staff. In fact, she hid evidence of bleeding from doctors.

- Have patients complained to you of either awareness or pain during an operation in the post-anaesthetic period?
- If so, how was this followed up?
- Does your hospital have a guideline on this issue?

....

In *Tucker,* the patient complained of excruciating pain during a caesarean section, despite an epidural block. The court found she had suffered an unacceptable level of pain at the outset and during the procedure.

In *Lunn,* the patient experienced extreme pain (and continued to suffer pain for years) after a doctor, within a few minutes of the birth, removed the placenta without anaesthesia. The court found the doctor's actions represented a departure from reasonable medical practice.

- Discuss the role of attending midwives, doctors and nurses if it becomes evident that a doctor is departing from reasonable standards of practice in the provision of pain relief.
- Does/could hospital policy provide guidance?

....

In *Ritchie v Chichester Health Authority* (Chapter 7 Medication) the judge questioned whether health professionals working in obstetrics could become 'somewhat immune' to cries of pain.[27]

- Discuss.

NOTES

1. Powers & Harris, *Medical Negligence,* Butterworths, London, pp.859–863 (1994).
2. *Ackers v Wigan Health Authority,* 2 Med LR 232 (1991).
3. Ibid., p.232.
4. Ibid.
5. Ibid.
6. *Taylor v Worcester and District Health Authority,* 2 Med LR 215 (1991).
7. Ibid,. p.215.
8. Ibid., pp.225-228.
9. Ibid., p.217.
10. Ibid., p.218.
11. Ibid.
12. Ibid., p.231.
13. *Tucker v Hospital Corporation Australia Pty Ltd & Ors* NSW Supreme Court, No. 12575/92, 18 Feb 1998 before- Hidden J. Case note: CCH Australian Health and Medical- Law Reporter, paras: 77–129.
14. Ibid., paras: 77–129.
15. Ibid.
16. Ibid.

17. Ibid.
18. Ibid.
19. Ibid.
20. *Lunn v Giblin,* Supreme Court of the Northern Territory (Aus) GRA 98008, 30 July 1998. Case note: CCH Australian Health and Medical Law Reporter.
21. Ibid.
22. Ibid.
23. Ibid.
24. Ibid.
25. Ibid.
26. Ibid.
27. Ibid.

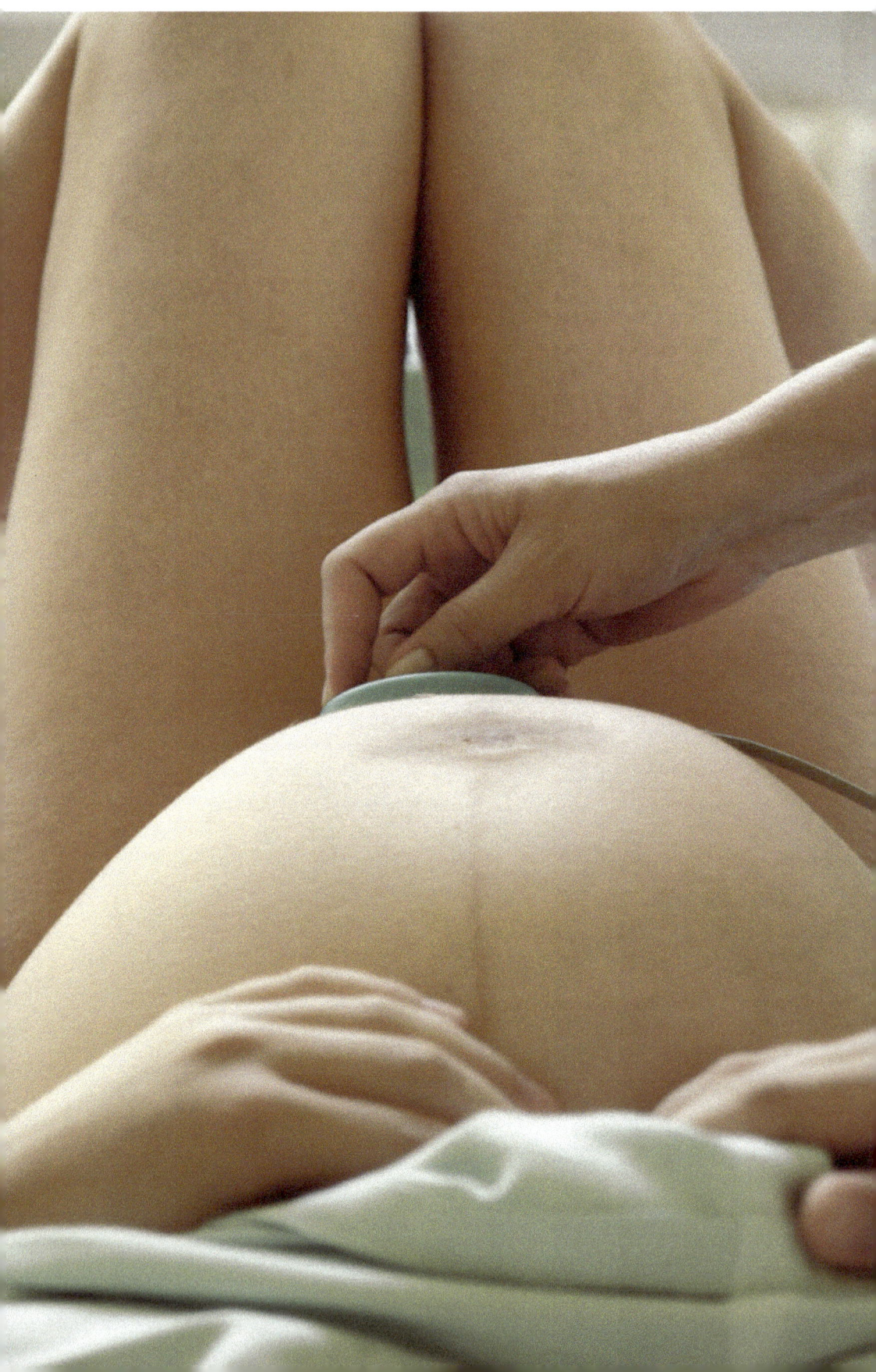

CHAPTER 9

Infection

Q: What happened next?

A: When she walked out, I was really shocked and I went straight over to Celia and I said, 'That sister didn't have any sterile gown, mask or gloves on.'

Q: What did Celia reply?

A: Celia just said, 'Yes, a lot do, a lot don't'.

—A patient's mother

Introduction

Despite stringent precautions, there is always a risk of infection in hospitals. As this is common knowledge, patients alleging sub-standard infection control face formidable obstacles in trying to prove their case. This may change as methods of typing organisms and identifying sources of infection become more advanced. But, at the present time, lawyers know that infection cases are notoriously difficult to win. Few are commenced and even fewer reach court. Nevertheless, from time to time patients contract infections, make complaints and consider litigation. A hospital's best defence will lie in good risk management: the implementation of state-of-the-art infection control policies, together with *convincing evidence* that they are enforced.

....

The first of the six infection cases in this chapter illustrates a) how a nursing care plan was vital to the hospital's argument that nurses had followed proper aseptic technique in the handling of a Hickman catheter, and b) how detailed hospital records describe the medical, midwifery and nursing responses to a developing infection in a pregnant patient who was already acutely ill.

Starkey v Connell, et al.
[Aus, 1994][1]

The facts

On 2 June 1987, Celia, aged 30 and eight weeks pregnant with her first child, was admitted to a maternity hospital with constant vomiting. An insulin-dependent diabetic, Celia also suffered from intermittent psychiatric disorders, including depression. Her father was the referring doctor. Celia came under the care of an endocrinologist and an obstetrician.

Discharge and readmission. Celia was discharged on 4 June, only to be readmitted the following day. She was given intravenous therapy with a number of drugs, including Largactil, and discharged on 13 June. Four days later Celia was admitted to a second hospital with vomiting, plus a urinary tract infection. The UTI cleared with antibiotics. A nephrologist found some evidence of mild diabetic nephropathy.

Vomiting and depression. The obstetrician remained Celia's treating doctor during her five subsequent visits to the second hospital. The medical team now included a psychiatrist and a gastroenterologist. No obvious cause or specific treatment for the vomiting could be found. Depression and weight loss continued. The endocrinologist, who specialised in diabetes, noted on 26 October that he had 'not seen a pregnancy behave like this'.[2] On 5 November: 'Again what more can we do? She is nauseated and vomiting, has a very flat affect and is not taking her Largactil.'[3]

Hickman catheter. Because of Celia's poor oral intake, difficulty with IV access and nutritional deprivation, a Hickman catheter was inserted under general anaesthetic on 20 November. Total parenteral nutrition commenced, using an IVAC pump.

Nursing care plan. The Nursing Care Plan read: '20.11.87 - Hickman catheter inserted, (Nursing Goal) - to maintain patency of catheter and prevent ascending infection; (Nursing Action) - strict aseptic technique when changing dressing and lines i.e. sterile gown, gloves, mask- maintain IV therapy as ordered by doctor - observe insertion site- observe temperature, pulse and respiration) for infection... maintain F(luid) B(alance) C(hart).'[4]

Celia was noted as very drowsy and lethargic over the next few days. Vomiting continued intermittently.
   From the record:

24 November: (am) TPN line changed; remaining lethargic.

25 November: catheter site (chest wound) dressed using Betadine, lines changed using sterile technique and faulty IVAC pump changed. The endocrinologist noted Celia looked 'more stunned', 'more Parkinsonian.'[5] The endocrinologist asked the psychiatrist to review the Largactil dose.

26 November: second pump not functioning. Burette installed. By evening, neck wound (checked and cleaned with chlorhexidine am.) was 'red and inflamed.' 'Shakes on and off.'[6] Full blood test and removal of the sutures ordered by obstetrician.

27 November: wound re-dressed. Sutures removed. Light gauze applied and steri strips. Complaining of tingling lips and legs, feeling cold and very shaky. A resident doctor believed her to be hyperventilating. At 6 pm temperature 38 C.

The obstetrician prescribed cephalothin (Keflin). Full blood examination and blood cultures. Creatinine level.07 mmol / 1.

28 November: 6.30 am. Flushed, with a rapid pulse. Temperature 39 C. Septicaemia suspected. Gentamicin administered. Catheter left in place.

Given the now serious risk to both mother and baby, a caesarean section was performed and a baby girl successfully delivered. High temperatures; Gentamicin 12 hourly. Oedema noted.

30 November: Hickman catheter removed.

1 December: gentamicin levels tested. General condition improved. Temperature 37.8 C.

2 December: the endocrinologist noted 'Settling well. I think the infection is coming under control but would like another 24 hrs more of intravenous antibiotics.'[7] Blood sample taken 8.45 am. Creatinine level of 0.17 mmol/litre - first abnormal reading. Gentamicin administered at 9 pm.

3 December: blood pressure rose. Evidence of protein in urine, output dropped markedly. Creatinine level 0.28 mmol/litre. Acute renal failure diagnosed. On the nephrologist's recommendation, gentamicin stopped, Lasix administered. Patient transferred under his care to the Nephrology Ward at a third hospital.

5 December: intravenous Lasix (250 mg) administered at 11.15 am. Complained am of deafness in right ear. Resident doctor detected slight deafness in both ears. 'Very withdrawn'[8] on the 5 and 6 December.

7 December: nephrologist ordered Lasix (250 mg) orally at 10 am.

By lunchtime hearing 'drastically decreased to the extent that she can barely hear. She is relying on lip reading and writing notes.'[9]

Celia's renal failure subsided. By 24 December she was transferred back to the second hospital until March 1988. Her near total deafness was now permanent.

Allegations. The case that followed was concerned with whether nursing staff, hospital or doctors were negligent in the management of a Hickman catheter, thereby causing infection and septicaemia; whether the obstetrician was negligent in the administration of an antibiotic (gentamicin), thereby causing acute renal failure and severe loss of hearing; and whether the nephrologist was negligent in the administration of a diuretic (Lasix), thereby causing or contributing to Celia's deafness.

The trial

Vulnerability to infection. The judge found Celia very vulnerable to infection because of diabetes, malnutrition, pregnancy and surgical wounds, as well as the central venous catheter. Possible causes included surgical infection, postoperative infection as a result of some unidentified event, or negligent handling of the Hickman catheter by a nurse.

Risk of septicaemia. It was generally agreed there was no alternative to the use of the Hickman catheter in so ill a patient. One of Celia's doctors (a specialist in hypertension, nephrology and endocrinology) explained that the catheter would carry a significant risk of infection and subsequent septicaemia 'whether Celia was treated at home, in hospital or in a hermetically sealed container',[10] gentamicin was agreed to be the correct prescription for septicaemia and the gentamicin levels taken on 1 December indicated satisfactory kidney function.

Lack of aseptic technique alleged. What was alleged was that the septicaemia (infective agent staphylococcus epidermidis) developed as a result of the lack of aseptic handling by nurses at the second hospital. It was further alleged there were no proper protocols or nursing care plans in place. Celia gave evidence, as did her parents, that they had seen nursing staff attend the central venous catheter and dressings without gloves or masks, or without washing their hands.

The father's evidence. Celia's father gave evidence that on one occasion Celia had been in a sitting room when the pump starting beeping. A nurse was called, who was unable to get it going. The nurse had then folded back the dressing of the catheter to arrange or adjust the junction of the line. She had worn a gown but no gloves or mask, and had not washed her hands. A second nurse who was walking by was called in and asked by the first nurse to assist in the adjustment of the drip or the intravenous flow. The first nurse again attended to the reservoir and the pump, then withdrew the covering dressing again, disconnected it, and in some way tried to manipulate the tube to get the drip flowing.

At the trial, the father was asked specifically about what he observed during the manipulation of the tube by the first nurse:

Q: With what success, if any, on this occasion ?

A: Apparently it started to flow again and she was satisfied with her efforts.[11]

Further questions followed about the second nurse :

Q: The second nurse, what, if anything, did she have upon her hands?

A: Nothing.

Q: What did she have upon her face?

A: No mask.

Q: What did she have by way of a gown ?

A: No gown.

Q: What precautions, if any, had you seen her take by way of cleansing her hands doing this?

A: She made no attempt to cleanse her hands.[12]

The mother's evidence. Celia's mother gave evidence that on 27 November a nurse had re-dressed the chest wound without gloves, mask or gown.

Q: What happened next?

A: When she walked out, I was really shocked and I went straight over to Celia and I said, 'That sister didn't have any sterile gown, mask or gloves on.'

Q: What did Celia reply?

A: Celia just said, 'Yes, a lot do, a lot don't'.[13]

Strict aseptic technique. A doctor giving expert evidence told the court that 'strict aseptic technique' meant no part of the human body can touch the lines running from the bag to the Hickman catheter unless it is either protected by sterile gloves or the line is being managed without touching the connections at the end. If a nurse was not going to use gloves, she should scrub her hands with an antiseptic for 30 seconds or so.

Gloves were not required for the installation of a new line or for bag changes. Washing hands and a 'no-touch' technique were sufficient, together with the painting or swabbing of the ends of the lines with disinfectant. However, gloves should be used when dealing with any disconnection or reconnection of an existing line. In the doctor's opinion, the wearing of gowns, masks or hats was less important than gloves and of little, if any, relevance to an infection resulting from staphylococcus epidermidis.

Findings

The judge accepted this evidence, but was not satisfied that it would be a failure to take reasonable care to omit the painting or swabbing of the lines with disinfectant in all the circumstances. As the judge noted 'It was hard to comprehend'[14] that Celia's father, as a medical practitioner, who must have understood aseptic technique and was aware of his daughter's high susceptibility to infection, had not complained at the time about the sitting-room incident.

Inconsistencies. There were inconsistencies in the father's evidence. The judge was not satisfied that any disconnection of the line or lack of aseptic technique had occurred. Further, the incident was probably too early to be the infecting event. The evidence showed that if bacteria entered the bloodstream through the lumen of the catheter, the onset of infection would be very rapid.

The mother's evidence. The reliability of the mother's evidence was also questioned. The judge accepted that the nurse would have observed aseptic techniques when re-dressing the wound on 27 November, even though she had no recollection of the incident.

Celia's evidence. There were good grounds to question the accuracy and reliability of Celia's recollection of events. The judge found that at the relevant time her memory would have been impaired by a major tranquilliser. In addition, she was very sick. She had been noted as drowsy and lethargic, as well as non-communicative.

Nursing care plan 'tailor made.' The judge found the nurses had been properly trained in the use of aseptic techniques. They had a nursing care plan which was kept at the foot of the bed. This plan had been described by medical witnesses as 'a tailor-made nursing care plan for a patient with a Hickman catheter';[15] it provided an adequate procedure and protocol.

Medical staff's reliance on nursing care plan. Medical staff were entitled to rely upon the nursing care plan as 'reasonably assuring'[16] proper handling of the catheter by the nurses. Although the possibility of isolated instances of negligence could not be excluded, the judge was not satisfied that it had occurred in the ways or to the extent alleged.

Medication issues

Gentamicin. Celia's condition had remained potentially life-threatening during early December. Blood tests had not yet determined the infective agent. Acute renal failure and deafness were side effects of gentamicin, but her condition could have deteriorated rapidly had it been stopped. The risk to her life outweighed these risks. The elevated creatinine levels had indicated significant renal dysfunction, but expert evidence had not established that a reasonably competent obstetrician ought not to have administered the 2 December dose. Though permanent, Celia's deafness had not been caused by the obstetrician's negligence.

Lasix. Celia also alleged that the nephrologist was negligent in ordering Lasix, which may have contributed to her loss of hearing.

The judge found Celia was close to needing dialysis, with its own associated risks, when the Lasix was administered. A high throughput of fluids was necessary to prevent further deterioration of kidney function. There had been no reasonable alternative. The likely cause of the deafness was not the diuretic (an extremely uncommon occurrence) but the gentamicin.

Review of evidence. The judge found, on a balance of probabilities, that a surgical infection (suggested by the neck wound) was the likely cause of the infection and septicaemia. But neither the nurses nor doctors had been negligent in their care.

Eighteen nurses who had been on duty at the second hospital were called as witnesses in 1994. Since this was eight years after the events, it was understandable that the majority could not remember Celia as a patient. The nurse, for example, could not recall re-dressing the wound on 27 November. Consequently, hospital records became decisive.

....

In the next two cases, pregnant women contract Cytomegalovirus (CMV). In the first, a United States court examines the standard of care for a doctor treating a patient with a communicable disease. In this instance, the foreseeable risk of infection was not to a particular person, but to a class of persons which included an in utero infant.

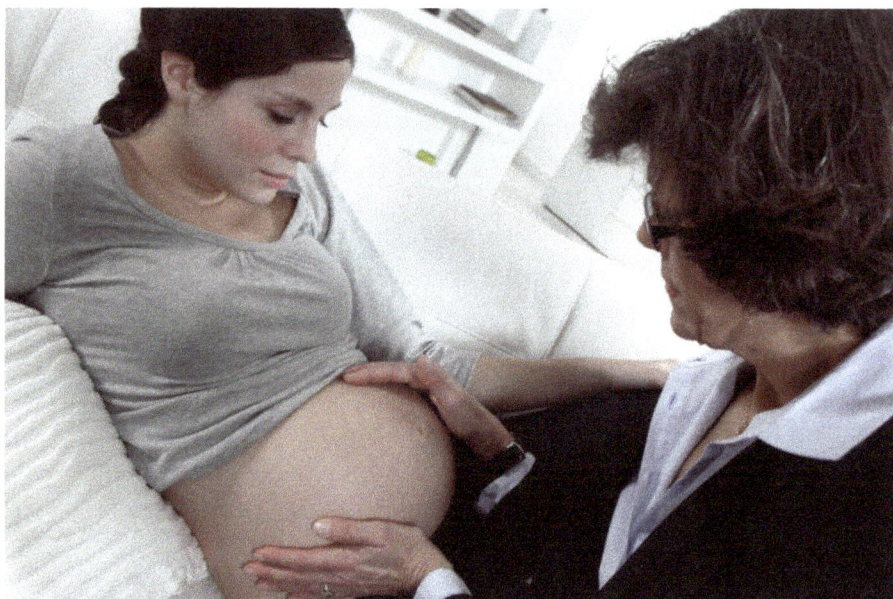

Troxel v AI Dupont Institute [US, 1996][17]

The facts

On 30 October 1987, Nerida gave birth to a baby girl, Jessica, with micro-cephaly and a pes cavus deformity of the foot. Jessica was examined at a medical centre by Dr Black, who suspected CMV and referred her to a sec-ond medical centre for additional tests. Jessica was seen at this centre by a neurologist, who confirmed the CMV diagnosis. In the meantime, the first medical centre discovered that Nerida was also suffering from CMV.

Involvement with baby. Nerida had a close friend, Maria, who become pregnant in November. Maria frequently visited Nerida and often fed and bathed Jessica, and changed her nappies.

Friend infected. In May 1988, Nerida learned (allegedly for the first time) that CMV was contagious and posed a special risk to pregnant women. By this time, Maria had entered the third trimester of her pregnancy and was al-ready infected. On 19 August, she gave birth to a son who had acquired CMV in utero and who died from the disease three months later.

The trial

Arguments and allegations

Maria and her husband sued the two medical centres for the wrongful death of their son. They alleged that Maria had acquired the condition through the negligence of Dr Black, who was then joined as a defendant.

Failure to warn. Maria and her husband claimed that the defendants had failed to inform Nerida of the contagious nature of CMV. In addition, they had failed to warn of the risk to pregnant women who might come into contact with baby Jessica. Dr Black's records contained a note that Nerida was looking for work and would be leaving Jessica with a friend.

The decision

The trial court held that a doctor has no duty to warn a patient with a highly contagious but ubiquitous viral infection that they should avoid contact with pregnant women whose unborn infants may be at risk of death, or debilitating birth defects. Maria and her husband appealed.

The appeal

Medical community aware. The appeal court found the medical community was well aware of the risks CMV poses to in utero infants.

A deadly risk. While the doctors had no way of knowing the identity of a particular pregnant woman whose infant would be at risk from exposure to Jessica (and therefore could not be expected to warn them), they knew, or should have known, that 'a class of persons' very likely to come into contact with a young mother and her baby were at risk, and that the risk was deadly.

'A class of persons.' Despite this awareness, neither of the medical centres nor Dr Black advised Nerida of the contagious nature of CMV. Nor did they warn her that she and Jessica should avoid close contact with pregnant women. As a result, Nerida continued to visit Maria, who would frequently feed, change, hold and kiss Jessica. It was clear that Maria's unborn son was 'within the class of persons'[18] whose health was likely   to be threatened by the patient and therefore within the 'foreseeable orbit of the risk of harm.'[19]

The doctors therefore had a duty to correctly inform Nerida about the contagious nature of the disease in order to prevent its spread to those within that foreseeable orbit of risk of harm.

Was CMV a 'contagious' disease in this context? Both sides conceded CMV was a contagious disease which exists in the general population. While CMV is generally harmless, going unnoticed in most individuals, it may have severe consequences for 'at risk' groups. These include those whose immune systems have been compromised, pregnant women and the newborn.

Common medical knowledge. The court found the risks were not obscure but well recognised in medical literature. It was argued that imposing upon doctors such a duty to warn in relation to infectious diseases would render them liable for the spread of any infection – even the flu and the common cold. The court rejected this. This type of information was common knowledge, in contrast to the case where risks regarding the spread of certain diseases may only be known to the medical profession. It was essential that correct information be disseminated.

AIDS/hepatitis. The court used the example of AIDS or hepatitis. In these cases a doctor has a duty to inform the patient how to avoid the spread of disease by avoiding specific at-risk conduct, even though the general population may not be otherwise at risk. The same could be said of the communicable nature of CMV.

Standard of care. The appeal court clearly spelt out the standard of care for a doctor who is treating a patient with a communicable disease :

1. inform the patient about the nature of the disease and its treatment,
2. treat the patient and
3. inform the patient how to prevent the spread of disease to others.

Appeal upheld.

....

In the second case, an Australian appeal court finds a child's disabilities have been caused by the mother's 'primary', rather than 'reactivated', CMV. Although concerned with a day care setting, *Hughes* contains warnings for the safe organization of staff in a neonatal nursery.

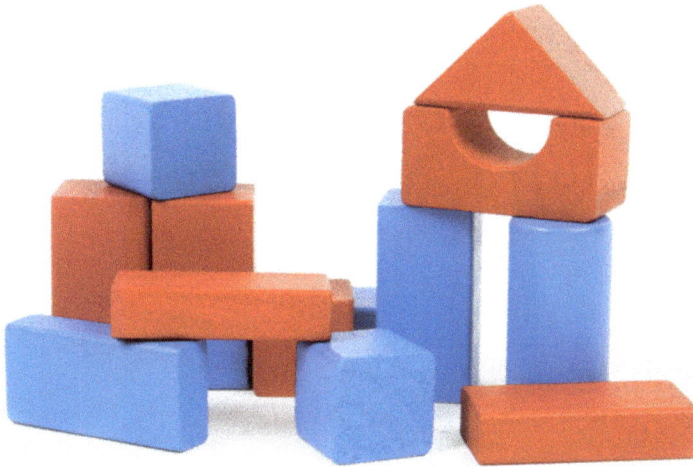

Hughes v Sydney Day Nursery [NSW, 2002][20]

The facts

Eve was employed as a child care worker by a day nursery when she became pregnant. Child care workers are considered to be exposed to an increased occupational risk of acquiring CMV infection. At three months, Matthew was diagnosed with CMV acquired transplacentally. He was later seriously disabled.

The trial

The trial judge found there was no causative link between the day nursery's negligent failure to warn staff and the baby's injuries.

Reactivated rather than primary infection. This decision was based on statistical evidence that the infection was a reactivated rather than a primary infection. Although the nursery was negligent in failing to warn Eve of the possibility of damage to the unborn baby if the CMV virus was acquired during pregnancy, the nature of Eve's occupation made it highly likely that she would have had CMV before her pregnancy commenced.

The appeal

The Court of Appeal overturned the decision of the lower court. The trial judge appeared to have disregarded the pattern of Matthew's disabilities. Eve had flu-like symptoms, typical of CMV infection, early in her pregnancy. The date of the fetal insult corresponded to a contraction of the virus early in the pregnancy. All this pointed, on a balance of probabilities, to the disabilities being caused by primary infection.

....

In the next case, a coroner investigates the death of a baby who contracted Group B streptococcus. The coroner makes a number of recommendations to ensure that pathology results reach the appropriate health professionals.

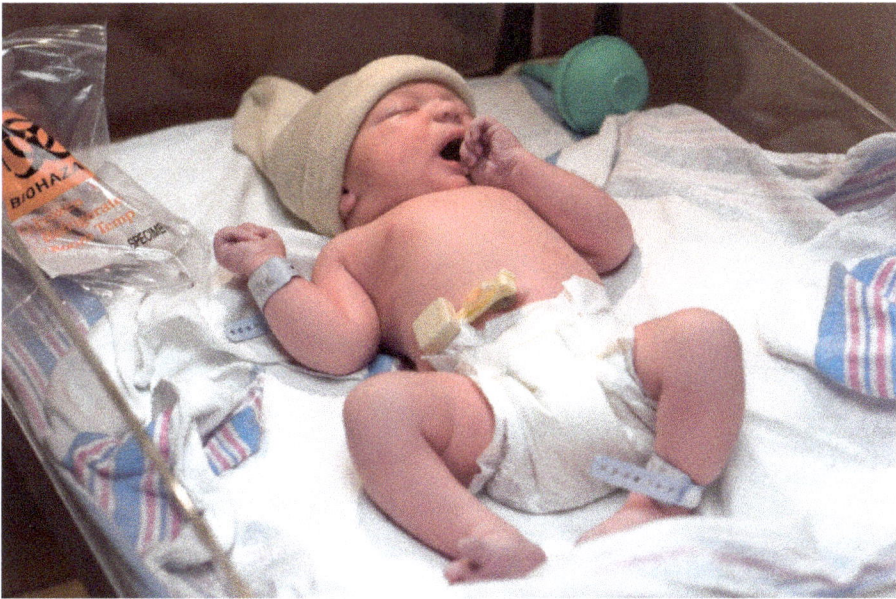

Coronial Investigation [Aus, 1998]²¹

The facts

On 5 October 1995, Eleanor, then 31 weeks pregnant with twins, was admitted to a public hospital for investigation of back pain on the referral of her obstetrician. As her private health cover had not yet come through, Eleanor was admitted as a public patient under the care of the hospital's medical staff.

Streptococcus agalactiae. A high vaginal swab and midstream urine sample revealed a growth of streptococcus agalactiae (also known as Group B streptococcus or GBS). These results took a minimum of three days to come back from pathology. Eleanor was discharged on 6 October, having had no contractions since 9 pm the previous evening. It was noted in the medical records that she was to be reviewed by her obstetrician the following week.

Birth of twins. Eleanor was induced at a private hospital at 35 weeks, owing to severe back pain. The first twin delivered, was floppy at birth, appeared to stabilize, and then deteriorated rapidly with the development of pneumonia and respiratory collapse. A paediatrician commenced IV fluids,

administered penicillin and gentamicin, then arranged for the baby's transfer to another hospital. Despite treatment and resuscitation after cardiac
collapse, the baby died 11 hours after birth. At autopsy, bacterial assessment
of tissue grew streptococcus agalactiae. The second twin survived without
complications.

The tests

The coroner heard that Eleanor's pathology results had never come to her
obstetrician's attention. Her obstetrician did not recall ever being advised
that tests had been undertaken, but guessed the tests had been explaining
that 'investigation of a patient in premature labour can include the taking of
swabs.'[22]

During Eleanor's admission to the public hospital, the obstetrician had
spoken to two doctors who were looking after her. The obstetrician was
asked at the inquest whether she had discussed with one of them (an RMO)
on 5 October as to whether he was going to order the tests (which were in fact
conducted). The obstetrician replied, 'He wouldn't need to have discussed it.
He was an extremely competent resident at that time and has subsequently
become a registrar.'[23] The obstetrician could not recall whether they had discussed the matter.

10 October review. Eleanor said that during the appointment with her
obstetrician on 10 October, she mentioned that she had tests but did not
know what they were for. Her obstetrician could not recall this conversation, but did not dispute that it could have taken place. Eleanor also said
she had been given a letter on discharge from the public hospital, but had
been confused at the time due to the medication she had been given. She
could not recall if the letter was a discharge summary or another letter to her
obstetrician.

Tests not communicated. The court heard that the original discharge
summary, dated 6 October, was still on the hospital file. It contained the
nature of the tests conducted. Her obstetrician could not recall seeing a copy
and said she was surprised that the positive results were not communicated
to her. She felt that adequate indication of her involvement could have been
included on the request form sent to the laboratory.

Frank manner. The obstetrician agreed it would have been prudent of
her to find out the results. She agreed that it was remiss not to have made

the inquiry, given her responsibility for Eleanor's on-going care. The coroner commended the obstetrician for the frank manner in which she gave her evidence.

Probability of positive test results. The obstetrician explained that had she known of the test results, taken at 31 weeks, she would probably have taken further swab specimens at 34 weeks when she admitted Eleanor to the private hospital for bed rest and analgesia. Knowing the outcome at birth, she agreed that it was probable the results would have been positive. The obstetrician said she would not have taken swabs routinely at 34 weeks and did not do so.

The findings

Routine testing not universally accepted. The coroner noted from the evidence that Group B streptococcus was recognised as a possible risk factor in pre-term labour at less than 34 weeks. Evidence had also been given that in 1995 routine testing at about 28 weeks was not, and was still not in 1998 (at the date of the inquest), universally accepted by the profession. The coroner considered that there should be no criticism of the obstetrician's failure to conduct swab or mid stream testing at 34 35 weeks.

The obstetrician said that had she known of the results of the tests at 31 weeks she would have administered penicillin to Eleanor after the commencement of labour. All medical witnesses agreed there would have been little value in administering antibiotics to the mother prior to labour.

Expert medical opinion

Antibiotics after delivery. An independent consultant obstetrician was engaged by the State Coroner's Office to review the file. The obstetrician said that in her practice when it was known that the baby might have been exposed to the bacteria, the attending paediatrician would also administer antibiotics to the baby soon after delivery.

Risk of death reduced. Another expert witness (with whom the consultant obstetrician agreed) referred the court to research findings. Of pregnant mothers carrying the bacteria, half the babies will have the organism on their skin. Of these, two per cent will become infected or show signs of infection.

Of those, 15-30 per cent, depending on immaturity, will die. Intrapartum administration of antibiotics reduced the risk of death by 80 per cent.

Protocol. The consultant obstetrician had designed the protocol in relation to screening and prophylaxis for Group B streptococcus (GBS) at the public hospital. The protocol provided for a low vaginal swab to be taken at 28 weeks routinely and tested for bacteria. Where a patient in labour has an unknown status, a list of risk factors are identified which require an antibiotic (penicillin unless an allergy exists) to be administered. The list included pre-term labour of less than 34 weeks.

The findings

Chance of survival greater. The coroner found that had Eleanor been given penicillin after labour commenced, it was likely on a balance of probabilities that the baby would have survived. It was also likely that the paediatrician who had treated the baby would have given an intramuscular injection of penicillin soon after delivery had he known of the earlier results. The paediatrician agreed that the baby's chances of survival might have been 20 times greater.

Mother within risk category. The coroner found that the medical treatment had been highly professional. The mother had been correctly identified as coming within a risk category, a fact borne out by the results.

Records archived. As Eleanor was in a public hospital at the time of admission and discharge the test results, after being seen by a doctor, would have been filed with her medical records. These would have been archived. Had she remained a public patient, and delivery taken place at the hospital, it was 'extremely likely'[24] that antibiotics would have been given after labour commenced. This would have occurred in reliance on test results attached to the file. However, Eleanor had been accepted for private health care under her obstetrician's care.

The error. The coroner found the error had then occurred in two ways:

1. The positive results were not communicated to the obstetrician, even though medical staff at the hospital knew she was the private doctor managing Eleanor's pregnancy.

2. Given the practice of inserting laboratory results in a patient's file, the doctor who ordered the tests should have noted that the obstetrician was to be informed of these results (there was a space on the form to indicate to whom the results were to be sent). The court heard that 'shared caring' (where a private patient of a doctor is admitted as a public patient), is not unusual and happens frequently, particularly in the case of patients from outlying areas.[25]

Results to go to appropriate people. The coroner found it 'disappointing'[26] that since the tragic outcome of the case, it appeared no policy had been introduced at the hospital to ensure that this would not happen again. The coroner commented:

If indeed, as suggested by Eleanor's evidence, she was given a discharge summary to take to the doctor, I do not consider that this relieves the hospital of responsibility in the sense that it might be argued that it was the obstetrician's sole responsibility to chase the results. When positive results of this nature are uncovered, I consider that it behoves the staff in possession of these to ensure that they find their way in the most efficient manner to the appropriate person, in order that their former patients get the benefit of them. [27]

Prophylactic measures. The coroner considered that it was highly likely that if the obstetrician had received the abnormal results, she would have taken prophylactic measures. This would have changed the outcome for the baby. There was consequently a direct link between the hospital's conduct and the baby's death.

Swabs not routine at 35 weeks. By the same reasoning, had the obstetrician been aware of the results, she would have administered appropriate antibiotic therapy at the commencement of labour. She had explained it would not be routine at 35 weeks to order swabs and she had no basis for suspecting the presence of bacteria, as no recognised risk factors were identified at the time of the induction. Multiple gestation was mentioned in the public hospital's protocol as a risk factor, but the obstetrician said that in isolation she did not recognise it as such. The paediatrician had agreed.

The coroner found that on the basis of direct factual, causal links, the obstetrician had also contributed to the baby's death.

Comments and recommendations

The following comments and recommendations were made to hospitals, pathology laboratories and medical practitioners to ensure that test results reach all relevant parties.

1. Introduce or encourage a culture in which the doctor ordering the tests, the laboratory performing them and any doctor who has an interest in the results must assume a joint responsibility to ensure the results reach the appropriate people.
2. The doctor ordering the tests should identify all people who have any interest in learning the results. These names should be noted on the request form. Those people should be notified by that doctor that the tests have been ordered.
3. The laboratory should disseminate the results to everyone noted on the request form. Abnormal results should be highlighted in some way. In some instances, a direct approach will need to be made to the doctor ordering the tests without the delay of waiting on the hard copy.
4. Doctors interested in the results will therefore have been told that the tests have been conducted. They should be responsible for informing themselves of the results. It should be no defence to argue that the laboratory did not initiate the communication of the results. Each person is jointly responsible for ensuring that the test results are known by all who need to know them, so that appropriate action can be taken.[28]

The last two cases, from the 1930s, raise issues that may resonate in contemporary settings. The first case poses this question: Does a hospital have a duty to warn patients and their doctors of a serious infection in the hospital prior to a patient's admission? A recent case of puerperal fever in Australia suggests that the infective agent in this case, though rare, can still pose a clinical risk.

Note why the court describes the risk as 'hidden.'

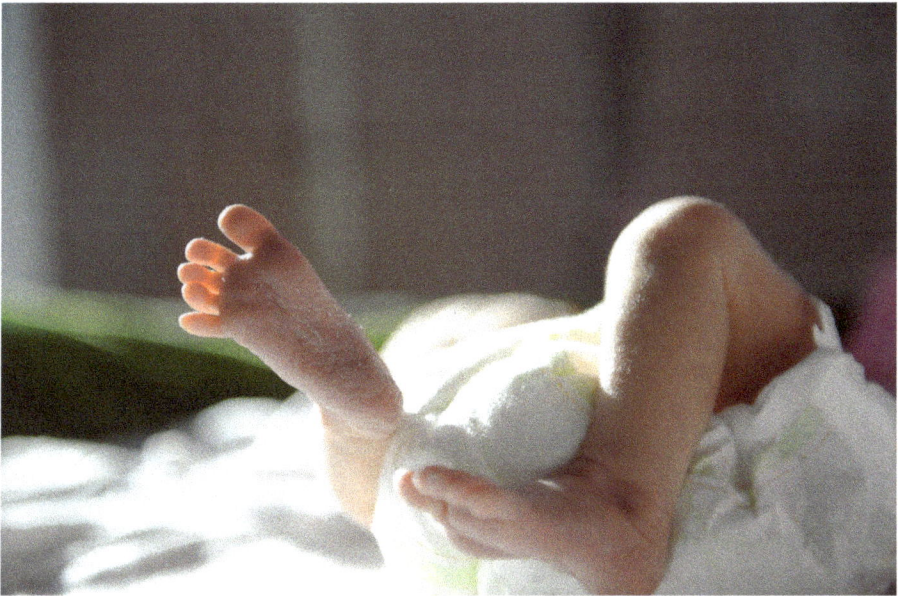

Lindsay County Council v Marshall [UK, 1936]²⁹

The facts

A county council in England provided a maternity home and midwifery staff which was administered by a committee advised by doctors. Patients engaged their own doctors. Beth, who was pregnant, booked a single room in January for an expected delivery in July.

On 30 June, another woman, Nora, was admitted to the maternity home. She delivered a baby on 1 July and developed a temperature of 100.4 F (38 C) on 4 July. When her temperature rose to 105 F (40.6 C) by evening, Nora was moved to the district hospital. Dr Black, who advised the maternity home, gave instructions for the disinfection and spraying of wards, clothes and linen. Staff took disinfectant baths and gargled with disinfectant. The midwife who had delivered Nora was put off duty for forty-eight hours; the ward Nora had been in was closed until 11 July.³⁰ These were usual precautions after a patient developed a high fever.

Staff not tested. At the second hospital, Nora was diagnosed with acute puerperal fever, 'a very dangerous and highly infectious disease.'[31] After the council at the maternity home was told by the hospital on 5 July that Nora was suffering from puerperal fever, a further disinfection took place. No swabs were taken from staff who had been in contact with Nora (who died at the hospital on 12 July), the view being that if there was a carrier present the disinfection process would have dealt with the problem. Dr Black considered it 'quite unnecessary' that the maternity home should be closed or any warnings given.[32]

Another high temperature. On 12 July, another patient, who had been admitted on 9 July and given birth shortly afterwards, had a high temperature. This was reported to Dr Black and again the usual disinfection precautions took place.

No information to patient or doctor. When Beth was admitted to the maternity home on 12 July, there was no single room available. She agreed to go into a ward on the understanding that she would be moved to a private room as soon as possible. Neither Beth, her husband nor her doctor, were given any information about either of the infection cases. Beth gave birth on 13 July. On 16 July, four other patients developed puerperal fever. On 17 July, Beth developed a fever and went on to suffer a very severe attack of the disease.

Negligence was alleged.

The trial

Admission should have been refused. The court found the maternity home should have refused admission to any patients after 5 July. Swabs should have been taken from all staff after it was known Nora was ill. Beth and her husband, as well as Beth's doctor, should have been told of the puerperal fever cases. The failure to take these measures was a breach of duty by the maternity home. Beth was awarded damages. The maternity home appealed.

The appeal
Duty to warn of hidden dangers

Both the Court of Appeal and the House of Lords upheld the jury verdict. The House of Lords acknowledged that there was no absolute warranty of safety, but that the maternity home did have a duty of care to make their premises reasonably safe for patients. This general duty of care to provide a safe environment included the duty to warn of any 'hidden danger'[33] of which the home was aware, or ought to have been aware.

Doctors should have been informed. The court's message was clear: doctors should have been informed of the infection, in order that to decide whether or not their patients should be admitted and, if they were admitted, what precautions against infection should be taken.

....

In the second of the 1930s cases, the patient alleges that the vaginal and rectal examinations she received without her consent constituted assault and battery. As such, this case could find a place in Chapter 2. But the circumstances of *Inderbitzen* (extreme even in a historical context) also contain two infection issues, rough examinations and the failure to wash hands. This may prompt discussion about the manner in which women were (and are) examined internally. Note the court's rejection of any need for expert evidence: the court could draw on its common sense.

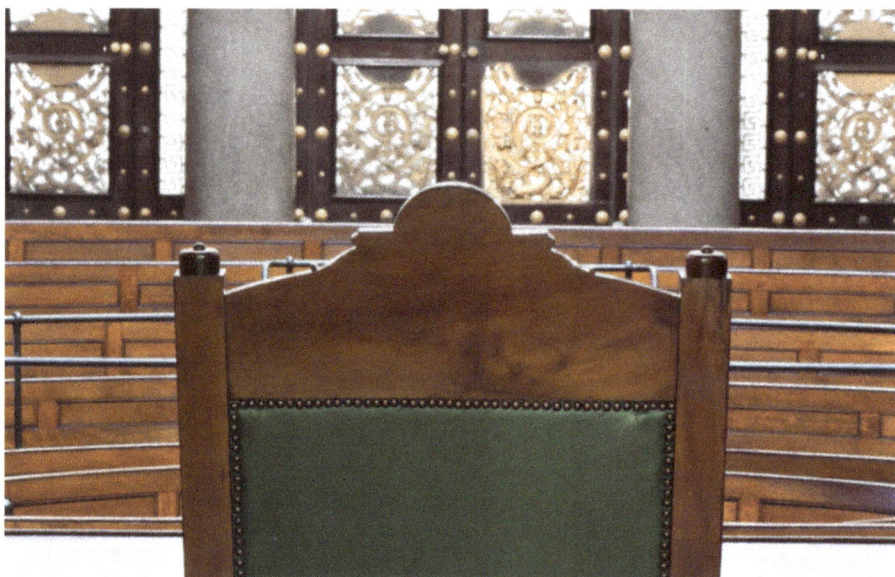

Inderbitizen v Lane Hospital [US, 1932][34]

The facts

Maisie was admitted to hospital for the delivery of her baby. She was examined by someone she presumed to be a medical student and demanded to be seen by a doctor. An older man then performed both vaginal and rectal examinations without washing his hands. The younger man examined her again without washing his hands. Maisie was taken to the delivery room 'where she was examined intimately two or three times by at least ten or twelve young men whom she took to be students.'[35]

Protests. Maisie said that the men had laughed, told her to shut up and repeatedly 'prodded and poked her' despite her protests and screams.[36] A doctor who examined her several months later found a torn uterus that was infected and profusely discharging.

The trial

The court rejected the hospital's argument that Maisie had failed to prove her treatment had been unnecessary and improper because she had not called expert evidence on that point. Instead, the court noted that 'common sense will tell any reasonable person that such treatment at the hands of so many is unnecessary and improper.'[37] Not only was scientific evidence not necessary to prove that point but the doctor and medical students had no more right 'to rudely and needlessly lay hands upon a patient against her will than has a layman.'[38]

This was an application by Maisie to proceed with a negligence action against the hospital and the court ruled that she could.

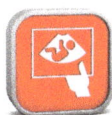

Discussion of Key Issues

In *Starkey,* the patient (pregnant, diabetic, vomiting and depressed) developed septicaemia and became deaf after being treated with gentamicin. Possible causes of the septicaemia were surgical infection when a Hickman catheter was inserted, postoperative infection as a result of some unidentified event or negligent handling of the catheter by a nurse.

The judge concluded that the most likely cause was a surgical infection (suggested by the neck wound), but that there had been no negligence. In a similar case, a different result could occur if hospital records revealed infection control standards had not been observed in the cleaning, disinfecting and sterilizing of instruments used during a patient's surgery. Records of these processes (packing, times, temperatures, etc.) tell their own story, as does the OR record.

The nursing care plan

As eight years had elapsed between wound care and the trial, many nurses understandably could not remember any details of their care. A nursing care plan became decisive.

The judge:

1. Accepted the plan as evidence that nurses had been *properly trained* in the use of aseptic technique,
2. drew an inference that the nurses had *followed* the plan and observed aseptic technique,
3. found the plan provided an adequate procedure and *protocol* for infection control and
4. found medical staff were *entitled* to rely upon the plan as reasonably assuring proper handling of the catheter by the nurses.
   - Although the nature of infection control and wound care may change, would your nursing care plans, as well as their implementation, stand up to similar scrutiny?
   - Do plans have input from appropriate staff; are they up to date and 'state of the art'?
   - How would you persuade a court what was 'state of the art'?
   - Is there time to read the plan ?
   - If you were asked in court whether you always read the care plan, what would you say? Why?

Progress notes and medication chart

Allegations by the patient and her parents of substandard infection control by the nurses were rejected by the court for a variety of reasons. Note in particular how the patient's allegations are rebutted by the documentation. Progress notes and the medication chart provided information of the patient's state of mind (major tranquiliser, drowsy, lethargic and non-communicative) and lead the judge to conclude her memory of events was unreliable.

....

Troxel and Hughes: The contraction of CMV, an infection described as 'generally harmless' to the general population, may have severe consequences for those with compromised immune systems, pregnant women and the newborn. In *Troxel,* the infection led to the baby's death; in *Hughes,* to a child's serious disability. The courts in both cases spelt out the duty to inform the patient/employee about the nature of a communicable disease and how to prevent its spread.

How do you inform patients/employees in your hospital?

....

Coronial investigation. Many women move between the public and private hospital systems. In this instance, the patient was admitted into a public hospital in premature labour for investigation of back pain, but delivered twins in a private hospital. Pathology results in the public hospital showed her positive to Group B streptococcus. These results were not transferred and one twin died after contracting the infection.

In your experience, can hospitals fail to transfer pathology results? If so:
- Are you aware when this has occurred?
- How/why has this occurred?
- Is an incident report made ?
- Is there follow up?
- In the absence of pathology results, what evidence would you put before a court to substantiate (a) giving a prophalactic dose or (b) adopting a 'wait and see' approach?
- Either way, do midwives and doctors hold different views? If so, discuss.
- Does your hospital have a policy to reflect responsibility to follow-up test results (pathology or otherwise)? By whom?
- Read the coroner's recommendations again. Have they been adopted where you work? If not, should they be?
- Could pathology results be *overlooked* where you work, for example, over a weekend? Discuss why/why not.

....

In *Lindsay,* a court found hospitals have a duty to warn doctors and their patients of the 'hidden dangers' of infection (of which they know or ought to know) in order that:

1. Doctors can decide whether to admit their patients (at all, or to specific areas) and,
2. if so, what precautions against infection should be taken.

Courts recognise that despite all care, there is always some risk of infection in hospitals. The court in *Lindsay* was concerned with the outbreak of a serious and specific infection.

- Choosing an infection, discuss this reasoning in relation to neonatal units.
- Discuss the risks of infection (and to whom) in situations where children are treated in adult wards and/or in proximity to midwifery units.

....

The patient in *Inderbitzen* did not consent to the repeated vaginal and rectal examinations she received. Assault and battery (for unauthorised touching) were proved.

In the early workshops I facilitated, some senior midwives recalled working in hospitals where women would be left in a cubicle, speculum inserted, for examination by 'numbers' of medical students.

- How is the dignity and privacy of women better protected today?

Damage in *Interbitzen* also arose from a tear in the uterus that became badly infected. Allegations were made that medical students (and possibly an older doctor) had examined the patient roughly and not washed their hands.

- Do some women still suffer unnecessary physical/emotional distress during internal examinations by trainee health professionals?
- Is there hospital direction on the role of the midwife in these situations?
- In your experience, is the protocol for hand washing always observed in your unit?
- Could you prove (a) your hospital has a protocol for hand washing and (b) how it is implemented?

NOTES

1.   On July 26, 1994 Justice Mandie delivered judgment in the Supreme Court of Victoria in *Starkey v Connell & Others*, No. 12477 (1990).
2.   p.3.

3. Ibid.
4. p.5.
5. p.6.
6. Ibid.
7. p.8.
8. p.9.
9. Ibid.
10. p.34.
11. p.22.
12. Ibid.
13. p.25.
14. p.23.
15. p.36.
16. p.60.
17. *Troxel v A1 Dupont Institute,* 6675 A.2d 314 (1996).
18. Ibid., p.321.
19. Ibid.
20. *Hughes v Sydney Day Nursery,* NSWCA 11 (2002).
21. *Record of Investigation into Death,* No. 903/96, State Coroner's Office, Victoria.
22. Ibid., p.2.
23. Ibid.
24. Ibid., p.4.
25. Ibid., p.5.
26. Ibid.
27. Ibid.
28. Ibid., p.6.
29. *Lindsay County Council v Marshall,* 2 All ER 1076 (1936); (1937), AC 97.
30. Ibid.
31. Ibid., p.102.
32. Ibid., p.110.
33. Ibid., p.107.
34. *Inderbitzen v Lane Hospital,* 124 Cal. App. 462, 12 P.2d 744 (1932), *reh. denied,* 124 Cal. App. 469, 13 P.2d 905 (1932).
35. Northrop, C.E. and Kelly, M., *Legal Issues in Nursing,* Mosby, p.169 (1987).
36. Ibid.
37. Ibid.
38. Ibid.

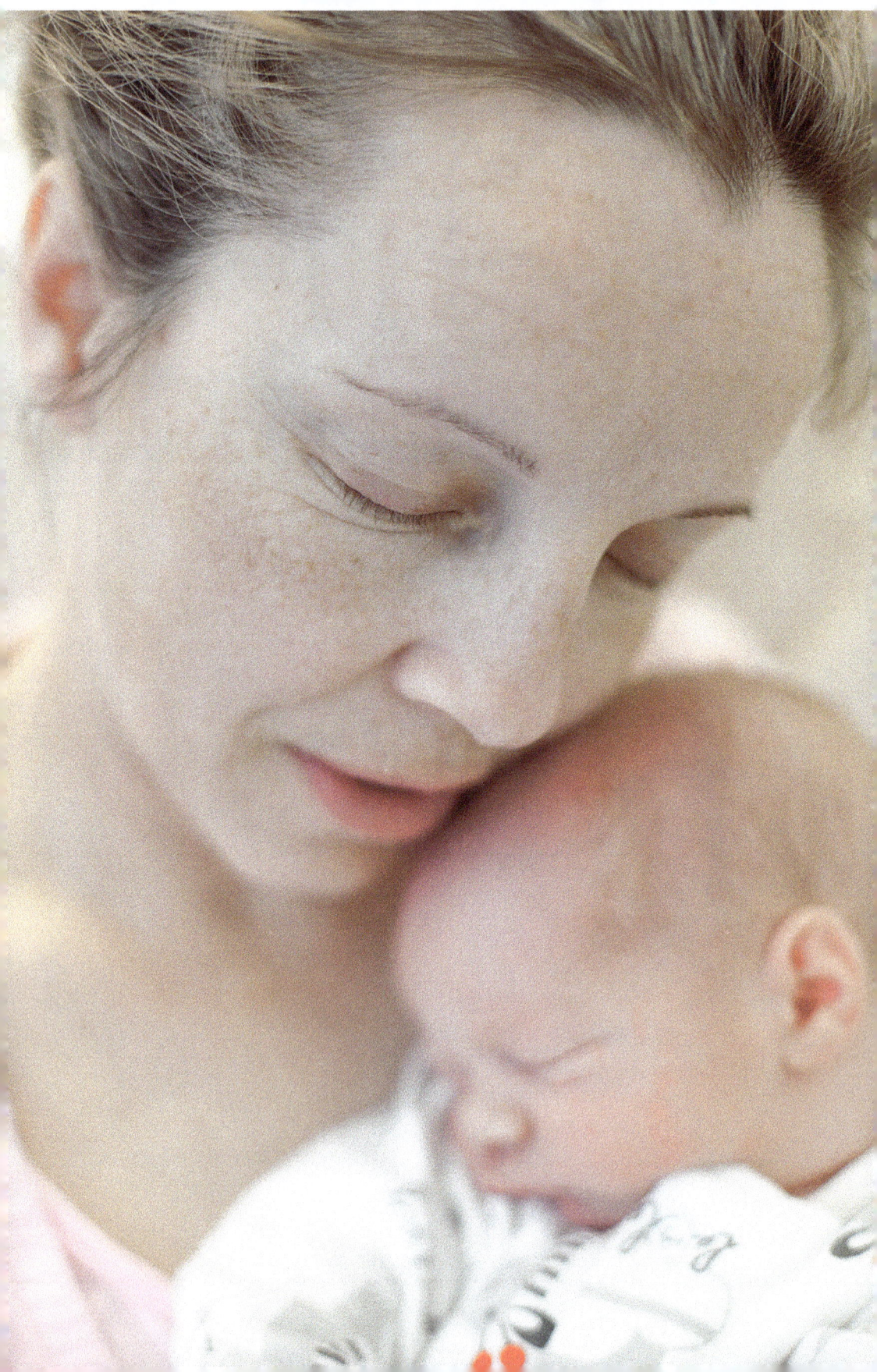

CHAPTER 10

Postpartum

'Two central questions emerged:

What was the probable cause of the postpartum bleeding?

Was the response to the bleeding adequate?'

— A coroner

Introduction

The cases in this chapter concern women who have suffered adverse out-comes in the postpartum period. The clinical issues (blood pressure, hae-morrhage, rupture of the diaphragm and pelvic fracture) contain warning signals for both doctors and midwives. The legal decisions provide a fertile field for the management of risk.

The first case is unusual in that it is an appeal from a coroner's decision *not* to hold an inquest. In a similar vein to Australian legislation, the Coroner's Act 1988 in England requires coroners to hold an inquest where there is reasonable cause to suspect that the deceased died an 'unnatural death.' In the case below, the coroner accepts that care at a private hospital in London 'appeared wholly inadequate,'[1] but concluded that the death was not contributed to by neglect and was therefore not unnatural. As you will see, two courts thought otherwise.

R v Inner London North Coroner, ex parte Touche [UK, 2001][2]

The facts

On 6 February 1999, Laura Touch delivered healthy twins at about 10.25 pm at a private hospital in London. The babies were born by caesarean section under spinal anaesthetic.

Headaches. Following delivery, Laura's BP was within normal limits at 120/60. At approximately 11.00 pm, she was transferred to the postnatal ward. She was complaining of headaches. The next note on BP was the following morning (7 February) at 1.35 am when it was recorded as 190/100. The headache was now severe and Laura clearly unwell. It was only at this stage that treatment began. BP recordings were taken regularly until normal limits were reached.

Hemiplegia. But damage had by now occurred. At 5.15 am on 7 February, Laura was diagnosed with a left-sided hemiplegia. At 6.15 am she was transferred to the Middlesex Hospital and from there to the National Hospital for

Neurology and Neurosurgery, where she died eight days later. The postmortem recorded brain swelling and tonsillar herniation (brain stem coning), as well as intra-cerebral haemorrhage.

Coroner informed. The coroner was informed by a doctor that Laura:

Gave birth to twins by caesarean on 6.2.99 at Portland Hospital. Collapsed three hours later. Admitted to National Hospital on 7.2.99. Examination indicated spontaneous brain haemorrhage unconnected with surgical procedure. No evidence of neglect nor complaints by family. No PM required.[3]

Not unsurprisingly the coroner did not consider an inquest appropriate. Laura was cremated.

Legal action. In July, Peter Touche sought an inquest into his wife's death. He referred the coroner to the two and a half hour period between 11 pm and 1.35 am when it appeared his wife had not been monitored.

In August, Peter Touche's solicitor wrote to the coroner complaining that a basic, fundamental failure to record blood pressure readings ...vitiated any opportunity to avoid the catastrophic events which led to Laura's death.'[4]

In September, the solicitor wrote saying that the private hospital had confirmed that it did not have a protocol to reflect the level of monitoring that should be given following a caesarean section. This was contrary to protocols in all NHS hospitals.

Lack of records. The solicitor also provided a report from a consultant anaesthetist (with a particular interest in obstetric anaesthesia) who was very critical of the lack of records relating to the period during and after surgery. The anaesthetist found the failure to monitor or record vital signs, including blood pressure, at a time when Laura was receiving pain relief 'astonishing.'[5] The level of neglect was described as 'starkly apparent.'[6]

The coroner also obtained a report from a doctor who said he had looked after countless numbers of pregnant and postpartum women who had blood pressure readings in the same range. None had ever had a stroke. This doctor described the death as 'extraordinary.'[7]

Substandard practice. In May 2000, the solicitor provided the coroner with a final medical report, this time from a doctor who ran a high-risk obstetric service. The report concluded that the failure to undertake BP readings during the postoperative period involved substandard practice and that Laura's severe hypertension was responsible for her cerebral haemorrhage. It was likely that more prompt identification and treatment of her hypertension would have prevented this haemorrhage.

Inquest refused. The coroner accepted that monitoring by the private hospital appeared wholly inadequate, but concluded that the defects complained of had not put the case into the category of 'unnatural death.' An inquest was therefore not required.

Peter Touche appealed.

The appeal

The High Court found the evidence provided clear grounds for suspecting that the hospital failed to monitor Laura's blood pressure as it should have done in the critical postoperative phase. This failure had been an effective cause of her death. Had she been monitored she would probably, or at least possibly, not have suffered the cerebral haemorrhage and died.

Neglect. On the material available, the coroner could have found reasonable cause to suspect that Laura Touche's death was at least contributed to by neglect and therefore 'unnatural.' The court concluded there were grounds for holding an inquest.

The coroner appealed the High Court decision, arguing that as he was entitled to decide that there was no reasonable cause to suspect that Laura Touche had died an unnatural death, it was not necessary to hold an inquest.

In upholding the High Court decision, the Court of Appeal made the point:

Where a death takes place in hospital and a failure to provide 'routine' treatment is a cause (even a secondary cause) of death, the coroner, for the purpose of deciding whether or not to hold an inquest, should conclude that the death may be unnatural and that an inquest should be held. The combination of the unexpectedness of the death, and the culpable human failing, are the factors which re-

sult in the death being considered as potentially unnatural ('should never have happened'; 'abnormal and unexpected') within the meaning of the Coroners Act 1988 (Eng).[8]

In a legal summary of the judgment an English lawyer commented:

Even if the court had decided that this was not an unnatural death in that sense, it would have held that these facts had the potential to be a 'neglect' case, where the evidence suggests that there may have been a gross failure to provide basic medical attention to a person in a dependent position, which may have caused or contributed to the death.[9]

In the next three cases, courts consider the causes of postpartum haemorrhage and whether responses to this emergency were adequate. In the first case, a medical witness questions whether women attempting vaginal delivery following a previous caesarean section should be assessed by a specialist before any decision is made, and then managed in hospitals capable of major surgery and resuscitation.

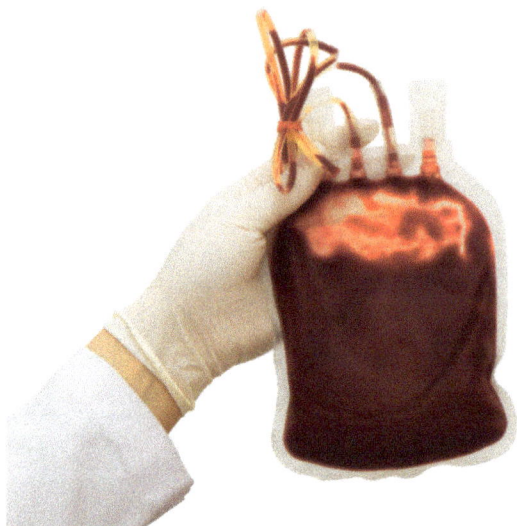

Coronial Investigation [Aus, 1994][10]

The facts

Louise, aged 24, was admitted to a rural hospital in 1991. She was under the management of Dr Atkins for a trial of labour with her second child. Her first baby had been delivered by caesarean section 12 months earlier. Despite Dr Atkin's misgivings, Louise was anxious to experience a vaginal birth with the second pregnancy.

Labour induced. Labour was induced on the afternoon of 19 December. Progress was slow. At 9.00 pm on 20 Dec, there were signs of disproportion. An emergency caesarean section was performed by Dr Atkins, assisted by Dr Cole, a GP credentialed as an anaesthetist at the hospital. As Louise would not consent to a general anaesthetic, she received a spinal anaesthetic block.

No abnormality. In the course of the caesarean section, Dr Atkins inadvertently incised the bladder, which was then sutured. At approximately 10.20 pm, a large female baby was delivered and the operation was completed by 10.50 pm. The last recorded blood pressure reading prior to Louise's return to the ward was 122/70 at 11.15 p.m. There was nothing to indicate any abnormality.

Blood loss. Then at 11.55 pm midwives noted that Louise was restless and confused for two minutes. A similar episode occurred at 12.05 am. Copious blood loss per vaginum was noted, accompanied by low blood pressure and a rapid pulse. Dr Atkins was notified. He immediately implemented uterine massage, plus a Syntocinon drip to contract the uterus. Dr Atkins called in Dr Masters, a GP, and later Dr Cole. Two lines of transfusion were commenced. Advice was sought from a maternity hospital and a mast suit applied.

Admission to ICU. At approximately 2.00 am, Dr Cole accompanied Louise to a large regional hospital, where she was found to be in a state of profound shock and too ill for surgery. There were no clinical signs of intra-abdominal bleeding. There was little sign of per vaginum blood loss, although blood pressure was extremely low. Louise was admitted to ICU in the hope that her condition could be stabilized sufficiently to enable a laparotomy and, if necessary, a hysterectomy to be undertaken.

Cardiac arrest. Between 5.30 am and 7.30 am, Louise was observed to have expanded abdominal girth suggestive of intra-abdominal bleeding. After discussion between an obstetrician and the senior ICU consultant, an emergency laparotomy and hysterectomy were performed at 7.45 am. The obstetrician was unable to locate any site of bleeding. A general surgeon was called in and performed a mid-line incision, with similar result. During surgery, Louise suffered many episodes of cardiac arrest requiring CPR and inotropic support. Approximately three litres of blood were found in the abdomen.

Louise remained unstable in ICU, suffering a profound episode of bradycardia at approximately 4.00 pm. Cardiac massage and resuscitation were abandoned after 30 minutes.

The inquest

Two central questions emerged:

- What was the probable cause of the postpartum bleeding?
- Was the response to the bleeding adequate?

The coroner believed there were two possibilities in relation to the bleeding :

1. It was caused by a failure of the uterus to remain contracted, so that blood was released into the large placental site (atonic uterus). In this context, the blood loss was so great it led to Louise developing Disseminated Intravascular Coagulation (D.I.C). This was the preferred view of the two obstetricians called as independent medical experts by Coronial Services to examine the case.
2. The second view was preferred by a pathologist who did not perform the autopsy but interpreted the autopsy report. This pathologist believed the source of bleeding was probably the caesarean section incision due either to incomplete suturing, or to suturing which subsequently broke down during the hysterectomy or between the caesarean section and the hysterectomy. This view was supported by the pathologist who had examined the uterus. Remnants of sutures along the right side of the incision were found and surrounding tissues were easily broken on handling. No one could say when the sutures had broken down. One expert said he was not convinced the wound had been mis-sutured.

The coroner said it was not possible to find which of these two scenarios had contributed to the blood loss, hypovolaemic shock, necrosis of the liver and kidneys and, ultimately, death.

Minimising the risk of atonic uterus. The coroner spent a good deal of time considering measures that might have been taken to minimize the risk of atonic uterus. One of the two medical experts believed the condition was more likely after prolonged labour, as had been the case. Both medical experts said it was their practice to administer Syntocinon by slow infusion after delivery, in addition to that administered immediately after removal of the placenta. Staff were instructed to regularly check to ensure the uterus was contracted.

Checking of uterus. Dr Atkins said it was not his practice to give Syntocinon after delivery other than 10 units at the time of the caesarean section. The coroner noted that it appeared that no instructions were given to check the uterus periodically, except to check for per vaginum blood loss, as well as general observation of the patient.

Syntocinon. One medical expert believed that it could not be said that administration of Syntocinon would necessarily have avoided the slackening of the uterus. It did not always work and postpartum haemorrhaging could still occur. The second medical expert was not prepared to say additional Syntocinon should always be administered by slow infusion. This was a matter of preference for the practitioner involved. There was no known ill effect from the drug.

Had the measures taken at both hospitals been adequate once blood loss had occurred? The coroner found Louise had received the best treatment available in the circumstances. With the benefit of hindsight, earlier transport to the larger hospital, or air transport to the city, may have led to a different result; it was not possible to speculate about this. It was at least as likely that the treatment she did receive could have led to a different result. Transport in the condition she was in immediately after midnight on 21 December would have been at least as risky as keeping her in the first hospital. The best efforts had been made at the first hospital, given the facilities and level of expertise available. Similarly, no criticism could be leveled at staff at the second hospital.

Assessments by specialist. One medical expert pointed out that, optimally, mothers attempting vaginal delivery following previous caesarean section should be assessed by a specialist before any decision is made. They should be managed in hospitals capable of major surgery and resuscitation. However, the coroner noted that Louise's husband described her as 'fanatical'[11] to have a vaginal delivery. She had wanted to see her baby born. The coroner did not find it clear that Louise's wishes had contributed to her death. According to expert medical evidence, the result could have been the same, even at a major hospital.

Unable to find what caused the postpartum bleeding, the coroner concluded that it was inappropriate to speculate whether anyone had contributed to the death.

....

The patient in the next case gave birth to twins by caesarean section. Following delivery, she developed a postpartum haemorrhage, later undergoing a subtotal hysterectomy. The patient had a very low haemoglobin level when she underwent surgery; cross-matched blood was not immediately available and she left theatre without a Syntocinon drip. Further blood tests were not organised, no routine palpation was made of the uterus and contingency plans for massive blood loss were breached. Questions before the court in this negligence action were the same as those considered by the coroner in the previous case: could the bleeding have been controlled, and, if so, how?

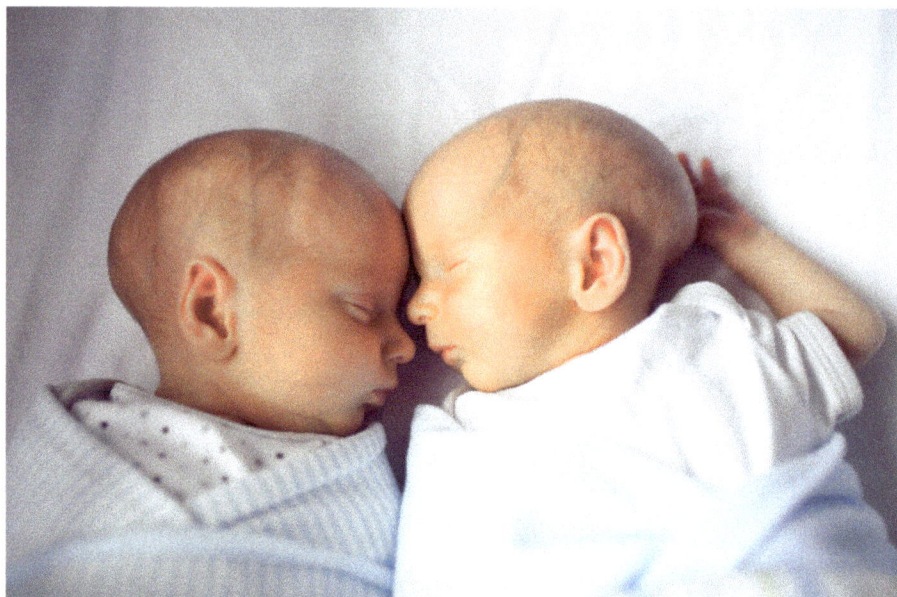

Le Page v Kingston and Richmond Health Authority [UK, 1997][12]

The facts

Christine, aged 22, was pregnant with twins, with 8 May being the estimated date of delivery. Because of concerns about the twins' development, she was admitted to hospital on 18 April. The membranes were artificially ruptured at 10.30 am on 30 April.

Possibility of surgical intervention. When labour had not progressed by midnight, the possibility of surgical intervention was noted by the doctor on duty. The senior registrar in obstetrics and gynaecology (the obstetrician) chose to wait. This decision fell within a broad range of competent obstetric judgment.

Exhaustion. At 12.40 am, the midwife recorded protein, blood and a very considerable presence of ketones in the patient's urine. This signified Christine was in need of fluid and approaching exhaustion. At 2.18 am, Christine complained of low back pain. A top-up dose of 8 mls of Marcane was administered.

Transfer to theatre. The obstetrician examined Christine some time after 3.00 am, then decided to proceed to a caesarean section. There was no record of a vaginal examination or of her transfer to theatre. Partogram and fetal heart records ceased at 3.30 am.

The anaesthetist started his anaesthetic sheet shortly after 3.30 am, recording administration of anaesthetic at about 3. 45 am.

Unavailibility of blood. Surgery was then delayed until 4.20 am due to the unavailability of cross-matched blood. The first twin was delivered at 4.32 am, the second at 4.34 am. Blood loss was estimated at 1250 ml, although originally recorded as 1350 ml. The court later heard that any quantity over 700-800 ml is excessive.

Records incomplete. Christine remained in theatre for longer than expected. While the operating record note by Dr H, the doctor on duty, did not record the time the operation concluded, the anaesthetic sheet suggested the patient left theatre at 5.15 am. The obstetrician later gave evidence that he observed a tendency for the uterus to fail to contract satisfactorily in theatre. There was no reference to this in the OR record.

Midwifery observations. Christine, in poor condition, was returned to the labour ward for close observation. Midwifery records began at 5.15 am. Gelofusin, a plasma expander, was being infused on return from the OR. The midwife noted that blood was available.

Blood loss and relaxing uterus. The obstetrician and the anaesthetist had written orders for 3 units of packed cell blood, plus an infusion of normal saline. Christine's BP at 85/ 40 was low.

Transfusions. The first unit of blood commenced transfusing at 5.30 am. BP fell to such an extent that the diastolic reading was unattainable. The transfusion was completed by 5.45 am; the second transfusion began.

Concern. The obstetrician, concerned at Christine's condition, remained with her until 6.00 am. He then rested in an adjoining room, having instructed the midwife to observe the patient 'because of blood loss and relaxing uterus.'[13] The midwife assessed Christine to be stable at 6.00 am.

BP falls lower. At 6.15 am, transfusion of the third unit of packed blood cells, designed to run over one hour, was started. A minimal blood loss per vagina was noted. At 6.30 am, BP was 100/60. The midwife noted that the patient was feeling better, was more responsive and was still receiving oxygen. By 6.45 am, the effects of the epidural anaesthetic were wearing off and Christine was feeling pain. BP had fallen again, so that no diasystolic pressure was discernable. The midwife brought the markedly increased pulse rate to the attention of Dr H, the doctor on duty. At 6.55 am, BP was noted at 100/50. The obstetrician attended at 7.05 am.

Blood loss. The midwife reported a heavy loss of blood per vagina. The obstetrician's contemporary note confirmed 'still had a watery pv. blood loss.'[14] An infusion of IV Prostin E2, via a second line, was ordered to assist the contraction of the uterus and control postpartum bleeding.

No recording of third unit. The third unit of packed cells, prescribed at the conclusion of the operation, ought by this stage to have been completely transfused (transfusion rate of one hour and fall in BP would have accelerated the rate of transfusion). No step was taken to administer any further blood until 9.35 am. The time when the third unit of blood was completely transferred was not recorded.

Prostin commenced. According to differing reports, the infusion of Prostin was commenced at either 7.15 or 7.30 am. At 7.30 am, a new midwife came on duty. The obstetrician went home to prepare for his outpatients' clinic at 9.15, but remained contactable. At 7.45 am, the midwife recorded Christine's BP as 115/70, which was satisfactory, as was her pulse. The lochia, normal postpartum vaginal discharge, which in excessive quantity would be described as 'bleeding' or 'bloodloss', was recorded as 'now satisfactory.'[15] Omnopon was administered for pain at 7.55 am.

PV loss heavy. The next observation was by Dr A, another doctor undertaking a routine ward round at 8.30 am: 'Uterus not well contracted, PV loss heavy, to continue Prostin infusion.'[16]

A critical situation. By 9.00 am, BP had fallen to 90/60. No record of pulse. By 9.15 am, there was a further fall of BP to 60/30. The midwife recorded 'lochia very heavy.'[17] The bed was elevated and the doctor on-call contacted. Dr P arrived at 9.15 am to find Christine breathless, panting for air, very pale and with a pulse of 160. The uterus was palpable, 4-5 cm above the umbilicus and described as 'boggy.'[18]

Gelofusin was administered and the infusion rate of Prostin increased. Further supplies of blood were ordered. Dr P contacted the obstetrician and at 9.20 am injected Ergometrine intravenously.

Blood clot expelled. The obstetrician arrived at 9.45 am. He palpated the abdomen and the uterus, and rubbed up a contraction. This expelled a blood clot, together with about 500 ml of blood per vagina. Arrangements for transfer to ICU were made. By 9.50 am, the third unit of the blood previously ordered was being transfused.

BP unrecordable. Christine's temperature was now 41 degrees C, pulse 160, BP unrecordable. The urine passed was blood-stained and limited (20 ml in an hour). The uterus seemed well contracted and was just above the umbilicus. The same record concluded with the observation that the pulse was 180+; BP "/85 (the judge later found this more probably 85 systolic – diasystolic was unattainable). At 10.15 am, the Prostin infusion was stopped and normal saline started. At 11.00 am Christine was transferred to ICU.

ICU. The registrar who had administered the anaesthetic for the caesarean section was now actively involved in the management of the postpartum haemorrhage. Dr D recorded: 'Uterus contracting reasonably. Wound satisfactory. Haemorrhage settling.'

Assessment (1) Haemorrhagic shock; (2) Prostin reaction [19]

Tachycardia. At 2.10 pm, the obstetrician recorded :

Condition improving apart from tachycardia. Continuing to lose blood pv. On examination fundus above umbilicus – reasonably well contracted. Situation: ? Blood in uterus or pelvic haematoma. Further procedures will require general anaesthesia and this would appear to be undesirable in her present condition but could be reviewed.[20]

Blood loss into uterine cavity. A haematologist assessed blood on a provisional basis at 3.30 pm. At 3.40 pm, BP was 105/70. A number of doctors, including the obstetrician and the obstetric consultant, examined Christine at 4.50 pm. The obstetrician found the uterine fundus height suggested blood loss into the uterine cavity. He noted that the patient needed an examination under anaesthetic when fit to do so.

Collapse. Within 10 minutes Christine collapsed. BP at 5.00 pm not palpable or recordable. Pulse 185. Resuscitation. Transfer to the operating theatre was postponed.

The next record at 8.00 pm noted Christine had been stabilised. BP was now 140/90, pulse had fallen to 130. She had been transfused with a further six units of blood plus additional units of plasma and platelets.

Hysterectomy. At 9.30 pm, an examination under anaesthetic commenced. The obstetrician performed a laparotomy, finding the uterus equivalent to that of a 30–week pregnancy in size. 1.5 litres of blood was evacuated. This included old clot and some fresh bleeding. It was decided to proceed to a subtotal hysterectomy, conserving the ovaries.

The OR record included: 'Bleeding from placental site. Uterus brought out. Would not contract despite Syntocinon plus PGE 2 (Prostaglandin). Floppy.'[21]

Return to ICU. Christine remained very ill until 7 May. She was then returned to the maternity ward and discharged from hospital on 19 May.

Continuing problems. Christine continued to experience blood loss per vaginum, possibly due to the presence of a small amount of endometrial tissue following surgery. As she was reluctant to undergo surgical removal of the cervix, the bleeding was expected to continue to menopause, itself accelerated because of the hysterectomy. She also developed a psychiatric illness, becoming depressed and angry. Her marriage eventually broke down.

Negligence was alleged.

The trial

Very thin posterior wall. The defence attributed the cause of the uncontrolled bleeding, and hence the hysterectomy, to a highly unusual feature of the uterus. It was contended that the thickness of the posterior wall of the uterus was little more than the peritoneum. The peritoneum was described to the court as 'a membrane whose thickness could be equated to domestic cling film.'[22]

Visit by obstetrician. The court heard that the day after surgery, Christine had been visited in the ICU by the obstetrician, who had informed her about the hysterectomy. She had been on a ventilator overnight, had a laryngeal tube in place and could not speak. The obstetrician agreed under cross-examination that his patient was entitled to a prompt, sympathetic and truthful account of what had occurred.

Contrasting view. The explanation given to Christine contrasted with the histopatholical report that measured the posterior uterine wall at 2 cm, compared with an anterior wall of approximately 3 cm. This report concluded that it was a normal uterus and that the coagulation disorder was largely, if not entirely, due to multiple blood transfusions given after a significant delay and after a severe blood loss occurred.

Criticisms. Medical experts explained to the court that the probable cause of uncontrolled postpartum haemorrhage generally lies in the case management.

Criticisms of Christine's care included the following:

1. It was negligent, when she had so low a haemoglobin level, to embark on a caesarean section without having available appropriate supplies of cross-matched blood for transfusion. Blood should have been transfused at the outset of the operation.

   (The obstetrician contended that he was unaware of the unavailability of cross-matched blood, and also unaware that the patient had a low haemoglobin reading of 8.5 g/dl. Evidence was given that a normal haemoglobin level with a twin pregnancy is 10-11 g/dl. The obstetrician said if he had known of these factors, he would not have started the operation when he did).
2. Given the known risk factors for postpartum haemorrhage and, specifically, a uterus which was known to be poorly contracting after delivery, it was negligent not to set up a continuous infusion of an oxytocic drug such as Syntocinon in a prophylactic dose when the patient left theatre.
3. Despite the express requirement for close observation of the patient, it was negligent not to organise blood tests; these would have revealed a gross anaemia.
4. In addition to observing any loss of blood, it was vital to measure the pulse, as well as, and in preference to, the blood pressure.
5. There was no routine palpation of the uterus, which would have identified the existence of bleeding into the uterine cavity. It was vital to ensure that the uterus remained contracted. The midwife should have kept her hand on the abdomen, palpating the fundus of the uterus, which would have alerted her to any relaxation of the uterus. Her omis-

sion to note the fundal height or the general tone or appearance of the uterus was only explicable if she omitted to palpate the uterus. When palpation was undertaken, it was not difficult to achieve.

6. Postpartum haemorrhage is a fairly common occurrence and can almost always be adequately controlled by a combination of appropriate uterine massage and the administration of oxytocic drugs.

7. The obstetrician ought to have undertaken an internal examination at 7.05 am and recorded his findings.

8. The actions of Dr A, the doctor on duty at 8.30 am, were wholly inadequate.

9. Dr A should have either undertaken a vaginal examination, rubbed up a contraction, expelled such clot and blood as was retained within the uterus and then adjusted the infusion rate of the Prostin. Or, if she was in doubt, she should have summoned the obstetrician. She took no action. This was in breach of the department's contingency plans for massive blood loss. These orders had been developed by the obstetrician.

The judge found these criticisms had been established, and that on a balance of probabilities, the following matters had been proved :

1. Christine should have received a transfusion of appropriately cross-matched blood at, or about, the commencement of the caesarean section.

2. The delay in transfusing her for over an hour, coupled with the excessive blood loss at the time of delivery, further compromised and prejudiced the capacity of her already anaemic system to withstand a falling blood pressure. This drove her system into shock, further depressing the natural contractibility of the uterus.

3. Routine palpation of the fundus of the uterus while the patient was under observation in the side ward ought to have detected the presence of an accumulation of blood and clot in the uterus.

4. Had such an accumulation been detected, it was likely that a clinician would have rubbed up a contraction. This would have expelled the blood and clot within the uterus. As an order for Prostin had already been written up, an infusion would have been immediately organised.

5. Had these steps been taken in combination, it was probable that the intra-uterine haemorrhage would have been brought under control.

These matters were the direct cause of Christine's gradual deterioration into a condition in which the haemorrhage became ultimately uncontrollable. Hysterectomy was the necessary and inevitable conclusion.

Damages awarded.

....

In the third case, the failure to take a full blood count, group and hold and/ or cross-match prior to an emergency caesarean section was again an issue, as was the failure to check fundal height, this time in the recovery room. The coroner was critical of the health professionals for their tendency to compartmentalize perceived areas of responsibility and for their failure to apply a holistic approach to the patient's overall care and treatment.

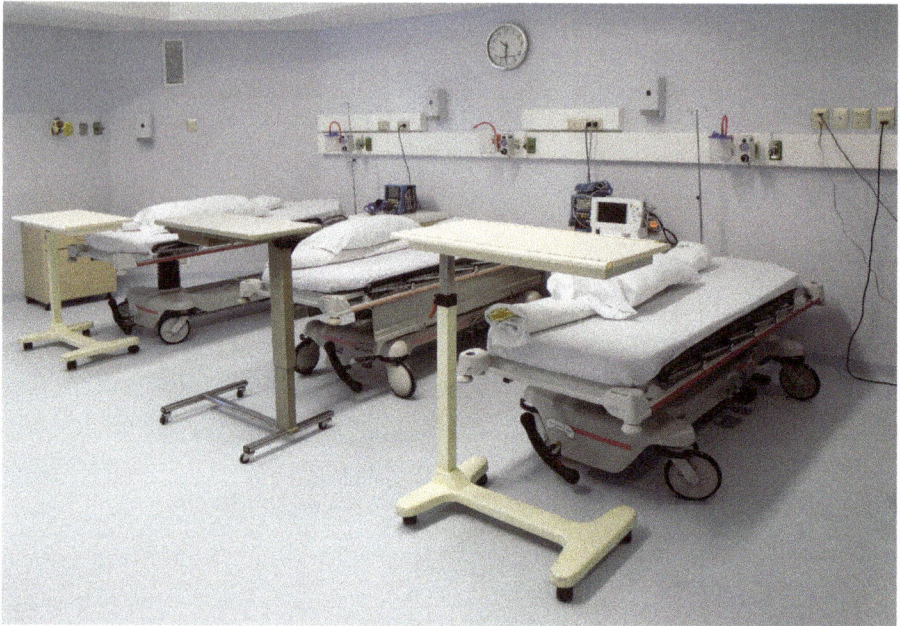

Coronial Investigation [Aus, 2009][23]

The facts

Rosalind, aged 29, was pregnant for the third time. During her first pregnancy it was known that she had low platelets (disc-shaped cell structures present in the blood which have several functions related to the arrest of bleeding). She had no history of postpartum haemorrhage and her first and second deliveries had been quite rapid. Antenatal care for the third pregnancy was shared between a major regional hospital and her GP. When it was confirmed that the baby presented by breech, Rosalind was referred to an obstetrician, who advised a caesarean section and noted her low platelets.

Admission to hospital. When her waters broke, Rosalind went to hospital, arriving between 4.30 and 5.00 am. After an assessment by a midwife, Rosalind was examined by Dr Rogers, a GP and VMO in obstetrics, and Dr Long, a locum obstetrician. It was decided to perform a caesarean section.

Staffing. On-call staff arrived between 5.30 and 6.00 am: anaesthetic nurse RN Taylor, scrub/instrument nurse RN Hall, scout nurse EN Fawkner and first-year anaesthetic registrar Dr Mitchell. The nurses had significant operating room experience.

Caesarean section. There was a discussion with Dr Long concerning Rosalind's preference for a vaginal delivery, then a spinal anaesthetic administered about 6.35 am. After fetal distress was noted, an emergency caesarean commenced at 7.01 am; eight minutes later a healthy baby girl was delivered. Following delivery, a small extension of the uterine incision on the left side was seen. The uterus was externalized, the tear repaired and the abdominal wall closed after a period of observation when Dr Long found no further bleeding.

Blood loss. The uterus, though initially slow to contract, was well contracted when returned to the abdomen. Dr Long ordered Syntocinon, of which 10 mls were initially given, followed by an infusion commenced at 7.20 am. The obstetrician 'generously' estimated one litre of blood loss (meeting the definition of severe postpartum haemorrhage) of which some 600 ml of blood (a usual loss during a caesarean) and fluids were collected in the suction bottle.

Postoperative instructions. Dr Long's postoperative instructions included Sytocinon to continue as charted, a left uterine tear repaired with haemostasis achieved and a 1 litre blood loss. She told Dr Simpson, a second GP obstetrician rostered on after Dr Rogers, about Rosalind's history of low platelets and asked him to perform a full blood count.

Recovery room. At 8.07 am, Rosalind was transferred to the recovery room, where she was the only patient. Nurse Taylor was the anaesthetic nurse in the operating room and had then (as was not unusual in rural hospitals) taken over duties in the recovery room. On handover, she was not told of the tear during the caesarean section or of the blood loss. Nurse Taylor obtained a copy of the operation report at about 8.15 am. Between 8.07 am and 8.36 am Rosalind's observations were fairly stable, although BP was low. This was communicated to the anaesthetist and the GP. Six sets of observations were recorded, but no fundal height was taken, nor any fundal massage performed.

Moderate ooze. At 8.15 am, a moderate ooze per vagina was recorded by nurse Taylor but not conveyed to any of the medical team. Between 8.15 am and 8.30 am, Rosalind was alert and talking to her husband, but at 8.36 am her BP dropped from the low 90s to 89/51. She was given 2 mg morphine, having received 1 mg 10 minutes earlier. At 8.41 am, there was little change in BP; pulse had risen from 74 to 79.

Dramatic change. At 8.46 am, Rosalind's pulse had risen to 94 and BP had dropped to 54/22. A large blood loss had soaked through two pads, blue sheets and bed linen. Nurse Taylor called EN Fawkner, who was in the operating room, for assistance in changing the pads and linen. This took about five minutes. Then, nurse Morgan, an experienced RN who was passing by and decided to call into the recovery room, came in as this process was being completed. Nurse Morgan observed the BP reading of 54/22 and obtained a further BP reading. (It was the coroner's view that this further BP reading was probably the 66/33 reading discussed below.) Nurse Morgan checked the fundal height, massaged the fundus, initiated 1000 ml of Hartmann's solution infusion, and momentarily ceased the Syntocinon infusion by attaching it to the Hartmann's solution in order for both fluids to be infused through the one cannula.

Telephone calls. Nurse Taylor telephoned anaesthetist Dr Mitchell and informed her of the BP of 66/33 and the blood clot passed. Dr Mitchell ordered a 500 ml bolus of Gelofusin IV.

EN Fawkner tried to locate obstetrician Dr Long, but she had left the hospital. A Dr Simpson, overhearing the telephone call, went to the recovery room to assist. Dr Simpson observed/was told the Syntocinon infusion had ceased. He inserted a second cannula, drew blood for a full blood count and to cross-match six units of blood, and took this to pathology. Consistent with hospital policy, there had been no blood taken for cross-matching or group and hold prior to the caesarean section.

Atonic uterus. Meanwhile, Dr Long, who had been contacted by telephone at 9.17 am, arrived at the hospital a few minutes later, at much the same time as anaesthetist Dr Mitchell. Dr Long instructed that the Syntocinon be re-started immediately, and diagnosed an atonic uterus. Large amounts of blood clots were expelled after uterine massage. Ergometrine and prostaglandin (to aid in uterine contractility) were administered sometime after 9.25 am, the prostaglandin being administered directly into the uterine wall. Neither drug was available in the operating room and had to be accessed from the maternity ward.

Surgery. After attempts were made to locate an experienced obstetrician, an experienced general surgeon arrived. At about 9.55 am (now one hour after the large blood loss was observed) the first unit of packed cells was commenced. At 10.00 am, Rosalind was transferred to the operating room for further surgery. A large blood clot was evacuated and her uterus found to be large and atonic. No obvious bleeding point was noted. Dr Long then performed an abdominal hysterectomy. About 14 units of packed cells were administered during and after the procedure, together with 10 units of fresh frozen plasma. A unit of platelets, which had arrived from another hospital, was transfused at about 12.30 pm.

Cardiac arrest. Rosalind had a cardiac arrest on the operating table and was resuscitated. She was then transferred to a metropolitan hospital, but died in ICU the following day.

The inquest

The coroner identified seven issues, the first five described as main issues:

1. Standard of obstetric services at the hospital

The hospital delivered between 500 to 600 babies each year, 25 per cent being deliveries by caesarean section. There was no evidence to suggest the standard of obstetric care was inferior to that of other regional hospitals. There was also little doubt that the same degree of expertise and access to highly skilled clinicians, midwives and nurses was more available and accessible in larger metropolitan hospitals. Invariably logistics and funding were factors in rural hospitals in terms of available care.

A fundamental difference. Unlike some larger metropolitan hospitals, the hospital had a policy of not undertaking a full blood count, group and hold, and/or cross-match prior to the operative procedure. Locum obstetrician Dr Long, who was not aware of hospital policy, stated it was her normal practice to order a full blood count, group and hold, and crossmatch. She had only become aware during the caesarean section that it had not been done. Expert witnesses agreed that group and hold/or cross match should be taken for an emergency caesarean section.

Benefit of hindsight. The coroner found that had a full blood count and group and hold been taken, even without cross-matching, blood transfusions could have been administered at an earlier time. This may have resulted in a different outcome for Rosalind.

2. Protocols for ordering a full blood count, group and/or cross-match

The coroner recommended the institution of a policy of ordering a full blood count and group and hold in regard to elective and emergency caesarean sections at the hospital, questioning why that policy should not extend state-wide.

3. Handover procedures from OR to Recovery

While opinions differed as to whether estimated blood loss in the operating room was lower due to its being mixed with liquor, there was little doubt that within the hospital guidelines Rosalind had suffered a postpartum haemorrhage during surgery.

Critical time. The period from when Rosalind left the operating room until her BP was noted to drop to 54/22 at 8.46 am in the recovery room was critical. While Dr Long had successfully repaired the tear, conducted a fundal massage and checked that bleeding had stopped, the internal bleeding most likely commenced within a very short time after Rosalind was received into the recovery room.

Dual role. Nurse Taylor (the anaesthetic nurse in the operating room, who was also the receiving nurse in the recovery room) said that when she was in the operating room she had not been aware of the blood loss or specifically recalled the repair of the uterine tear. Neither detail had been communicated to her at handover.

Assumption

The coroner found that there was an assumption by medical staff that nurse Taylor was experienced and trained in all facets of postoperative care following a postpartum haemorrhage. However, she had never previously experienced a postpartum haemorrhage; was unaware of the hospital protocol for that condition; and had not been trained in recognizing symptoms of haemorrhage, checking fundal height or performing a fundal massage that would cause the uterus to contract. She had not read the operating report in its entirety and was unaware of the estimated blood loss of 1 litre and the uterine repair. Nurse Taylor understood her responsibility was to monitor vital signs, set up the Syntocinon infusion and provide pain relief.

Verbal handover. Anaesthetist Dr Mitchell's verbal handover to nurse Taylor was limited to ensuring that Syntocinon was administered and BP checked. There were no clear instructions as to why BP and pulse needed to be checked carefully in the light of the known blood loss and the uterine tear. Dr Long, who had not given a verbal handover but had completed the operation report, said that had she known that nurse Taylor had no experience in nursing a postpartum haemorrhage patient, she would, as the surgeon responsible for Rosalind, have attended to her.

Other staff available. The coroner concluded that had a full and proper handover been given (including the need to check fundal height) it may have been ascertained at an early stage that nurse Taylor was not trained nor experienced in the area. Other staff were available to come to the recovery room.

4. Level of training and experience of nurses caring for obstetric patients in recovery

Employment history. Nurse Taylor's employment history over approximately 13 years indicated only limited exposure to duties in the recovery and postnatal areas. It was unreasonable to expect her to properly identify and adequately deal with a medical situation for which she had not been properly trained. Had she been informed of the loss of blood or been aware of the hospital's postpartum haemorrhage guidelines she may have been more acutely aware of the need to closely monitor vital signs. The moderate ooze she recorded at 8.15 am may have resulted in her contacting medical staff straight away had she been told of the blood loss in theatre.

Hospital responsibility. The coroner maintained that the responsibility to ensure appropriately skilled staff are available to deal with patient care rests squarely on the shoulders of hospital administrators. Hospital administrators have the responsibility to ensure that rostered staff possess the skills and training to identify and deal with a particular crisis. Nurse Morgan, for example, who had 'popped in'[24] while passing the recovery room, was a very experienced nurse who had recognized and responded to the crisis. A staff member with these skills should at least be able to identify a particular crisis and seek assistance.

5. Policies in regard to identifying and treating patients with postpartum haemorrhage

Appropriate hospital guidelines are of little significance if not known or understood by staff. They must be accompanied by appropriate training, especially in country regions where nurses may be infrequently rostered in particular areas. Some staff did not know of existing guidelines.

6. Availability of certain drugs

The drugs Misoprotol (highly effective as a contracting agent) and No-voseven (with coagulating properties) were not available at the hospital but available at certain other rural hospitals. The coroner found these drugs may have assisted in Rosalind's recovery. While it would be highly desirable to have immediate access to the full range of appropriate drugs at all hospitals, the coroner said he was not sufficiently informed to make formal recommendations. But he suggested that the Director General of Health should review and formulate a policy as to the minimum requirement for hospitals to stock a particular drug or range of drugs, having regard to availability, demand and shelf life.

7. Documentation

The inquest had suffered in not being able to determine with precision what actually took place at certain times, for example:

1. Time that elapsed between 8.46 am, when nurse Morgan detected an emerging medical crisis, and 9.17 am, when she called Dr Long was over 30 minutes. While the progress notes recorded the observations made by Dr Simpson following his examination of Rosalind, there was no specific time when he attended other than the date on the pro forma document, which prompted recording of dates and times. Similarly, it was difficult to determine when certain medical staff arrived or left the recovery room or the OR.

2. It was known that the Syntocinon drip was in place when Rosalind arrived in the recovery room, but there was conflicting evidence as to when it was turned off and re-commenced. Since there were no notations in the nursing notes or medication charts as to when the Syntocinon drip was turned off or back on, the coroner had been unable to determine for what period she was without a drug that was effective in assisting uterine contraction

3. Hospital administrators were reminded that coroners had commented on these matters in the past. There was a need to reinforce to all medical staff the need to make accurate and timely notes. When critical incidents occur, there should be an appreciation that a root cause analysis, if not a coronial inquest, may take place. Staff should be instructed to make detailed notes, even if these are made retrospectively. Nurse Morgan was commended for having written vital observations on her uniform and then completed a detailed note later while her memory was fresh.

Findings

Three factors in particular contributed to Rosalind's preventable death:

1. *The failure to take a full blood count, group and hold, and/or cross-match prior to an emergency caesarean section.* This failure was due to hospital policy and a belief by the locum obstetrician that it would be routinely done. Had these measures been taken, Rosalind would have received blood transfusions at an earlier time and her death would have been prevented.

2. *The failure to provide nursing care for a woman who had suffered a postpartum haemorrhage.* Allocated staff had no experience in identifying a continuing postpartum bleed or had not understood the significance of fundal height; nor had they been trained or skilled in massaging the fundus in order to achieve contraction of the uterus.

3. *The failure of all health professionals to apply a holistic approach to Rosalind's overall care and treatment.* There was too great a willingness between the disciplines to compartmentalize their perceived area of responsibility. Rosalind appeared to have fallen into a gap between the various medical and nursing roles. There had been a failure to identify individual or collective responsibility for the primary task of providing appropriate care and treatment from admission to discharge.

The individual failures of nursing and medical staff were more of a systemic nature.

Recommendations

The implementation of a uniform policy (in all NSW hospitals) that a full blood count and group and hold be undertaken for all elective and emergency caesarean sections.

....

The last two cases identify the risk of failing to properly investigate complaints of pain in the postpartum period. In the first case the patient is complaining of chest pain.

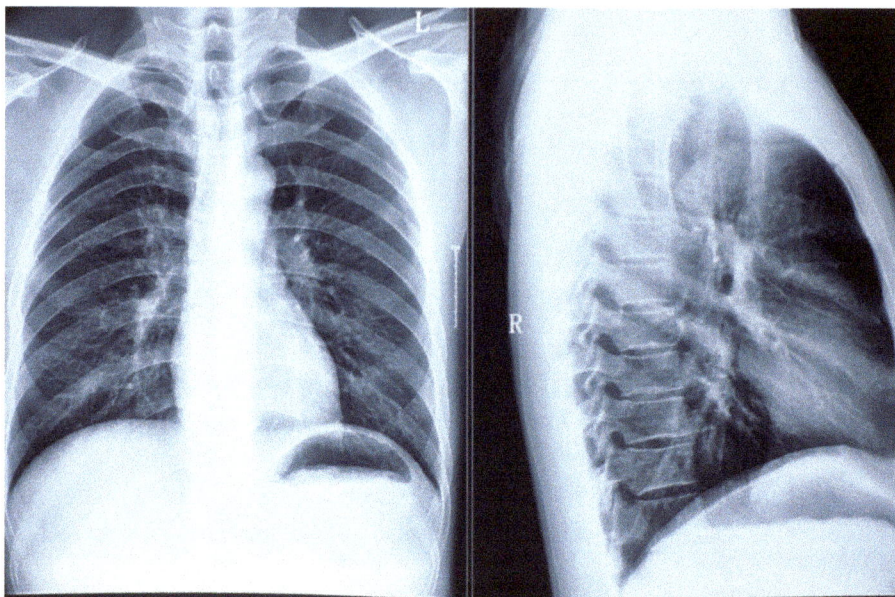

Gregorie v Spencer [Can, 1991][25]

The facts

Late in her pregnancy, Elsa complained of abdominal pain and blood in the urine. After an examination, the GP referred her to an obstetrician, who found nothing seriously wrong. The symptoms stopped.

Pain and nausea. The day after a difficult delivery, Elsa complained of pain in the upper left quadrant. The doctor found no abnormality, but after he left the hospital Elsa continued to complain of severe pain and nausea. An on-call doctor prescribed an anti-nausea drug. Some time later a midwife telephoned Elsa's doctor. Further medication was ordered over the phone, and a chest X-ray ordered for the following day. Soon after, Elsa suffered a cardiac arrest.

Diaphragm rupture. An X-ray showed that the diaphragm had ruptured and that the abdominal contents were in the chest cavity. Elsa was rushed to theatre for emergency surgery but did not survive.

The decision

The court found the doctor negligent in failing to examine his patient. This would have led to an earlier X-ray, diagnosis of the torn diaphragm and potentially life-saving surgery.

Damages awarded.

....

In the second case, the patient complained of severe pelvic pain and discomfort in the postpartum period. The hospital's physiotherapist believed the symphysis pubis had separated, but no immediate X-rays were taken. In fact, the pelvis had been fractured during childbirth and remained undiagnosed for six month after the birth. The patient alleged negligence against her GP and the hospital.

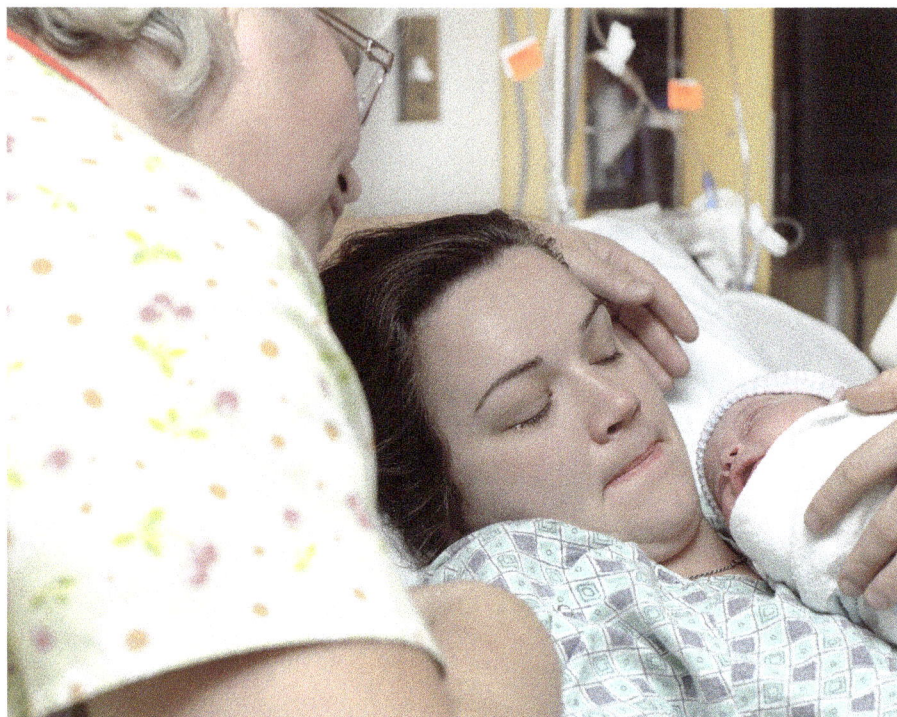

Eagle & Anor v Prosser [Aus, 1999][26]

The facts

When Lucy consulted her GP during her second pregnancy, in January 1988, the baby was found to be unusually large. In February, a sharp pain in the abdomen was diagnosed as a hernia. Lucy expressed concern on a number of occasions that as this was likely to interfere with the birth, she would prefer to have a caesarean section.

Violent contraction. Labour began spontaneously on 11 September. Before the baby's head was delivered, Lucy felt a violent contraction, and reported both hearing and feeling 'popping, snapping and tearing'[27] inside her. The baby's head was delivered, but the shoulders became stuck. The GP then rotated the shoulders, enabling the baby to be born.

Pelvic pain. Following the birth, Lucy experienced pain in the whole pelvic area, with grinding in the area of the symphysis pubis. The pain was so severe she could not mobilise. The GP said that she could expect to be sore after giving birth to a big baby.

Physiotherapist. The hospital's physiotherapist believed that given the nature of the birth and the big baby, the symphysis had separated. Lucy was discharged home five days later, but still felt unwell.

Vaginal haematoma. The GP diagnosed a haematoma between the vagina and the rectum. Antibiotics were prescribed and the haematoma was surgically removed one week after the birth. Lucy asked the GP to take X-rays of the lower spine and pelvis, but was told they were not necessary. A further evacuation of a vaginal haematoma was carried out by an obstetrician, who prescribed Pethidine for the pain.

Further surgical procedures. Lucy had a long history of constipation. Further, a sexual assault fifteen years earlier had included anal penetration. (The GP denied being told this.) During December, she was admitted to hospital for several surgical procedures, including anal stretch, sigmoidoscopy and haemorrhoidectomy. Loss of bowel function and pelvic pain continued.

X-rays. In February 1989, Lucy and her family moved interstate. She consulted a gastroenterologist and X-rays of the chest and pelvis were taken. The report noted :

Disalignment at the symphysis pubis with the left pubic bone being 2 or 3 mm higher than the right. There is also a little erosion of the left side of the symphysis and widening and evidence of erosion of the left sacro-iliac joint. The appearances would be consistent with trauma to the left sacro-iliac joint and to the symphysis pubis.[28]

Instability of pelvic rig. An orthopaedic surgeon reported that the orthopaedic problems were related to the antenatal period and delivery. This surgeon referred Lucy to a second orthopaedic surgeon, who ordered stress X-rays and a bone scan. These tests confirmed the instability of the pelvic rig at the symphysis pubis and the sacro-iliac joint. Both surgeons agreed surgery was necessary to stabilise the pelvis. In September, contoured plates were inserted and the symphysis pubis was internally fixed with a compression plate and screws.

Further pelvic pain. In December, Lucy saw the second of the orthopaedic surgeons again. She complained of discomfort in her right groin and pain
in her right proximal thigh and leg. Stress X-rays showed no movement of
the symphysis pubis. Pelvic pain continued through the first half of 1990.
During surgery in June to remove the pubic plates and screws, an inadvertent cystostomy (entry into the bladder) occurred due to the presence of scar
tissue. The tear was repaired and a suprapubic catheter, and later a urethral
catheter, inserted. Lucy was discharged in mid-July. By this stage she was
passing urine without difficulty.

Lucy was then referred to an obstetrician/gynaecologist in November
1991, by which time she was experiencing difficulty in passing urine and also
suffering from constipation.

Cystoscopy. This specialist referred her to a urologist for an opinion as
to whether hysterectomy would relieve her discomfort. A cystoscopy and an
ultrasound of the lower urinary tract were performed. By December 1991, a
cystocoele and a rectocoele had developed.

Hysterectomy. A hysterectomy was performed in January 1992, the urologist performing a bladder elevation at the same time. (According to a medical expert witness, this surgery may not have been indicated in the absence
of urodynamic evidence of genuine stress incontinence.)

In July 1992, a surgeon specialising in gastroenterology repaired the rectocoele. Lucy continued to experience problems with her unstable symphysis
pubis, urinary incontinence, and general pain and discomfort for the next
year.

Colostomy. In 1994, a colorectal surgeon diagnosed a rectocoele and a
fistula-in-ano. In July 1995, Lucy was admitted to hospital for a colostomy
to deal with her chronic constipation. In September 1995, the urologist reviewed her continuing problems, noting pain when any pressure was exerted
on the symphysis, even when walking.

Lucy alleged negligence against her GP and the area health service.

The trial

Expert medical evidence for the patient:

Obstetric opinion. If a caesarean section had been performed at 37
weeks, Lucy would not have had the severe diastasis of her symphysis and no

significant rupture of the anterior left sacro-iliac joint. Even if the diastasis was not diagnosed in the immediate postnatal period, it should have been diagnosed at the six-week postnatal check-up.

Gastroenterology. The court heard that pelvic disruption during a vaginal delivery and nerve damage to the pelvic floor muscles during prolonged and difficult deliveries was well documented. In the gastroenterologist's opinion, it was more probable than not that the patient's continuing bowel symptoms related to the pelvic disruption at the time of delivery and in the postpartum period.

Expert medical evidence for the defendants:

Gynaecology. A gynaecologist said the urodynamic study conducted in September 1995 revealed a pelvic plexus injury which was almost certainly caused by surgery and not by childbirth. Neither the pelvic haematoma's development nor its drainage would have caused a pelvic plexus injury. The specialist found that incontinence in women is very common and has many causes. The diagnosis made in 1991 of genuine stress incontinence could not be made without a urodynamic study, which was not conducted at the time. Even if that diagnosis was correct, childbirth was not a specific cause of genuine stress incontinence. The bladder injury occurring during surgery had been immediately repaired. In the gynaecologist's opinion, such injury does not cause incontinence and an anterior bladder tear does not cause pelvic plexus injury.

The decision

The trial judge preferred the expert evidence that the injuries were the result of childbirth. The GP had been in error when she informed Lucy that a caesarean section was not an option. Lucy would not have sustained the injuries had there not been this breach of duty. The GP should have referred Lucy for a caesarean section when she had requested one. The GP appealed.

The appeal

The central issues at appeal were (a) the GP's alleged negligence for failing to deliver the baby by caesarean section and (b) the meaning the judge attached to the GP's statement that a caesarean section 'was not an option.'[29]

Differences in medical opinion. On the first issue, the court found that the trial judge had relied on written reports from the expert witnesses and found they proved that the caesarean section was an option which should have been pursued. The court found these reports had then been substantially qualified under cross-examination when the doctors gave oral evidence in court. Expert evidence had in fact illustrated that there were medically legitimate differences of opinion about whether the GP should have arranged to have a caesarean section performed or should have referred the patient to a gynaecologist for advice.

Non-interventionist practice. In the court's opinion, the GP's treatment and discussion with Lucy constituted an acceptable 'non-interventionist practice.'[30] While other doctors may have opted for the caesarean section, the evidence did not suggest that a doctor who disagreed with such treatment was unprofessional. Considering the evidence as a whole, there was insufficient evidence to support the trial judge's finding that the GP had been in breach of her duty.

Caesarean preferable. On the second issue, the court found that the trial judge had understood the words 'it is not an option'[31] to imply that under no circumstances could the patient have had a caesarean section. The appeal court considered the words to imply that it was not practical to consider an elective caesarean when Lucy could have gone into labour at any time. The words should have been considered in the light of all the circumstances of that particular consultation. The possibility of a caesarean section was raised in the context of that procedure being preferable to an induced birth. Lucy wanted a caesarean section in order to avoid being induced, but went into labour spontaneously. The GP's advice did not relate to the events during and after labour. For these reasons, the GP had not breached her duty of care to the patient.

Insufficient evidence to act on physiotherapist's report. However, Lucy had also alleged negligence against the hospital. The trial judge found the GP and hospital negligent for failing to act on the physiotherapist's report of diastasis of the symphysis pubis and for not reporting it. The appeal court held there was insufficient evidence on which the judge could have reached this conclusion. A new trial was ordered to decide whether there were any breaches of duty by the GP or hospital in the care and treatment of the patient from the period of birth to the time of the postnatal check.

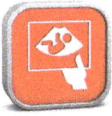

Discussion of Key Issues

In *Touche,* postoperative monitoring by a private hospital was described as 'wholly inadequate.'[32] BP readings were not taken regularly, despite the fact the patient was complaining of headaches following delivery of twins by caesarean section.

Midwives who attended workshops I have facilitated reported that on rare occasions a patient has suddenly and unexpectedly died in the postpartum period. Documentation of how the patient was monitored will become critical evidence in any investigation. In this case, the private hospital did not have a protocol to reflect the level of monitoring required following a caesarean section.

- Would your protocols provide such evidence to a court?

....

Coronial investigation. (1) An inquiry into a maternal death following a postpartum haemorrhage will investigate the most likely cause of the bleed and whether response to it was adequate. In this case, a coroner was unable to determine the cause, finding the patient had received the best care available at both hospitals.

Two doctors told the court it would be their practice to instruct staff to regularly check that the uterus was contracted. The coroner found that it appeared no instructions were given to check the uterus regularly, except to check for per vaginum blood loss, as well as general observation of the patient.

- What would you inform a court was usual practice in your unit ?

One doctor told the court that, optimally, mothers attempting vaginal delivery following previous caesarean section should be assessed by a specialist and managed in a hospital capable of major surgery and resuscitation. The patient in this case was described by her husband as 'fanatical'[33] to have a vaginal delivery and see her baby born.

- How would you advise a patient in similar circumstances?

....

Page: In this second example of postpartum haemorrhage, the focus of inquiry was again whether, and how, the bleeding could have been controlled. The court heard expert medical evidence that uncontrolled postpartum haemorrhage generally lies in the case management.

Discuss whether any of the following events could occur where you work?

a) A caesarean section was embarked upon when the patient had a low haemoglobin level and appropriate supplies of cross-matched blood were not available.

b) The uterus was known to be poorly contracting after delivery, but the patient was not receiving a continuous infusion of an oxytocic drug (such as Syntocinon) when she left the OR.

c) Despite the express requirement for close observation of the patient, blood tests were not organised or progressed.

d) In addition to observing blood loss, the pulse was not measured, as well as, and in preference to, the blood pressure.

e) There was no routine palpation of the uterus to ensure it remained contracted. This remains a contentious issue. Note that in this case the court accepted evidence that the midwife should have kept her hand on the abdomen, palpating the fundus of the uterus. Her omission to document the fundal height or the general tone of the uterus led to the inference she had not done so.

f) Would you agree with the view that postpartum haemorrhage is fairly common and can 'almost always' be controlled by appropriate uterine massage and oxytocic drugs?

g) Evidence of times was critical to the story of this patient' s care. When specific times were lacking (for example, when the patient went to theatre), the court had to infer a time.

h) Blood loss in theatre is vital to later midwifery care. 1250 ml was estimated, originally recorded as 1350 ml. The court heard evidence that anything over 700-800 ml is excessive. In what way, if any, do such estimations cause you concern?

....

Coronial investigation. (2) was concerned with factors contributing to a patient's death following the continuation of a postpartum bleed.

- Does your hospital have a policy of taking a full blood count, group and hold and/or cross-match prior to elective and emergency caesarean sections?
- Would you expect details of blood loss/uterine tear to be given at handover to the recovery room nurse?
- Are recovery room staff aware that internal bleeding can occur again in a very short time after a patient who has had a postpartum haemorrhage has left the operating room?

The obstetrician and anaesthetist assumed the recovery room nurse was experienced and trained in caring for a postpartum haemorrhage case:

- Do you think this was a reasonable assumption?

The nurse understood that she was to monitor vital signs as well as set up a Syntocinon infusion and provide pain relief:

- In your experience, are recovery room staff always, mostly or seldom experienced in recognizing the symptoms of haemorrhage and in recognizing the need to check fundal height or perform fundal massage?

Where do you think the final responsibility should fall:

- On the hospital to provide trained staff who are experienced for the tasks they are asked to undertake in the recovery room or
- On nurses to state their limitations?
- Would you agree that a nurse may not be aware of her/his limitations?

Particular drugs with coagulating properties were not immediately available at the hospital but available at a number of other regional hospitals.

- What recommendations would you make in the formulation of policy as to the minimum requirements for hospitals to store a particular drug or range of drugs, having regard to their availability, demand and shelf life?

The inquest had not been able to determine precisely when certain events occurred during this critical stage, for example when the Syntocinon drip was turned off and re-commenced. Accepting that care of the patient takes priority, is there sufficient emphasis placed on:

- locating a scribe in an emergency?
- making detailed notes after the event when memories are still fresh?

This case was concerned with areas of responsibility. The coroner commented on :

(a)   the willingness of disciplines to compartmentalize their areas of responsibility and

(b)   the failure to identify individual and collective responsibility.

- Do you agree?
- Does this happen where you work?
- How could change be effected?

....

In *Gregorie* and *Prosser,* the common factor was severe pain in the postpartum period. How pain is assessed and responded to should be reflected in the documentation. While the GP in Prosser advised the mother she could expect to be sore after giving birth to a big baby, the physiotherapist believed the symphysis had separated.

- How would you respond to a patient's concerns if a GP and physiotherapist held seriously divergent views?

NOTES

1.   *R v Inner London North Coroner, ex parte Touche,* 60 BMLR 170, at p.179 (2001).
2.   Ibid.
3.   There is an apparent contradiction as the previous paragraph notes results of a post-mortem.
4.   Ibid., p.173.
5.   Ibid.
6.   Ibid.

7. Ibid.

8. For an analysis of the Court of Appeal judgment: http://alexanderharris.co.uk /article/touchecoronerappea ldismissedlegalsummary153.asp

9. Ibid.

10. *Record of Investigation into Death*, No. 4210/91, State Coroner's Office (NSW).

11. Ibid., p.3

12. *Le Page v Kingston & Richmond Health Authority*, 8 Med LR 229 (1997).

13. Ibid., p.233.

14. Ibid., p.234

15. Ibid.

16. Ibid., p.235.

17. Ibid.

18. Ibid.

19. Ibid.

20. Ibid.

21. Ibid., p.236.

22. Ibid., p.237.

23. *Record of Investigation into Death*, Case No: 615/2007, State Coroner's Office (NSW).

24. Ibid.

25. *Gregorie v Spencer*, 300 APR 1 (QB) (1991).

26. *Eagle & Anor v Prosser*, NSWCA, No. 20460 (1994). Case note in 2000 CCH Ltd: Australian Professional Liability, Medical, paras 8-840.

27. Ibid.

28. Ibid.

29. Ibid.

30. Ibid.

31. Ibid.

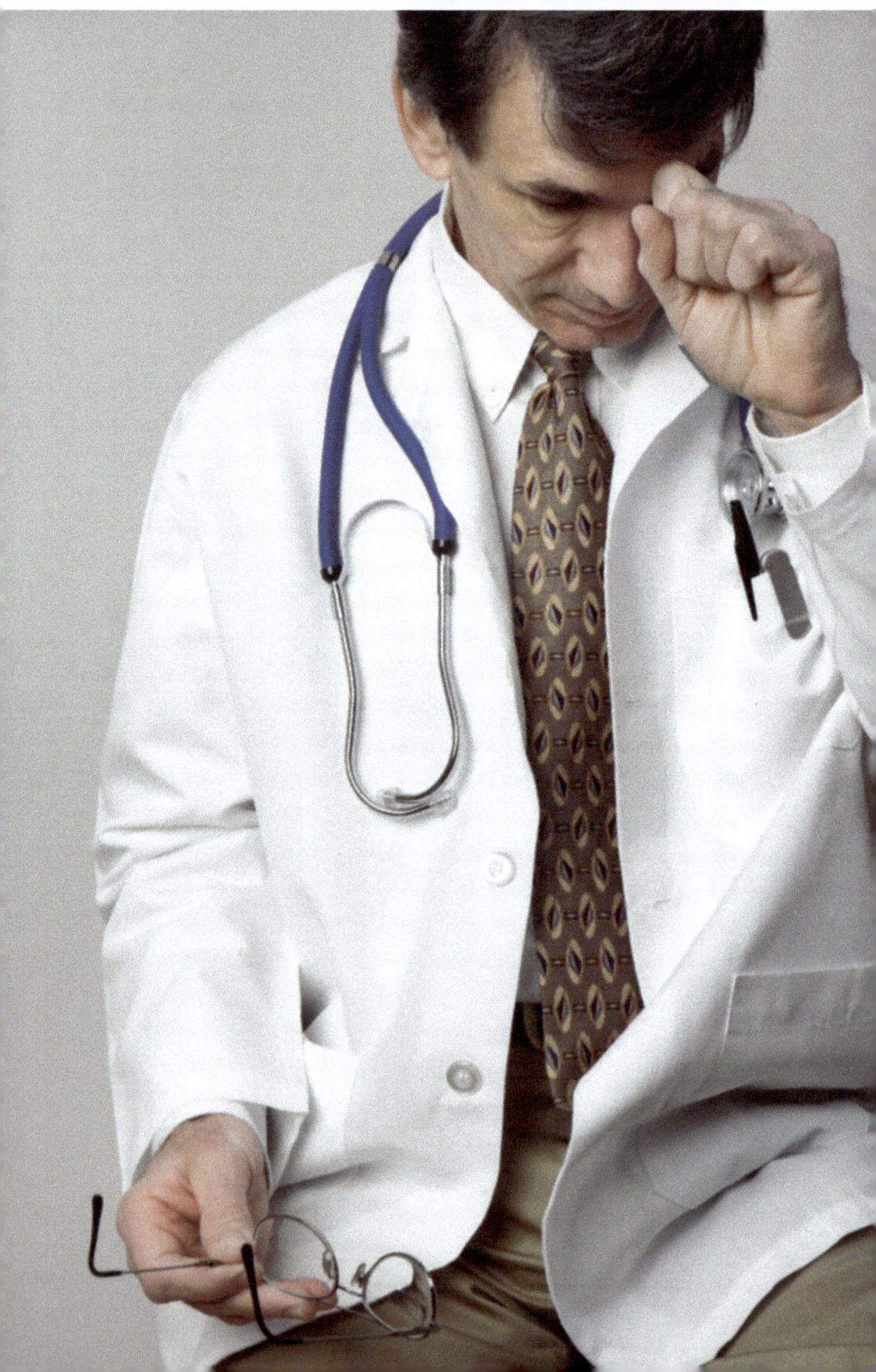

CHAPTER 11

Nervous shock

'I have never cried so much in my life. To me, my son was the missing part of my life .... It is what I believed then and still do now.'

—A father

Introduction

So far, the cases in this book have focused on adverse outcomes suffered by mothers and babies in hospital. Occasionally, fathers have appeared briefly in the story as witnesses because they were present during labour and birth. But in two of the four cases in this chapter, both parents tell of lives radically altered by the development of nervous shock when their child was severely injured during the birth process.

Nervous shock is mental illness arising from negligence. It is not an emotional or grief reaction, but a lasting condition affecting mental health. Such damage also deserves compensation. The following excerpts from the *Australian Health and Medical Law Reporter*[1] explain the concept.

In *McLoughlin v O'Brian* in 1983, Lord Wilberforce said:

Although we continue to use the hallowed expression 'nervous shock', English law, and common understanding, have moved some distance since recognition was given to this symptom for liability. Whatever is unknown about the mind - body relationship, it is now accepted by medical science that recognizable and severe physical damage to the human body and system may be caused by the impact, through the senses, of external events on the mind.[2]

In 1970, the High Court of Australia awarded damages to an employee who suffered a schizophrenic reaction after he witnessed a fellow employee's electrocution caused by the company's negligence. *(Mount Isa Mines Ltd v Pusey).*[3] One judge found that an illness of the mind set off by shock is not the less injury because it is functional, not organic, and its progress is psychogenic.

In *Jaensch v Coffey,*[4] another High Court judge explained that it is not necessary for psychiatric illness to result from a sudden sensory perception:

The notion of psychiatric illness induced by shock is a compound, not a simple, idea. Its elements are, on the one hand, psychiatric illness and, on the other, shock which causes it. Liability in negligence for nervous shock depends upon the reasonable foreseeability of both elements and of the causal relationship between the two.[5]

Proximity

Under earlier law, when there was less knowledge of psychiatry, courts would permit recovery of damages for nervous shock only if plaintiffs were within sight or sound of an event caused by negligence, or in very close *proximity* (a term you will encounter a number of times in this chapter). It is now recognized that a plaintiff may suffer nervous shock even if not present at the scene. As one judge explained in *Jaensch,* emergency services act quickly to take the injured to hospital. Consequently, the aftermath of a scene (caused, for example, by negligent driving) and the resultant shock could take place not only at the scene of the accident, but in an emergency department when a parent first sees her seriously injured child.

....

Against this background of legal principle, consider the clinical issues and the management of risk in the next four cases, where the adverse outcome in each instance was the death of a baby.

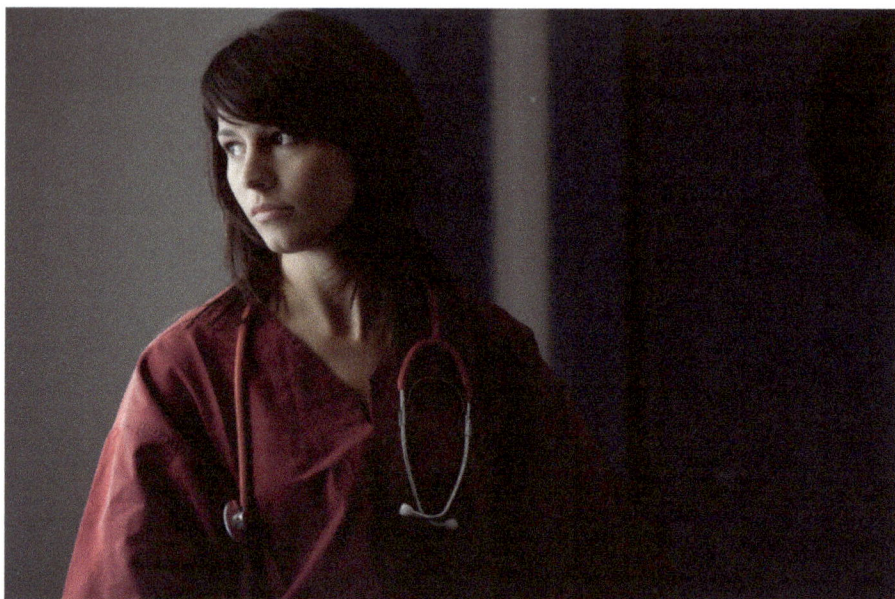

Kralj v McGrath [UK, 1986][6]

The facts

Felicity, aged 35, had one child following a normal birth in 1977 and planned a family of three. In 1979, she became pregnant with twins. An examination showed one twin in the correct position and the second in a transverse position. The obstetrician reassured Felicity, explaining he would be able to turn the second twin.

Felicity was admitted to hospital at 5.15 pm and a midwife determined the twins were still in the same position. The obstetrician set up a Syntocinon drip at 8 pm and returned at 10 pm, by which time the cervix was fully dilated. At 10.05 pm, the first twin was born. A paediatrician, house doctor and two, possibly three, midwives were present. There was no anaesthetist.

Pain. Felicity described what she then experienced: 'After Peter's birth, there was a slight lull, then the contractions started again. The obstetrician told me to push and the next thing I experienced was dreadful pain.'[7] Realizing the obstetrician had put his arm inside her, Felicity said: 'I tried to push him off … and asked him to stop … but others were holding me down.'[8] Felicity said she had almost gone mad with the pain and was then taken to the operating theatre where the second twin, Mark, was delivered by caesarean section.

No explanation. Felicity said she was given no explanation of what the obstetrician was intending to do. At one stage of her struggles she remembered taking the drip out of her arm and it being put back. She recalled being lifted back on a trolley after the operation. She had not seen the second baby for two days. Initially she was told Mark was 'a bit poorly,'[9] but Felicity then discovered he had been resuscitated.

The baby's condition. Felicity saw her son convulsing, twisting and unable to cry or swallow. Even when he was later able to swallow, he could not retain body heat. A paediatrician explained that 'progress was uncertain.'[10] Staff told her that Mark could be 'a vegetable.'[11] By this stage, Felicity said, 'When we knew that we hoped he would die.'[12] When Mark died at eight weeks, Felicity said that the death had prompted almost a sense of relief, as well as a sense of guilt. The guilt was because she and her husband had hoped their son would die. She believed this guilt would never leave them.

Compensation. Negligence was admitted. The case then proceeded on the amount of compensation for pain, injury and financial loss.

Medical evidence. Medical notes described a spontaneous rupture of the second sac and the second twin in the transverse lie. External cephalic version was not possible and: 'Internal cephalic version attempted but not possible.'[13] Mark's scalp showed marked oedema. An expert on neonatal pathology was unequivocal that the baby suffered, then died, from anoxic ischemic brain damage. There was no evidence of old internal injury or haemorrhage. Another medical expert contended that the anoxia occurred after the birth of the first twin and before the caesarean section.

Physical injuries. Felicity had a 'relatively uneventful'[14] recovery from the physical injuries of her labour. There had been an episiotomy without anaesthetic, vaginal bleeding for three months, a caesarean scar, and pain during sexual intercourse. As a result, she found it quite impossible to have intercourse with her husband for the following 18 months and would 'break down'[15] if she tried. Though she wanted three children, Felicity remained terrified of another birth. She could only envisage a caesarean delivery.

Review of records

A medical expert reviewed the records and concluded:

1. The drip was not advisable, as the acceleration of labour would have made external rotation of the second twin more difficult. There was no call for its use unless the obstetrician had some commitment later that day. If the drip had not been used, the first twin may have been born approximately two hours later.

2. Internal rotation should not have been tried without an anesthetist, and an anaesthetist should have been present before the attempts were made to deal with the internal rotation. If the mother had been undergoing contractions, rotation would be more difficult. The fear and pain involved would have made the mother contract more vigorously, making the task more difficult.

3. A podalic version should have been done. It was quite wrong to try cephalic version in any circumstance. The medical expert explained that if by cephalic version the head was brought down, it would be above the rim of the pelvis; then there would be the need for forceps. However, in order to safeguard the child and mother, it was a rule that forceps should never be applied when the child was above the pelvis. If the child was moved in this way, there was a danger the umbilical cord could be compressed.

4. The mother had received completely unacceptable and horrific treatment that broke all the rules made to safeguard a mother and child. She had undergone an excruciatingly painful experience that indicated a very bad and totally surprising practice. The caesarean section would have been unnecessary if the twin had been turned in an appropriate way.

A slightly increased risk. The medical expert believed Felicity could become pregnant again without difficulty, but that there would be a slightly increased risk to mother and child.

The decision

Felicity received compensation for nervous shock as a result of learning what had happened to her son, and of seeing him in his brain-damaged condition.

....

In the next case, the parents claimed damages against the health authority for psychiatric illness, which contributed to the breakdown of their marriage. This illness followed their son's death, which the hospital admitted had been caused by its negligence. In order to succeed, the parents had to prove the 'shock'[16] of the event caused their pathological grief reactions, in addition to normal 'stress, strain, grief or sorrow,'[17] (which could not be compensated). This case identifies the psychiatric problems that can follow when a mother experiences a poorly managed labour and both parents witness the aftermath of a very difficult birth, resuscitation and eventual death of their baby.

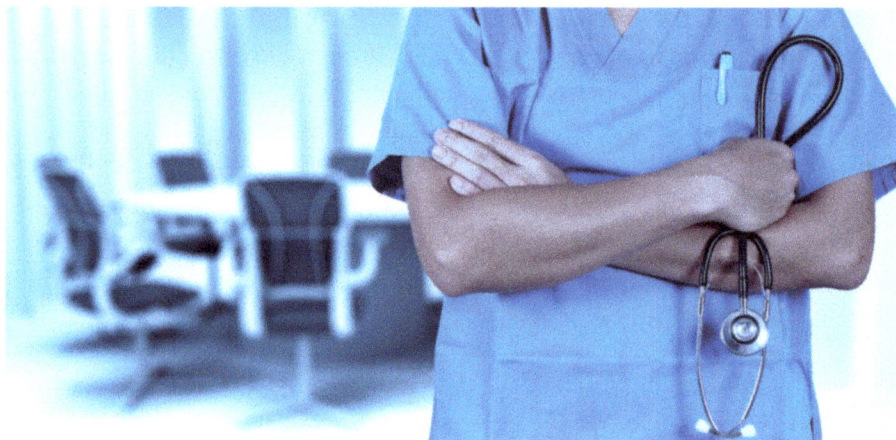

Tredget and Tredget v Bexley Health Authority [UK, 1994][18]

The facts

Gillian (no age given), an insulin-dependent diabetic since the age of 11, miscarried after ten weeks in 1984. In 1987, she was suffering from polyhydramnios and delivered a daughter by caesarean section. A third pregnancy was terminated because of herpes labialis. In February 1989, Gillian conceived again. This pregnancy was normal, but having been distressed by the earlier caesarean section, Gillian was now very anxious to have a vaginal delivery.

Admission for normal birth. Because her obstetrician would not have agreed to a vaginal delivery, Gillian's GP referred her to an obstetrician prepared to perform vaginal delivery. Gillian was admitted to hospital for an induction on 5 November, at just under 38 weeks. Strong contractions started during the evening of 7 November. No excessive hydramnios was present, but scans revealed that the baby was larger than average.

Slow labour. Labour progressed normally until 2.00 am, when the cervix was noted to be 7 cm dilated. The waters had broken an hour or so earlier. Labour then slowed. By 8.30 am, there was cause for concern and an attempt made to stimulate the uterus. The fetal heart showed deceleration. Oxygen was administered.

Complications of delivery. The obstetrician saw Gillian at 9.45 am. As there had been no progress since 9.30 am, the obstetrician pushed the anterior lip of the cervix over the baby's head to allow it to come down. Gillian pushed for half an hour from 10.30 am without success. A vacuum extraction was begun. When the baby's head appeared, the umbilical cord, which was around his neck, was clamped and cut. When the shoulders became caught within the pelvis, a shoulder bone had to be broken.

Resuscitation. When finally delivered at 11.32 am (birth weight 4.365 kg), the baby was in a severely asphyxiated condition, with no detectable heartbeat. He was resuscitated and taken to the special care nursery, but died two days later.

Negligence was alleged.

The trial

The mother's evidence. Gillian recalled a 'long, painful and traumatic experience.'[19] After labour had slowed at 2.00 am, she was not told what was happening. She recalled trying to force the baby down, but by then being too tired. Then 'all hell was let loose'[20] when there was difficulty in getting the baby out. She remembered someone saying, 'it's out',[21] of two midwives pushing on her abdomen, of someone shouting 'push' and of someone trying to assist the delivery internally. She commented 'My feeling at the time was of fear.'[22] (It had taken four minutes from the time the head emerged to deliver the rest of the body.)

Exhausted. By then, Gillian had been in labour for 15 hours. She said she was exhausted. She had not seen the baby because of the state she was in, but as she 'regained her senses,'[23] had become aware he was being resuscitated behind her. She sensed that things were wrong. Her husband, Anthony, who had been present throughout, had looked 'stunned.'[24]

The father's evidence. Anthony recalled that at this point his legs were shaking. He had to sit down. 'I was in a state of disbelief. I didn't know what was going on, but I knew there was a problem. I sat down and cried. I was not prepared for it.'[25]

Anthony described the atmosphere in the delivery room as 'casual' until about 10 am. He then sensed there were problems and described 'pandemonium'[27] when the delivery was taking place. He was asked to keep saying to his wife that she should push while staff were physically trying to complete the delivery. The four minutes it had taken to deliver the baby had seemed 'an eternity.'[28] He saw that his son was black and mauve, observed him being resuscitated and watched him being taken to the special care nursery. He did not realize how bad things were until a doctor said, 'The good news is that he is alive, but the bad news is that he has a 60 to 70 per cent chance of brain damage.'[29]

Photograph. Gillian recalled being given this same information and had been shocked. 'I had no idea the situation was so bad.'[30] When a midwife later gave Gillian a photograph she had been distressed by the image of her son with tubes in place. Although the photograph had been put by her bed, she could not recall looking at it again. 'The events at the time were more important than the photograph.'[31]

Special care nursery. Both parents saw their son in his incubator the following day. Gillian spent one or two hours alone with him. The baby was described as 'in a bad way'[32] and appeared to be crying. Gillian was distressed for him as well as for her husband, who was crying. They received upsetting and conflicting reports about their son's chances of survival and the degree of possible brain damage. The baby then appeared to improve, but deteriorated overnight.

Life support discontinued. Anthony was called from home urgently early on 10 November. The decision was then taken to turn off the life support. The baby was christened and held by his mother before he died.

Confusion for the mother.

'For me the time between his birth and when he died was very traumatic. There was uncertainty; neither of us was prepared for what happened. I had shock and disbelief. Physically, I felt unable to do anything. Mentally, there was confusion. I wasn't sure what had happened. We had different explanations. I didn't understand what had happened or why. I subsequently became obsessed with the loss of the baby.'[33]

Confusion for the father.

'I remember being distraught and confused. I was distraught because of what I saw was chaos. It left me confused. I have never
cried so much in my life. To me, my son was the missing part of my
life, albeit a profound statement. It is what I believed then and still
do now.'[34]

Arguments and allegations. Despite Gillian's evidence to the contrary,
the court accepted that the obstetrician had warned her of the possibility of
intra-uterine death and that this risk was to be countered by inducing labour
before term.

Negligence admitted. The health authority admitted negligence in the
management of Gillian's labour. A decision to perform a caesarean section,
or at least advise it in very strong terms, should have been taken at about
4.45 am. It was agreed that the parents' suffering may have gone beyond the
consequences of normal mourning.

Grief not shock. However, the health authority contended that it was
grief, rather than shock, which had caused the psychiatric illnesses. No single event justified the nervous shock necessary to find them liable.

Findings

Relationship changed. The judge found the relationship between Gillian and Anthony, which had been happy, was immediately affected by their
son's death.

Mixture of anger and guilt. A consultant psychiatrist gave the only
medical evidence. From his reports and the parent's evidence, the judge
found that the parents were left blaming themselves, each other and any-
body else who might possibly be culpable. This bewildering mixture of anger
and guilt left them psychiatrically disturbed as their marriage and lives were
torn apart.

Birth of a daughter. Another child, a daughter, was delivered by elective caesarean section in January 1992. This did not stop the deterioration of their relationship. The psychiatrist explained to the court that, far from producing anticipated relief, the birth of another baby could exacerbate the parent's symptoms.

Aftermath

Anthony continued working until 1992, then had a nervous breakdown. At the time of the trial, he was a full-time psychiatric patient. Before the final breakdown of the marriage, he had two extra-marital affairs, one of which (as this judgment records) led to Gillian suffering a further miscarriage. A prosperous household with good prospects had now broken up.

Psychiatric evidence

Normal mourning process. The psychiatrist described Gillian and Anthony as each having plunged into a complicated reaction riddled with grievance and blame, common hallmarks of pathological unresolved mourning. Pathological grief reactions are not just slight exaggerations of the normal mourning process, which is part of human experience for everyone at some time. The normal process is self-limiting. Although there is some disability, it passes with the re-establishment of a realistic perspective of life.

Pathological mourning. By contrast, pathological mourning may be mild, moderate, severe or catastrophic. It is marked by its duration, which can last months or years. It is also marked by an exaggeration of the normal features of mourning, often to a bizarre extent. This can manifest in extreme preoccupation and attachment to grievances or idealization of an attachment to the deceased, as well as an underlying mutual or self reproach.

Difficult to mourn neonatal death. The psychiatrist explained to the court that a neonatal death was intrinsically difficult to mourn because of :

1. the bewildering nature of the experience,
2. the lack of a clear sense of a known child whose loss can be remembered and mourned,
3. the sense of birth and death mixed up and

4. the fact that so often the circumstances are confused.

Aggravated reaction. In the psychiatrist's opinion, each parent had susceptibility towards an aggravated reaction to their son's birth and death. Firstly, there had been the prior loss or termination of pregnancies. Secondly, they had perceived grounds for grievance from the outset, but the circumstances of the death were confused. Finally, the experience of the birth was, in different ways, traumatic for each parent. The period in which the staff were making desperate efforts to release the baby from his mother's body and resuscitate him had been 'frightening and horrifying'[35] for them.

Degrees of severity. Each parent had continued to suffer from pathological unresolved mourning of the baby's death, but with different degrees of severity. The suffering was serious and persistent, but not florid, in Gillian's case. It was florid and very severe in Anthony's case.

The decision

The judge found that the parents had established the necessary points to prove nervous shock:

- They were both deeply emotionally tied to the birth of their child, therefore a proximate relationship clearly existed.
- The problems which beset the difficult and prolonged labour, the traumatic delivery and the short period of their son's life in intensive care were effectively 'one event' in which each parent had been a principal rather than a passive witness. Anthony had been in full view of what was happening and actually participating at the request of staff. It was unrealistic that a distinction should be drawn between him and Gillian because she was labouring, in pain, sedated and suffering from exhaustion. Although not fully conscious, Gillian had been aware something was wrong.
- Both experienced not merely grief, distress and sorrow, but suffered (for all the reasons given by the psychiatrist), a reasonably foreseeable psychiatric illness resulting from shock.

Damages awarded.

Aggravated and exemplary damages

In some jurisdictions, in addition to special damages (medical expenses, loss of earnings, economic loss) and general damages (pain and suffering, loss of enjoyment of life, loss of expectation of life and so on), aggravated and exemplary damages may be awarded in certain circumstances.

Aggravated damages. Awarded over and above special and general damages when the harm done was aggravated by insult and humiliation.

Exemplary damages. Awarded to punish and to deter others from acting in a similar way. Such damages also reflect the court's view that the action complained of is 'detestable.'

....

Exemplary and aggravated damages are claimed in the next case where the baby suffered asphyxia during a shoulder dystocia delivery and was later removed from life support without her parents' consent.

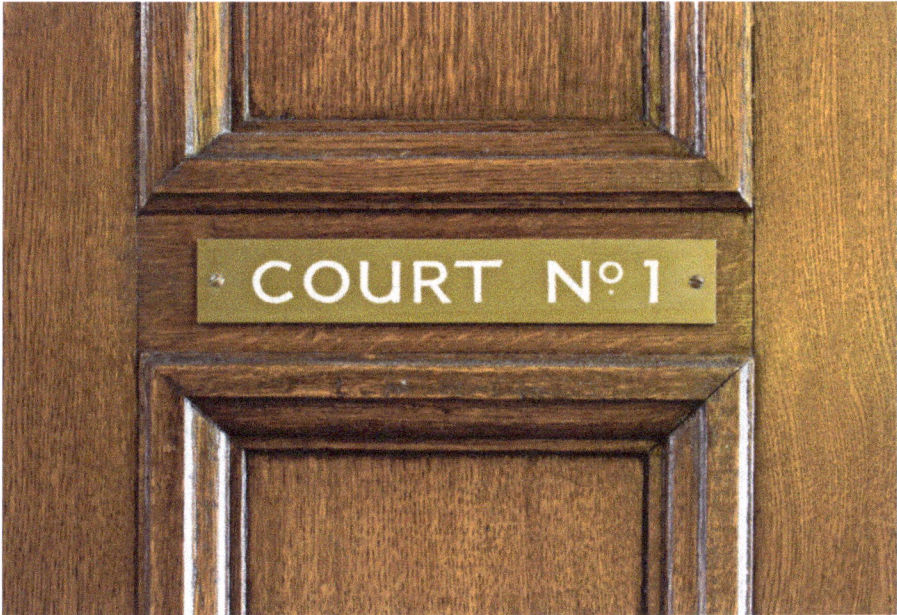

Hunter Area Health Service v Marchlewski & Anor [Aus, 2000][36]

The facts

Lea's first pregnancy went to full term with no difficulties, but the baby was very large in comparison with the mother. During a second pregnancy, Lea was scheduled for an ultrasound, but went into labour and was admitted to hospital on 29 September 1992. Labour proceeded normally, with strong contractions and no sign of fetal distress. When delivery was imminent, two nurses and a midwife were joined by the RMO.

Shoulder dystocia. At 11.30 pm, the baby's head emerged, but the shoulders did not, indicating shoulder dystocia. The emergency procedures set out in the hospital's *Guidelines for the Management of Impacted Shoulders* were followed, but failed to resolve the problem. Approximately nine minutes later, the senior midwife and senior registrar were called. The midwife cut a large episiotomy and the registrar directed that the patient be made ready for the McRoberts manoeuvre. This succeeded and the baby was delivered at 11.50 pm.

Removal from life support. The baby was born clinically dead and re-suscitated. Her brain damage was caused by cerebral hypoxia resulting from asphyxia during delivery and she was placed on life support. The parents specifically directed the hospital that their daughter not be removed from life support without their consent. This decision was made despite neonatologists giving them a grave prognosis that continuation of life support was not in the baby's best interests. Both parents spoke little English, having only recently arrived in Australia.

On 16 October, the hospital decided, without any consultation with the parents, that the baby should not be re-ventilated in the event that she deteriorated. On 27 October, a respiratory arrest occurred that did not respond to resuscitation. The baby, who was not fully ventilated, died.

Allegations

The parents alleged that the hospital breached its duty of care as well as the terms of its contract with them, arguing that:

1. Had an ultrasound been performed as soon as was practicable after 23 September, it would have revealed the size of the baby in relation to the mother. A senior registrar would then have been present at the birth.
2. The hospital failed to summon help within a reasonable time after the obstetric emergency occurred.
3. The Hospital Guidelines were deficient in that they were not amended to include the McRoberts manoeuvre, a recognized procedure since 1983.
4. Their daughter's life support was terminated without their consent despite their specific instructions that she not be taken off life support.
5. Had they appreciated what was involved in an autopsy, they would have refused consent on religious and cultural grounds.

Admission of negligence. The hospital admitted negligence, conceding the parents had suffered nervous shock caused by negligence in the delivery. It was agreed that general damages be awarded.

Denial of responsibility. The hospital denied that the differing factors impinging on the parents' lives since the baby's death were its responsibility. It submitted that any damages should be moderate, considering the parents would be able to continue with their lives, and were doing so (they had since had a son).

Aggravated and exemplary damages. The parents also claimed exemplary or aggravated damages, arguing:

1. That they did not appreciate what was involved in an autopsy and coronial inquest. If the hospital had explained the procedure, they would not have consented. The court heard that the mother had fainted when given details of the autopsy.
2. That the decision by the hospital not to reventilate their daughter contravened their express directions to continue with life support.
3. That they had both suffered a pathological grief reaction, post-traumatic stress disorder, delusional disorder, mood swings and other problems.

The decision

The autopsy. The judge said it was not submitted that the hospital had acted unlawfully, but that owing to the 'exacerbated sensibilities'[37] of both parents, and their religious beliefs, some degree of care should have been taken to ensure that the consent or instruction to have a coronial inquiry was based on proper knowledge of what was involved, in particular as to the way an autopsy is carried out.

The failure of the hospital to ensure the parents understood the nature of an autopsy did not constitute a basis for aggravated or exemplary damages. The negligence that gave rise to the damages related to the baby's death. Although a coronial inquest was the result of the hospital's negligence, there was no evidence of any contumelious (insolent, contemptuous, insulting) disregard for the parents.

The extent of suffering. Even though the decision not to reventilate was in deliberate disregard of the parents' wishes, the judge found this did not warrant moral retribution or deterrence deserving exemplary damages. However, the hospital's actions after the baby's death did aggravate the damage suffered by her parents.

Abnormal predisposition. The father had a history of personal problems since arriving from Europe. He had been in and out of employment owing to a work injury, subjected himself to mutilation, and previously had been diagnosed with reactive depression. The hospital argued that he had a very clear predisposition to an abnormal psychiatric condition. The judge referred to *Jaensch*[38], which held that even where an abnormal predisposition to shock or 'nervous injury' exists, liability must also extend to such people. They should also be able to recover in the same circumstances.

An ordinary person would have suffered the depression and grief disorders. The father had suffered in this way but to a greater extent.

Damages

The following breakdown shows the way damages were awarded:

The father

Special damages

- $94,342 loss of earning capacity
- $188,071 future loss of earnings
- $86,192 intensive therapy and medication likely to be necessary for more than ten years

General damages

- $180,000 for the likely distortion of a life affected by grief plus 20 per cent for aggravated damages
- The judge described the damage the father had suffered as 'cruelly exacerbated'[39] by the decision not to reventilate his daughter

The mother

The court heard that the mother held strict Buddhist beliefs and spoke very little English. The judge found that she was suffering from a pathological grief reaction and a post-traumatic stress disorder that was likely to persist for years. She was unlikely to ever return to the workforce. Had it not been for the trauma suffered, she would have done so for economic reasons arising from her husband's employment problems and injury. The judge doubted she would ever recover from the trauma.

Special damages

- $60,000 was awarded for future economic loss
- $25,000 for future therapy costs

General damages
$200,000 for pain and suffering
An additional $40,000 for aggravated damages

Damages were not awarded to a child who was three and a half at the time of the baby's death. The judge acknowledged that while she may have suffered directly or indirectly due to the events surrounding the death, she had not suffered nervous shock in the manner defined by the law.

The following is a brief report on the coronial inquest into the baby's death.[40]

The coroner found that the hospital guidelines were outdated and had correct procedures been known and followed by the delivery staff, the infant would probably have been born alive and well. The coroner found that the delivery staff should have summoned help much earlier than they did. There were also many clinical indications of an increased risk of obstructed labour and an obstetrician ought to have been present at the delivery. Those indicators included the fact that the mother was small of stature; had previously delivered a large baby; was large for dates; and had an elevated fundal height, polyhydramios and symptoms of pre-diabetes. The parents refused to accept that their newborn daughter would not survive. When she was extubated and breathing spontaneously, they believed she was improving.

Frivolous claims

Courts are unlikely to be sympathetic to 'frivolous' claims, as the United States case of *Bro v Glaser*[41] illustrates. During a caesarean section, an obstetrician nicked the baby's face with a scalpel. The laceration did not result in any permanent injury and neither parent was aware of the injury until told by the obstetrician. The parents later alleged that the negligent and casual manner in which the bandaged baby had been presented to them had resulted in emotional distress.

The Court dismissed the claim as bordering on the frivolous. During the trial, the mother admitted she had expected the baby's face to be bandaged and would have wanted the obstetrician to do whatever was necessary to repair the damage.

Post-traumatic stress disorder

New mothers can perceive lack of communication with staff as a lack of caring. This sensitivity can act as a powerful trigger to consider litigation when parents are trying to deal with the trauma of a birth injury or death.

....

In the final case in this chapter, a breakdown in communication took a particularly poignant twist. The mother claimed she developed post-traumatic stress disorder following a difficult delivery when hospital staff told her that her daughter had died, but six hours later a paediatrician informed her that the baby had in fact survived.

The judge described the case as difficult, complex and very unusual. A midwife who cared for the mother and her baby said the event was one of the most traumatic in her career.

This case carries a clear pointer to the safe management of risk. Staff owe a duty of care to communicate accurately, and in a timely manner, not only with the patient, but also with each other, so that misinformation does not occur at highly sensitive times.

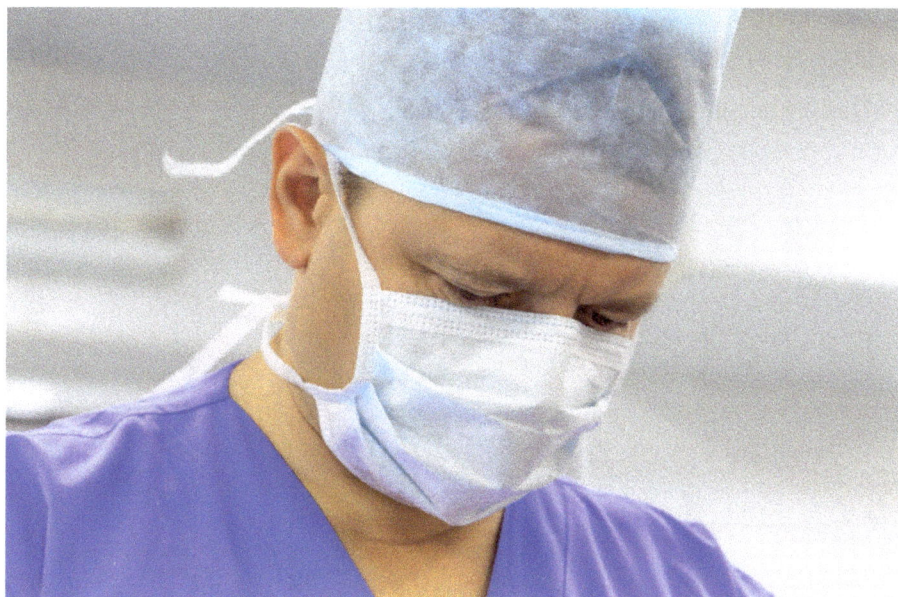

Allin v City & Hackney HA [UK, 1996][42]

The facts

Rosemary was thirty years old when she became pregnant in July 1990. She had been divorced some years earlier, had suffered a miscarriage and was now in an unhappy and unsupportive relationship.

The pregnancy, jointly managed by her GP and antenatal staff at the hospital, did not proceed smoothly. There were concerns about the baby's position, as well as the size of its head. By 16 April, some doctors believed Rosemary was suffering from placenta praevia, and would require an elective caesarean section. The consultant obstetrician disagreed. As a result, Rosemary was admitted, allowed to go home and then re-admitted.

Haemorrhage. On 4 May, there was discussion about inducing the baby by the use of prostaglandin. Rosemary was linked to a CTG to monitor the baby's heart, which began to behave erratically. By the early hours of 5 May, the baby was very distressed. Dr Taft decided to artificially rupture the membranes but the procedure resulted in a copious haemorrhage. The consequent emergency rush to the operating theatre was described by Rosemary's mother as 'all hell let loose.'[43]

Support discontinued. At 3.13 am, Amy was delivered by caesarean section in a poor condition, having suffered an 80 per cent blood loss. Paediatricians took her to the special care nursery, where cardiac massage was attempted. The various scores by which the baby was being monitored were 'very, very low indeed negative'[44] and it was not until 22 minutes after the birth that a heartbeat was detected. Nobody thought Amy would survive. By 4.10 am, both the consultant paediatrician and paediatric registrar decided all support should be discontinued and the baby left to die. A nurse cared for Amy and comforted Rosemary and her mother; Rosemary's mother saw her granddaughter in a cot. A Catholic priest was called. It was now the shared view of all medical staff that the baby could not and would not survive.

Recovery. But by 5.20 am, Amy was giving irregular gasps. By 7.00 am, these were described as 'gasping respirations.'[45] By 8.00 am, her heart rate was 120 and there was warmth in her body. She was given a facial mask. At 8.30 am, she was transferred to an air-shield. It was now feared that survival would be at the expense of considerable brain damage.

Amy did recover and, although suffering some disability, went on to attend school. Six years later, a judge was to describe her as 'a treasured member'[46] of the family.

The trial

Rosemary's case focused on two issues:

1. Had she been negligently misinformed that her baby was dead when, in fact, Amy was alive?
2. If so, had this misinformation caused the development of her post-traumatic stress disorder (PTSD)?

The bad news. Rosemary said that after the rush to the operating room she woke from the anaesthetic back in the ward to find no cot beside her. She was then taken to a side room, again with no cot, away from the other mothers and babies. She was frightened, fearing that Amy was dead or seriously damaged. The two doctors who had attended the delivery visited her, both in tears and repeatedly apologising. They told her the baby had been a girl, who, despite all their efforts, had died after 22 minutes. They said the crucial condition had been vasa praevia. The baby's placental blood vessels had been ruptured, causing heavy bleeding which had exsanguinated her. In their opinion, if Amy had survived, she would probably have been brain damaged. Rosemary said she had been told in plain terms that her baby had died. Her mother said she had been told the same thing shortly before.

The good news. Rosemary remained in the ward without receiving any communication about the baby for six hours. Then a nurse asked her if she would like to see and hold the baby. Rosemary said she had not wanted to, as the baby was dead. Then, at 11.15 am, a paediatrician arrived. While talking of Amy in the present tense, the paediatrician suddenly realized that Rosemary, as well as members of staff, thought the baby had died.

The paediatrician's note of this visit read: 'Sister Dow, Dr Mee, mother's mother present. Family and staff under impression that the baby had died.'[47]

Nursing notes. The hospital argued that Rosemary and her mother were not misinformed, although both were told in plain terms, at the appropriate time, that there seemed no chance of Amy surviving. It was further contended that the following entry in the ward records was a mistake:

> 1. am   Transferred from the theatre following emergency. [Details of the mother and Rosemary's condition] then: Baby in poor condition at birth. Subsequently died in Special Care Baby Unit.[48]

The judge believed this second and untimed entry was made shortly after Rosemary returned to the ward. He did not accept the hospital's suggestion that a nurse had either made a mistake or acted on erroneous information given by Rosemary or her mother. A gynaecologist giving expert evidence described the second suggestion as 'astonishing.' No nurse, in his opinion, would act on such an authority, given the seriousness of the matter.[49]

No misunderstanding. The judge acknowledged that Rosemary was frightened, traumatized and recovering from the anaesthetic, but did not find it probable that either she or her mother had misunderstood what was said to them by the two doctors who had delivered Amy. The judge accepted that this highly emotional visit would not be normal or usual behaviour from trained doctors, but could be explained by their extreme distress, together with the long and tiring sequence of events since the previous evening.

Duty to communicate accurately. The judge held that hospital staff have a duty of care to give accurate information to a mother about whether her baby was dead or alive. On a balance of probabilities, Rosemary had been told her baby was dead when in fact she was not.

Psychiatric evidence of post-traumatic stress disorder. Psychiatrists called by both parties agreed that Rosemary was suffering from PTSD. She was generally unhappy, cried very easily and had irrational fears that Amy would die or be taken away. Rosemary also could not bear to let Amy out of her sight; she slept during the afternoon, when her mother minded Amy, then stayed awake at night to watch over her. She also had frequent nightmares that her daughter was falling over cliffs or being pulled away by some force and was obsessed with events at the hospital, fearing people would dislike her for 'going on about it.'[50]

Rosemary became very upset by anything to do with hospitals or sick children, and her concentration had deteriorated to the extent that she did not feel she could cope with work.

Additional elements. The psychiatrists agreed that Rosemary had suffered from PTSD for an unusually long period. They agreed there was probably an additional element of either post-natal or reactive depression involved. It was recognized from the GP's notes, and Rosemary's own evidence, that she was a worrier with an anxious personality and a tendency to fear she might be ill. She suffered from asthma, migraines and panic attacks. There had been an unhappy marriage followed by a very unsatisfactory violent relationship with another man who had been particularly unsupportive during the pregnancy and hospitalization.

Pre-admission medical experiences. An additional factor was Rosemary's pre-admission medical experiences. These included warnings of the likely abnormality of the baby and disagreements between doctors about the position of the baby and the appropriateness of a caesarean delivery. Further uncertainties and disagreements occurred after admission. Pain and panic accompanied the rupture of vasa praevia vessels and the rush to the operating room.

Post-delivery. Rosemary had developed a growing belief that something had gone wrong. This was followed by misinformation, then the accurate information, together with warnings that if the baby survived it would probably be severely damaged. Rosemary had seen her 'precariously'[51] surviving baby looking battered, with tubes in place, suffering fits over the following 24 hours. She had returned home, a single mother having to cope with a 'hugely active'[52] baby. The death of a much-loved father occurred six months later.

Separating out the strands. Each medical witness acknowledged the difficulty in distinguishing between these different strands and processes in Rosemary's total experience. It was agreed that most mothers with handicapped children, or people whose fathers die, do not develop PTSD. Both psychiatrists, who had special experience in maternity matters, gave considerable weight to the evidence of the gynecologist whom the judge described as having 'enormous'[53] experience of mothers suffering unhappy events during and immediately after childbirth.

Deepening the trauma. The gynaecologist did not doubt that the misinformation was a severe matter. The discovery that Amy was not dead might, contrary to the expected reaction of relief and happiness, in fact deepen the trauma. He described the intricate machinery of human thoughts and emotions to the court, explaining that a mother, hearing that a baby had died or might be severely damaged, could quite quickly begin to adjust to the situation as she understood it. Being then asked to put the process of adaptation to the death into reverse could constitute a serious element in the development of PTSD.

The decision

The judge accepted that misinformation had been a substantial cause of the PTSD, but also heard evidence that recovery would occur quite rapidly when the case was over.

Damages awarded.

Further allegations

Rosemary also alleged that the hospital had been negligent in not arranging appropriate counselling or psychiatric assistance after the birth. The judge held that the hospital had been entitled to assume that her GP would do so. The GP had jointly managed the pregnancy, was well known to the hospital and had shown great care and commitment after Amy's birth. The hospital knew Rosemary would be discharged into his care. To ask more of the hospital was to demand a duty of care that was too high in the circumstances.

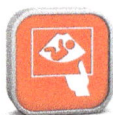

Discussion of Key Issues

The legal explanations at the beginning of this chapter and those reiterated by each judge contain the broad common law principles about nervous shock. In human terms, you have read about lives distorted by grief.

But each case contains the clinical story of how and why one parent, and sometimes two, was so traumatised.

- Identify the risk management issues in each case.
- How would you have managed the communication with the mother or both parents following the birth in each case?

....

In *Kralj,* the patient suffered severe and prolonged pain during unsuccessful attempts by an obstetrician to turn the second twin, who was in a transverse lie. This baby, delivered by caesarean section, later died from brain damage. The patient suffered nervous shock and remained terrified of another birth.

- A medical expert claimed that the Syntocinon drip was not advisable, as the acceleration of labour would have made external rotation of the second twin more difficult. Do you agree? If so, and if you were the midwife, how would you have responded when Syntocinon was ordered?
- The medical expert then commented that he would see no call for the drip 'unless the obstetrician had some commitment later that day.'[54] How would you explain this to a court?
- The patient was described as having received 'completely unacceptable and horrific treatment.'[55] The treatment 'broke all the rules to safeguard a mother and baby.'[56] The court also heard that a paediatrician, a doctor and two, possibly three, midwives were present. If this situation occurred at your hospital, what would you expect of these health professionals?
- The patient said she saw the baby in a very distressed state. Staff had commented on the probability of brain damage. It had been 'almost a sense of relief, but also a sense of guilt'[57] when her son died eight weeks

later. What can staff do, if anything, to assuage guilt in a patient endur-
ing such circumstances?

....

In *Tredget,* the psychiatrist explained to the court that a neonatal death is
intrinsically difficult to mourn because of:

1. the bewildering nature of the experience,
2. the lack of a clear sense of a known child whose loss can be remembered and mourned and
3. the sense of birth and death mixed up.

Parents who seek legal advice after a neonatal death sometimes describe a
sense of isolation in a hospital after the baby's death. Some feel hurt by the
way tragic news was delivered. Others sense staff 'move away' rather than
draw near. A legal consultation is often focused on these grievances rather
than on any meaningful move towards litigation.

- In terms of the psychiatrist's explanation, do you consider that there
  is either adequate training or adequate time to care for parents experiencing the possible onset of a complicated grief reaction? What
  literature would you recommend parents or lawyers read about this
  interaction?

....

In *Hunter,* the hospital's actions after the baby's death were found to have
aggravated the damage suffered by the parents.

- Who explains the nature of an autopsy to parents in your hospital?
  Are parents adequately supported?
- Do midwives and doctors have adequate training about religious and
  cultural differences?
- Discuss possible reasons for failing to re-ventilate in disregard of the
  parent's express wishes.
- How would you document such a decision?

....

In *Allin,* the emergency rush to theatre was described by the patient's mother as 'all hell let loose.'[58] The actions and communication between staff may be misinterpreted as being 'out of control' by patients and support people at such times.

- Do you think that there is the time/opportunity to de-brief the patient, and, if possible, the carers who were present?

The gynaecologist giving expert evidence explained that good news following bad news can, contrary to popular belief, *deepen* trauma. He described the machinery of human thoughts and emotions as 'intricate.'[59]

- Do you think courses leading to registration of health professions or ongoing professional development programmes adequately address the issues raised by these cases?

NOTES

1. CCH Australian Health & Medical Law Reporter, paras: 16–660.
2. *McLoughlin v O'Brian,* AC 410 Lord Wilberforce (1983) at p.418.
3. *Mt Isa Mines v Pusey,* 125 CLR 383 (1970).
4. *Jaensch v Coffey,* 155 CLR 549 (1984).
5. Ibid., pp.566–567.
6. *Kralj v McGrath,* 1 All ER 54 (1986).
7. Ibid., p.57.
8. Ibid.
9. Ibid.
10. Ibid., p.58.
11. Ibid.
12. Ibid.
13. Ibid.
14. Ibid.
15. Ibid.
16. *Tredget and Tredget v Bexley Health Authority,* 5 Med LR 178 (1994).
17. Ibid., p.182.
18. Ibid.
19. Ibid., p.180.
20. Ibid.
21. Ibid.

22. Ibid.
23. Ibid.
24. Ibid.
25. Ibid.
26. Ibid.
27. Ibid.
28. Ibid.
29. Ibid.
30. Ibid.
31. Ibid.
32. Ibid.
33. Ibid.
34. Ibid., p.181.
35. Ibid., p.183.
36. *Hunter Area Health Service v Marchelewski & Anor,* NSWCA 294 (2000). Case note based on CCH Australian Health and Medical Law Reporter, paras. 77–138.
37. Ibid.
38. Ibid.
39. Ibid.
40. Ibid.
41. *Bro v Glaser,* 22 Cal. App. 4th 1398, 27 Cal. Rptr. 2d 894 (1994)
42. *Allin v City & Hackney,* 7 Med LR 167 (1996).
43. Ibid., p.168.
44. Ibid.
45. Ibid.
46. Ibid.
47. Ibid., p.170.
48. Ibid.
49. Ibid.
50. Ibid., p.172.
51. Ibid.
52. Ibid., p.171.
53. Ibid., p.172.
54. *Kralj* at p.58.
55. Ibid.
56. Ibid.
57. Ibid.
58. *Allin* at p.168.
59. Ibid., p.171.

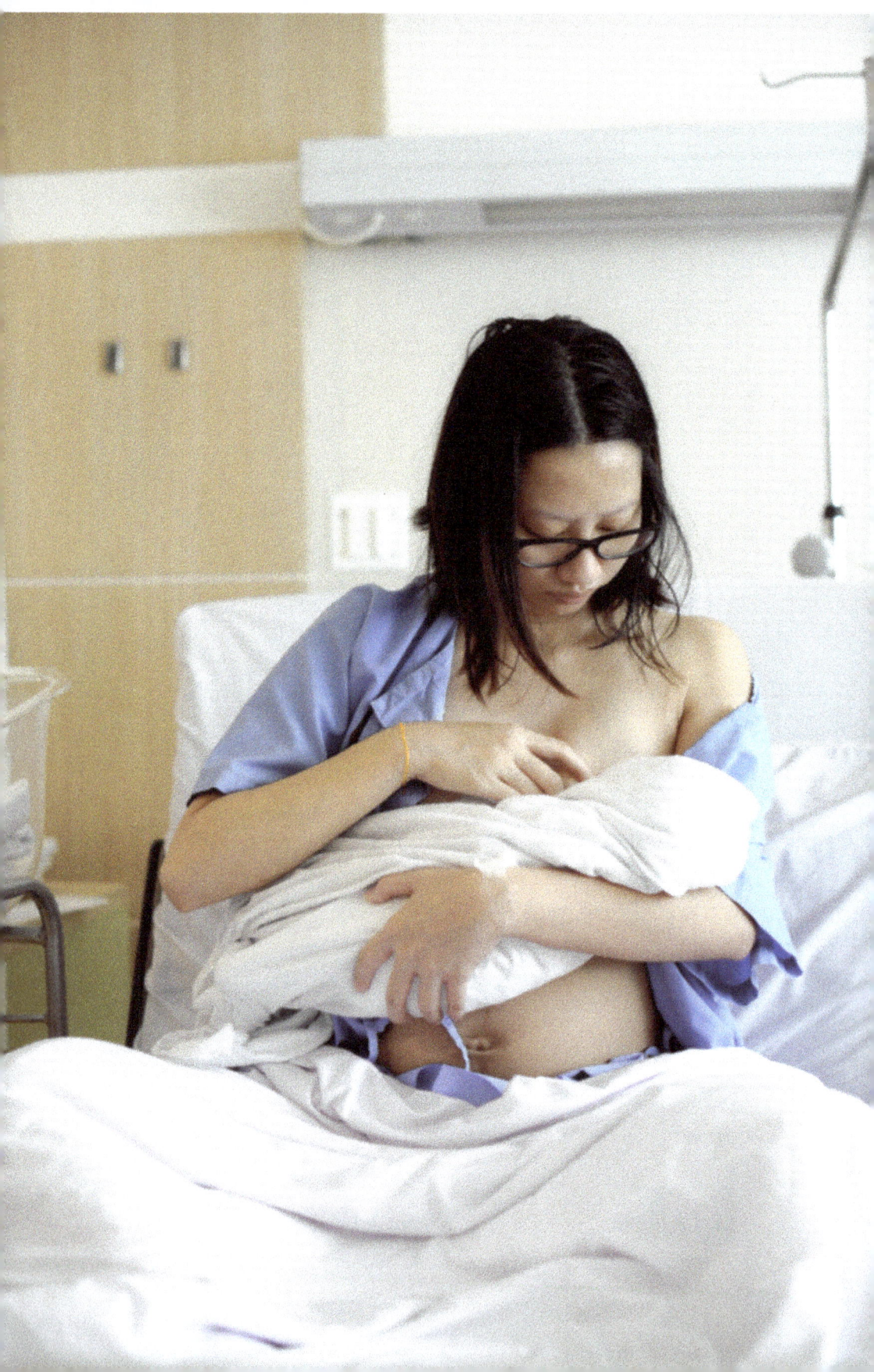

CHAPTER 12

Lactation

'My whole body felt numb when my daughter was brought in to be fed. I could not see the midwife properly and told her I could not feed the baby.'

—A mother

Introduction

Lactation would seem an unlikely area to find legal problems. But in this chapter breastfeeding in hospital becomes an issue in a number of coronial inquests; a coroner considers the dangers of a breast-milk substitute; and two judges are faced with the problem of mothers who are HIV-positive, one of whom intends to continue to breast feed against medical advice.

In the first two cases, coroners investigate the deaths of babies who suffered hypoxic episodes while being breast fed in hospital by mothers who were extremely tired. A paediatrician in the second case[1] explained to the coroner that in the past, mothers would stay 4 to 5 days in hospital, and if a mother was very tired, a nursery was available to care for the babies. Mothers now stay in hospital an average of 2.1 days and staff levels have not been maintained nor midwives transferred back onto wards when nurseries closed. Tight staffing levels and the consequent difficulty in monitoring mothers who are breastfeeding for the first time became an issue in both cases.

Coronial Investigation [Aus, 1993][2]

The facts

The baby was a breech presentation, with Anne's labour progressing slowly until a caesarean section was performed. From birth, the baby established regular respirations. The initial Apgar score was low, but normal by five minutes; cord blood pH was normal; and half hourly observations were normal. The baby was bathed at 5.30 am by a midwife, who described her as awake, alert, sucking on her fist and crying. At 6.20 am, the baby was given to Anne to be breast fed. Anne had received Pethidine at about 7 pm the previous night, an epidural at 10 pm, pentothal at about 12.15 am and Pethidine by IV at 4.am. Anne's husband saw her in the recovery room at about 3 am or 3.30 am. She was awake but very drowsy and unable to have a proper conversation with him. Anne later recalled feeling 'semi-conscious and very numb'[3] at that time.

The breast-feed. Anne said that her whole body had felt numb when her daughter was brought in to be fed. She could not see the midwife properly and told her she could not feed the baby. She said that the midwife had insisted, and put the baby to the breast without explaining what to do, then left the room. Anne had moved her right arm around the baby, as her left arm was immobilised by the drip. She said that she had not been attended to again and had fallen asleep, but was woken by crying. She tried to re-attach the baby to the breast, but could not do so. Nor could she find the buzzer to call for someone to take the baby. When the baby stopped crying, she had fallen asleep again.

Resuscitation. At 7.10 am, Anne was woken by a midwife who asked if she still wanted the baby with her. It was then discovered that the baby had stopped breathing. Resuscitation was commenced and the baby intubated, but gross neurological abnormalities consistent with severe hypoxic isch-aemic damage had occurred. This condition was considered irreversible and assisted ventilation ceased two weeks later.

The inquest

The court heard that it was hospital policy that newborn babies were given to mothers as soon as possible, although a caesarean section could delay this.

Insufficient supervision. The coroner found that despite the mother's drowsy state, it was appropriate for her to be given the baby to feed at 6.20 am, but from that point on there had been insufficient supervision. The mid-wife had not returned until 7.10 am. A second midwife, hearing crying, had gone in at 6.45 am, found nothing abnormal about either the mother or baby, and re-attached the baby to the breast.

Expert evidence

Speculation. A medical expert said it was conceivable that the baby was accidentally smothered by the mother or by the bedding. This was specula-tive and possible if the baby had in fact suffered some asphyxia at the time of birth (which was not observed by staff nor revealed by tests) or if Anne's consciousness was more clouded than the midwives' judgments led them to believe.

Findings

The baby's death remained unexplained. The coroner was not sat-isfied that the baby had suffered any substantial asphyxia at birth and even if Anne's consciousness was considerably clouded, there was not a strong possibility the baby had suffocated; the preferred conclusion was of Sudden Infant Death Syndrome (SIDS).

The coroner's comments included:

1. Mothers on Pethidine drips feeding newborn babies were not to be left unsupervised for more than a few minutes at a time; it was acknowledged that financial constraints might make such a high level of supervision unsustainable.
2. An experienced midwife's judgment as to the mother's fitness to breastfeed remained the best measure.
3. Until SIDS was better understood, the possibility of blame being directed towards carers remained.

....

Thirteen years later, a coroner found the risks relating to safe sleeping practices and SIDS were now better understood, the incidence of SIDs having declined from 2 per 1000 to 0.4 per 1000.[4] This investigation clearly illustrates the tension experienced by midwives trying to monitor breastfeeding mothers as well as cope with the demands of a very busy shift, in this instance a night shift. The coroner emphasizes the vital importance of hospitals not only requiring but *enabling* staff to keep up to date with changing policies relating to patient safety.

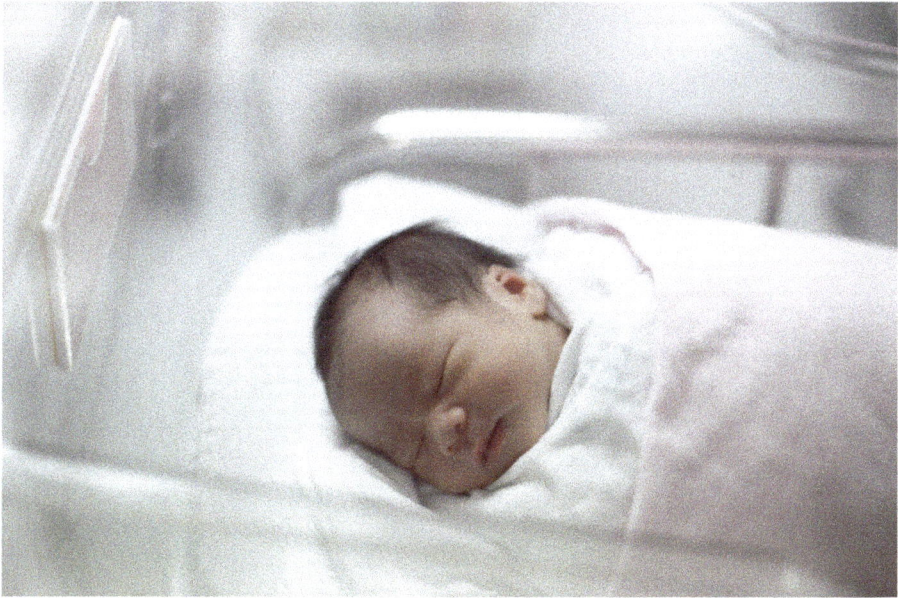

Coronial Investigation [Aus, 2006][5]

The facts

Yoko attended hospital at about 10.30 pm after her waters broke. As the delivery suite was very busy, she was told to go home and wait for a call to return. At about 4.40 am, Yoko returned to the hospital in significant pain. During the day an epidural was administered following signs of fetal distress and a baby girl delivered at 3.43 pm. The baby appeared to be in good condition at birth, with Apgar scores of 8 and 9 at one minute and five minutes respectively. Yoko required sutures and was given antibiotics for fever. The paediatric registrar recommended four-hourly observations of the baby in case the fever had been passed on.

Post-delivery

Recollections of the mother. Yoko and the baby were moved to a two-bed ward, with a cot next to the bed. Yoko, who had not slept the previous night, was tired and anxious, and felt affected by the medication and the noise of the other mother's visitors. She had difficulty sitting up because of her sutures and did not feel confident to respond to her baby's crying. She asked for assistance to attempt breastfeeding.

Breastfeeding. During the evening a midwife came in after Yoko buzzed, helped put the baby to the breast, then left. Yoko recalled the baby being left in the bed, and that she attempted to breastfeed several times and comfort the crying baby. A different midwife came in around 11.00 pm and placed the baby next to the breast. The baby was then put back in the cot.

Tiredness. Yoko recalled her sheets being changed in the night and a midwife being there at various times. At about 3.30 am, the baby was crying and a midwife instructed her to lie on her side so the baby could access the left breast. She felt exhausted. The light had been switched off and the baby left beside her. She thought she may have fallen asleep and remembered waking up, lying on her side with the baby's face beneath her breast and feeling her arm around the baby and the baby's body up against her.

Resuscitation. Yoko said that as she moved the baby up to feed her, a midwife came into the room and suddenly took the baby away. She recalled this occurring at about 6.45 am and that she must have been asleep. Another midwife came into the room and began to cry. She said the baby was not well and offered comfort. Yoko had then been taken by wheelchair to the baby, who was being resuscitated. Her husband arrived shortly afterwards and they saw the baby in the intensive care unit. The following day a decision was made to discontinue life support.

Yoko said she had not been warned of any danger to the baby by having her in the bed. Her husband later said that in Yoko's homeland, Japan, babies were looked after in nurseries.

The inquest

Possible cause of death. A paediatrician believed it unlikely that an autopsy would have found a cause of death other than suffocation and acknowledged that Yoko's tiredness may have been a contributing factor.

Recollections of the registrar

A registrar recalled explaining to the father (after the decision was made to turn off the respirator) that though not recommended by the hospital, it was not an uncommon practice for babies to be in bed with their mothers in the first few days after birth. The registrar also recalled Yoko saying she was exhausted after the birth and not in a fit mental state to be looking after a crying baby

Recollections of the senior midwife

Midwife A (of some twenty years' experience) had responsibility for approximately ten women and four babies overnight, including one post-caesarean mother. She made the following points:

11.30 pm. When she went into Yoko's room at about 11.30 pm, the baby was asleep in the cot and Yoko was awake. She administered antibiotics, discussed pain relief and then went to get medication. This was recorded.

2.30 am. The observations for the baby were within the normal range, other than a low temperature of 36 degrees. Yoko was awake and looking exhausted but said she would feed the baby, who was then placed by her right side. Feeding commenced successfully. Midwife A returned at about 2.45 am, wrapped the baby in two blankets and put her back in the cot.

3.30 am. When Yoko's buzzer sounded, midwife A and another midwife found her in bed, holding out her crying baby. Midwife A settled the baby, but could not recall any conversation or whether she had put the baby back in the cot or with the mother. She recorded the observations at 3.30 am.

4.30 am. Midwife A administered the antibiotics to Yoko intravenously over 20 minutes. She said that the baby (whose temperature had improved to 36.8 degrees) was 'still beside her in the bed.'[6] She asked Yoko if she wanted to try to breast feed again. As the baby was sleepy, she was laid down next to her mother.

6.00 am. Before completing her shift, Midwife A checked on Yoko, and saw that she was asleep on her back but that there was something wrong with the baby, who was also on her back. She ran with the baby to the resuscitation trolley, handed her to a midwife and ran to the staff room for help. Shocked and distressed, she was not involved in the resuscitation but went to support Yoko.

Findings

Midwife A could not later recall whether Yoko was awake at 4.30 am when she administered the antibiotics. She thought Yoko would have been awake because her usual practice was to check the patient's identity and put the baby back in the cot if the mother was asleep.

Rationalization. The coroner found this was 'rationalization after the event,'[7] drawing the inference from midwife A's earlier evidence that she had settled the baby after both midwives entered the room at 3.30 am, then 're-turned the baby to the mother's bed.'[8] The next time she came in she had recorded the baby was 'still in bed with the mother.'[9]

Policy. Midwife A said she was unaware of the hospital's policy (available to staff via the intranet) that 15- to 30-minute observations were required of a mother breastfeeding in bed; more frequently if the mother was sedated. She had checked to the best of her ability, but was unaware of specific time frames.

There was no designated time for staff to keep themselves informed of updated policies, nor had she kept herself updated. Documentary evidence showed that she had attended two educational sessions on breastfeeding.

Sleep inevitable. Despite midwife A saying she would not have left the baby with Yoko at 4.30 am if she had thought she would fall asleep, the coroner found that it was 'inevitable'[10] the mother would fall asleep, given the number of times she had been attended to and the fact that she was in pain and had had 'little or no sleep'[11] the previous night during labour.

Unaware of duration of labour. Midwife A had not read the chart in detail and was unaware of the nature and duration of Yoko's labour. While acknowledging that it had been a very busy shift, the coroner found that mid-wives play a crucial role in explaining and demonstrating appropriate and safe methods, and that night staff still had an obligation to inform them-selves about the needs of particular patients.

Handover. Midwife A said that despite policy changes requiring the re-cording of bed-sharing in the notes, this was often not done because of work pressures; such information could be handed over at the end of a shift, but in her experience it was not. If monitoring and recording of bed-sharing mothers was to occur, significant increases in staff levels would be required. The coroner noted that it was quite clear that whatever the official 'policy'[12] was, mothers did feed their babies in bed.

New policy

Following the baby's death, a new policy defined:

- **Bed-sharing** as the practice of the mother having the baby in bed with her for breastfeeding requiring the mother to be awake.

- **Co-sleeping** as the practice of placing mother and baby in the same bed, with one or both asleep. If the mother falls asleep when breastfeeding in bed, the situation is defined as co-sleeping. While it would be impossible to prevent co-sleeping absolutely, it was to be discouraged.

Breastfeeding in bed was unsafe if the mother:

   a. was sedated,
   b. was extraordinarily tired,
   c. had a condition that may alter the state of consciousness. (e.g, epilepsy),
   d. had a condition that may affect spatial awareness,
   e. is very obese,
   f. has multiple babies,
   g. is a smoker,
   h. is a known substance abuser,
   i. is known to consume alcohol or
   j. has a baby with a fever or an illness.

The paediatrician did not consider that post-epidural levels of sedating opiates would be particularly high in Yoko's case. While Pethidine would effect drowsiness, the fact that a patient is awake and asking for pain relief (as Yoko was) is an indicator that she is not currently sedated.

Workload. The coroner heard of the long-standing problem of inadequate staff-patient ratios to properly supervise new mothers, with extra demands occurring when the mother was very young, drug affected or suffering from mental illness. The fact that mother and baby are counted as one patient reduced an appreciation of the volume of work and care required. Evidence was given that the work load on the shift in question was 'extremely heavy.'[13]

SIDS. The coroner also heard that information on SIDS was available in antenatal classes, then reinforced and demonstrated by midwives during the period of hospitalisation. This evidence-based, best practice model supported babies being in the same room as the mother to maximize bonding and facilitate breastfeeding. However, there was also a 'continuous and variable'[14] demand on staff to move between rooms and patients with conditions of varying acuity to deliver care as well as deliver important educative information.

Comments

The coroner was clear that 'the safety of the child and the reduction of the risks of accidental suffocation must be paramount.'[15] He made the following key points:

1. The mother had a very disturbed night in the postnatal ward, following the previous night's labour and early morning admission. Although there was no evidence that the mother was sedated, she was 'clearly exhausted.'[16]
2. No specific warning was given to the mother before the baby was placed with her for breastfeeding. Educational programmes were available to mothers, but there should have been some advice given by the midwife to a new mother to take care and call for assistance if either she or the baby were becoming sleepy.
3. The midwife was very experienced, and neither incompetent nor avoiding work. She was aware of the risks of SIDS, but not specifically aware of the hospital policy, and did not follow the protocol of monitoring at 15 -to 30-minute intervals. She had exercised her judgement in considering whether the mother and baby should be in bed together. The problem was that due to pressures of work on a very busy shift, she did not get back to the mother and baby who were left unobserved for one and three quarter hours.
4. The coroner supported the proposed review of patient/ staff ratio where babies are counted as patients rather than grouped with the mother as one patient.
5. The practice of care pathways being documented with various prompts and guides had taken over from detailed chart notes. Extra cues could

assist staff and family: for example, 'cot card' placed externally on cots reminding parents and staff of risk factors and best practice to promote a safe environment for the baby.

6. Another safety measure would be an 'easy to use' section in the care chart to record the time and physical location of the baby each time there is observation/interaction with the mother.

7. There is a risk when mother and baby are asleep in the same bed, but much to be gained by breastfeeding in bed, provided safety can be assured. Safety requires an informed choice. Some factors are too risky: when the mother is obese, a smoker, alcohol, drug or medication affected or exceedingly tired. The hospital had adopted a safe position by not recommending co-sleeping, but supporting breastfeeding in bed when it is safe to do so.

8. Hyper-linking the policy documents for staff, so they can associate/consider both risks and benefits of having the baby in bed with the mother, would be helpful.

9. Education of parents and medical and midwifery staff was critically important. Education should commence in the community before the child is born, be reinforced and physically demonstrated in hospital, and be available postnatally in the community. Resources need to be available to support this process.

....

In 2008, a Tasmanian coroner,[17] summarising the findings of investigations into the deaths of four infants in Australian hospitals, made the following comments in relation to bed-sharing in hospital:

1. Major public and private maternity hospitals require staff to reinforce the correct and consistent safe sleeping message to parents through demonstration and discussions.

2. All hospitals require documentation of such discussions. One hospital required that staff complete an Incident Report form if a parent is noted to be bed-sharing with the baby.

3. The policy of one private hospital was that parents do not sleep with their baby in hospital, nor later when they take the baby home.

4. In at least two hospitals safe sleeping instructions were attached to the cot.

5. Hospitals identified the need for adequate funding to ensure staff are educated regularly, informed of new developments and research, and

are fully trained and equipped to provide correct and consistent information to parents.

6. SIDS information indicated that 30-33 per cent of midwives in two
states incorrectly placed babies on their sides to sleep.

Multiple activities. The coroner said that new mothers not only need to
recover from birth but have to undertake multiple activities and tasks in hospital. They are provided with a large amount of information in a relatively
short time. As some mothers are young, have substance abuse issues or are
not well educated, and may have literacy problems, information and advice
may not be absorbed.

Removal of risk factors. Therefore, despite demonstration and repeti-
tion of correct safe sleeping practices by hospital staff, there is a need to
ensure that the same information is correctly and consistently repeated both
antenatally and post-discharge.

By removing known risk factors and providing a safe sleeping environment, most sleep-related deaths are preventable.

....

The following case concerns the discharge and post-discharge care of a premature baby who had lost weight on two occasions when solely breastfed in
hospital. The coroner emphasised the need for clear and unambiguous written and verbal communication between hospitals and the nursing agencies
taking over care. Note that in a case so focused on lactation issues, there is
no evidence that midwives (as lactation consultants) were called as expert
witnesses.

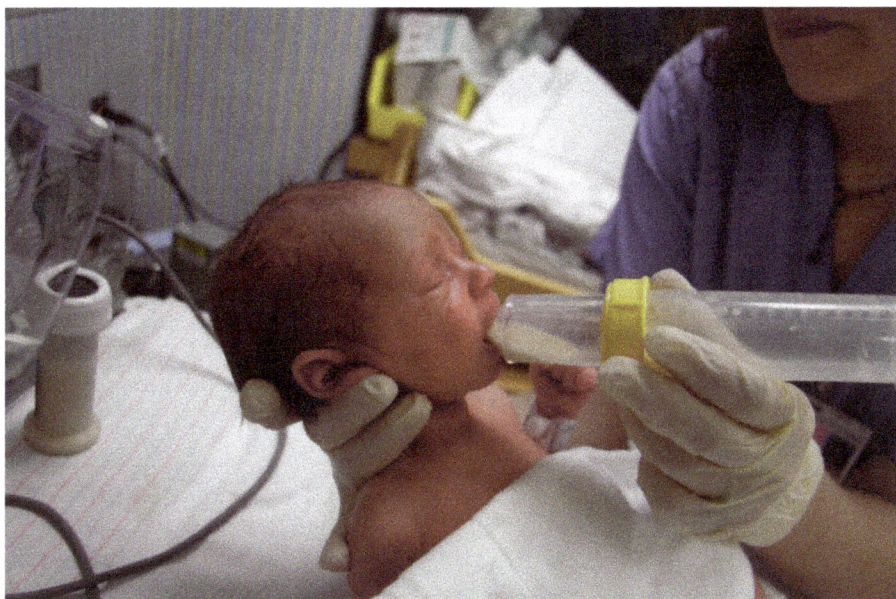

Coronial Investigation [Aus, 2002][18]

The facts

Catherine's baby, a girl, was born on 22 April 1999 with an estimated gestation of 32 weeks, 6 days. Hospital records showed the baby's weight as 1852 g, length 42 cm. The baby was transferred to the NICU, becoming mildly jaundiced the following day. The baby was discharged from hospital on 18 May with a weight of 2175 g, having lost a small amount of weight during two rooming-in periods, when she was solely breastfed.

On 29 May, the baby was breast fed at home at about 4 am. Shortly afterwards Catherine found her to be cold and unresponsive. Resuscitation attempts by paramedics were unsuccessful.

Autopsy

The cause of death could not be ascertained, but the pathologist's findings included prematurity, failure to thrive and aspiration of stomach contents into lungs. The autopsy weight was 2136 g.

The inquest

It was submitted that the baby's death was due to:

1. premature discharge from hospital.
2. failure of the hospital to put a proper discharge plan in place and failure to communicate with community agencies.
3. failure of treatment by community agencies.

Premature discharge. Having heard detailed expert medical opinion, the coroner concluded that the discharge from hospital was premature but 'whilst less than optimal,'[19] had not of itself contributed the baby's death. Had adequate post-discharge follow-up arrangements been instituted, it was unlikely the baby would have died.

Follow-up arrangements

The post discharge plan. A social worker had arranged for visits by a number of nursing agencies and telephone contact with a social worker, plus a medical follow-up at the hospital on 31 May.

How the plan was implemented

Tuesday 18 May.	The baby was discharged from hospital at approximately 1pm.
Wednesday 19 May.	The Royal District Nursing Service (RDNS) visited and was advised by Catherine that a maternal and child health nurse (M&CH) had arranged a home visit the following day. RDNS made a decision not to admit the family to their service and no physical examination of the baby was carried out, nor was she weighed. The RDNS nurse said that had the appointment not been made with M&CH, the following day she would have asked for consent for a full check-up with mother and baby, with a plan to come back in a couple of days. The baby would have been weighed and a baseline established.

Thursday 20 May.   Catherine returned to the hospital to collect an iron supplement. A midwife employed by a community health agency visited at approximately midday, stripped the baby and observed her in the natural light. A further visit was arranged on Thursday 27 May. An appointment was arranged for a M&CH home visit on Monday 24 May.

Friday 21 May—
Sunday 23 May.   No health professionals visited.

Monday 24 May.   M&CH telephoned Catherine to cancel the home visit. A further appointment was arranged for Tuesday 25 May at 3.30 pm.

Tuesday 25 May.   M&CH visited at 3.30 pm. Baby remained asleep and was not weighed. A visit to the M&CH Centre was planned for Friday 28 May at 4.30 pm.

Wednesday 26 May.   No contact with any health professional.

Thursday 27 May.   Visit by community health agency.

Friday 28 May.   Baby examined at M&CH Centre. Baby weighed 2150 grams.

Saturday 29 May.   Baby found unresponsive at approximately 5.30 am.

Review of evidence about implementation of plan

The paediatrician. The hospital paediatrican said that she expected the RDNS to look after the baby over the first week until the M&CH service became involved. She expected both agencies would be involved in making sure the baby was weighed, but did not ask who would do the weighing.

The discharge co-ordinator. The discharge co-ordinator at the hospital said she understood that the RDNS would provide service until uptake by M&CH. She expected the baby to be weighed by the RDNS on 19 May and anticipated a base weigh would be established and thereafter regular weighing would take place.

The mother. Catherine said she believed that she would be receiving care from both the RDNS and the M&CH, and that these services would communicate with each other.

The coroner found that:

- The mother was not aware that the engagement of RDNS was a matter to be negotiated between herself and RDNS, and that she would be liable for RDNS fees.
- A referral had been made to the RDNS, but after their initial visit and in the belief that care was to be assumed by M&CH within 24 hours, the baby had not been admitted to that service. (The court heard that the RDNS protocol provided that the two agencies did not run a duplicate or parallel service.)
- The M&CH nurse was aware that as of 20 May, RDNS were not to be further involved.

Telephone call. The coroner found that individual accounts of a telephone conversation between the discharge coordinator and the M&CH nurse on the day of the baby's discharge varied.

The discharge co-ordinator. The discharge co-ordinator said it was normal practice to try to contact the M&CH nurse by telephone to say that a baby would be discharged in a couple of days. She had telephoned the M&CH nurse about the baby on the day of discharge and expressed 'our concerns'[20] about the weight after breast-feeding; she had stressed the need to support the mother in her desire to fully breast feed her baby.

> *Having made known these concerns, I expected that [the M&CH nurse] would visit early in the week following discharge and weigh the baby as that was her responsibility.*[21]

The discharge co-ordinator said she had told the M&CH nurse that the baby was having breast-feeding difficulties and that weight gains had been static or poor.

> *I actually told her, I think, that the baby had lost 25 grams or some-thing like that.*[22]

There was no record of this conversation.

The M&CH nurse. The M&CH nurse said she was advised by the discharge co-ordinator by telephone on 18 May, that the baby was to be discharged that morning. She recalled being told that the baby had feeding problems, but was not given any details, nor had there been any mention of weight loss. An early home visit had been suggested. Had there been mention of weight loss, she would have asked why the hospital was sending the baby home, as there were not adequate community resources to deal with such a baby. She agreed that a request for an early home visit within a day or two indicated the hospital had concerns. There was no record of this telephone conversation, as the M&CH nurse's daily running sheets had been lost due to the closure of the Centre.

The plan and its communication

The coroner found that the success of the discharge plan was dependent upon the nature of the information provided, as well as the manner in which it was provided. Nurses in the community examining the baby should have been provided with a detailed copy of the discharge summary, the weight and what was expected of the baby in terms of weight gain. Specific changes in weight leading up to discharge should have been included in the summary, along with specific problems associated with feeding. Telephone contact was important.

> *This was a baby losing weight and clearly not established on a sole-ly breast fed regime. … Too much weight was placed on detection by the community nursing agencies and they had not been provid-ed with a full feeding history or weight changes.*[23]

The visit to the M&CH Centre on 28 May

The M&CH nurse. The M&CH nurse said Catherine had arrived late for her 4.30 pm appointment. She had appeared anxious, saying the baby was due for a feed. On examination, the nurse had found the baby sleepy, heart rate of 140 regular, lungs clear; pupils equal and reacting to light. Reflexes were consistent with a premature baby. Catherine said the baby was feeding six or more times over 24 hours, and had wet and dirty nappies.

Weight decrease. There had been a weight decrease of 25 g since discharge (ten days earlier) but the nurse said she was not concerned as the baby was due for a feed. This could make a difference of 100 g in weight in small babies. There had also been plenty of nappies and adequate skin turgor – both indicators of adequate nourishment.

Early visit arranged. The nurse said she had arranged to see the baby in four days instead of the normal seven in order to assess weight and feeding. She had recorded 'nil gain' in her records, and a weight loss of 25 g in the *Child Health Record Book.* She did not inform the mother of the weight loss.

The mother. Catherine said that the M&CH nurse had explained that premature babies often have a slow start to life and to 'feed her up and it will be fine.'[24] She had asked the nurse whether the baby should be tested for jaundice and suggested driving immediately to the hospital. The nurse had insisted that there was nothing to worry about and that she would make an earlier appointment. As the baby had sneezed and was due for a feed, the nurse had urged her to 'go straight home and feed (the baby).'[25] She had done so, then fed the baby again between 5.30 pm and 7.30 pm, at 10 pm, at midnight, and lastly at 4 am. Catherine said no one told her the baby had lost weight.

Conversation between discharge coordinator and M&CH nurse

The discharge co-ordinator said she had telephoned the M&CH nurse following the baby's death. The M&CH nurse said that she had noted the heart rate to be normal, but also that the peripheral circulation was down. The baby had been very sleepy. There had been a weight loss of 25 g after discharge. She thought the mother might have been overhandling the baby and that it had some reduced responsiveness.

Medical expert. A doctor giving expert evidence said that the baby, who had not been weighed between discharge on 18 November and 28 November, should have been weighed at least within three days of discharge. There should have been regular follow-up visits. The post-discharge weight loss should have alerted the M&CH nurse that urgent medical attention was required and the baby returned very rapidly to hospital. The comments that the baby was 'due for a feed'[26] and that 'this could make a difference of 100 g'[27] were assumptions. The infant had lost weight. 'Peripheral circulation down'[28] could mean that the infant was cold, or being debilitated from having to work hard to maintain its adequate nutrition. The baby, in the medical expert's opinion, was becoming exhausted.

Having acknowledged that the test of causation is solely a factual inquiry and questions of blameworthiness or culpability do not enter into it, the coroner found:

1. The premature discharge, whilst less than optimal, did not of itself contribute to the baby's death.
2. The discharge plan and communication of that plan were plainly inadequate. Had adequate post-discharge follow-up arrangements been instituted, it was unlikely the baby would have died.
3. Had the discharge plan included medical review at the hospital, perhaps within three days and certainly no more than seven, the failure to thrive would have been detected.
4. Had arrangements been made for weight results to be returned to the hospital within the first 48 hours and thereafter at regular intervals, the same result would have been achieved.
5. Had greater attention been paid to ensuring each of the agencies was aware of their specific roles and functions, and all relevant information provided to them, the failure to thrive would likely have been identified.
6. Had the mother been informed of the weight loss prior to discharge, had she been aware of the importance of weighing her baby and counselled as to signs indicative of failure to thrive, she would have taken steps to ensure the baby was weighed and sought medical advice.
7. Had the M&CH nurse weighed the baby on 25 May and recognised that it needed immediate medical attention on 28 May, it was likely death would have been avoided.

....

In the last of the coronial cases a baby was weaned from the breast and then fed on rice milk and dietary supplements. The coroner, investigating why the parents delayed seeking medical assistance when the baby was clearly critically ill, found the baby's death represented 'from any perspective, a tragedy beyond comprehension.'[29] This case supports the necessity for early education of mothers in relation to breast milk substitutes.

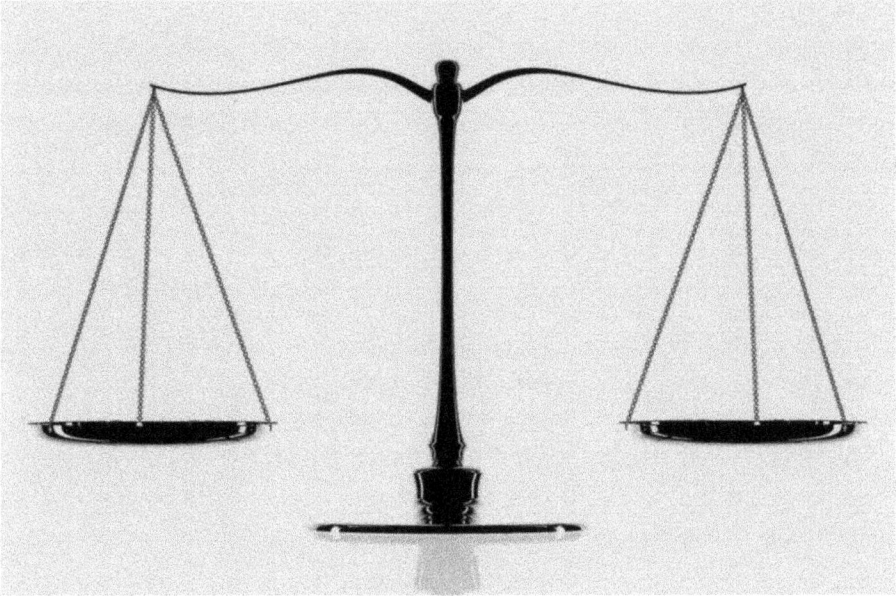

Coronial Inquest [Aus, 2003][30]

The facts

Hannah gave birth to her first child on 8 July 2000, then returned to work immediately at her husband's chiropractic clinic. A M&CH nurse visited mother and baby at the clinic, finding that the development of the baby, who was breastfed, was satisfactory on the first two visits.

The substituted feed. On the 9 August visit, Hannah told the nurse that she had concerns about baby formula. She explained that she was allergic to the traditional formula, so had begun substituting one breastfeed per day with an imported American rice milk product.

Hannah also told her doctor on a routine visit about the substituted feed. When people expressed reservations about the nutritional value of the rice milk, Hannah replied that on advice from a naturopath associated with the chiropractic clinic, she was adding vitamin and mineral supplements to the product.

Good developmental growth. On 4 September, the M&CH nurse examined the baby, who was still being breastfed, again noting good developmental growth.

Rice milk warning. Around about mid-September, a friend who was a doctor told Hannah that the label on the rice milk warned that the product contained 0.002 per cent barley protein and was not appropriate as an infant formula. Hannah said she was still breastfeeding and adding nutritional supplements to the rice milk.

M&CH visit. On 16 October, the M&CH nurse examined the baby for the last time. Again she found her progressing well. Hannah said she was feeding the baby breast milk, expressed breast milk and also the rice milk product.

Weaning. In late October, Hannah's milk supply diminished and the baby was weaned. It appeared she was then fed solely on rice milk and two herbal additives – Life Spring Colloidal Minerals and Lifestart Original Powder. About this time, Hannah sought informal advice from a kinesiologist as well as a naturopath associated with the clinic (no details of their advice were given in the coronial report).

Thrush. On 30 October, Hannah took the baby to a doctor, who found she had thrush at the mouth, neck and under the nappy. The doctor advised Hannah to bring the baby back if the thrush did not clear up in five days, as there could be an underlying condition of which thrush was just a symptom. She did not return.

Pharmacist concerned. A pharmacist said that during the November to early December period she had been concerned about the amount of anti-fungal cream purchased for what Hannah had described as 'nappy rash.'[31] The pharmacist said she could not recall suggesting that Hannah seek medical advice for the apparent persistence of the rash.

Deterioration. By the end of November, both parents noticed their baby had ceased smiling and laughing, and no longer made baby noises. Then Hannah's father-in-law, with whom they stayed early in December on an interstate visit, expressed concern that the baby appeared somewhat malnourished. A mothers' group to which Hannah belonged also noticed a deterioration in the baby's condition during December. These mothers were to later describe the baby as pale, inactive, lethargic, quiet and generally unwell.

Emergency. On 16 December, at approximately 10.40 pm, the parents took the baby to the emergency department of a regional hospital. A doctor found the baby, who had a widespread weeping rash and was patently oedematous, to be critically ill. A consultant paediatrician was called in. The paediatrician considered that the parents did not seem to appreciate how ill their daughter was, even though he told them she was very weak and could die.

By 18 December, the doctors, now gravely concerned, arranged for the baby's transfer to a children's hospital, where her care was co-ordinated by a consultant paediatrician.

Child protection. On 21 December, the paediatrician who had originally seen the baby at the regional hospital made a child protection notification. The basis of concern was that the baby had suffered significant harm as a result of inappropriate infant feeding and there had been an unexplained delay in seeking appropriate medical attention. This led to her presentation at the emergency department in a critical condition.

ICU. During the period in ICU at a children's hospital, the baby developed renal failure requiring haemofiltration, septic shock requiring high dose inotropes and continuing mechanical ventilation. She was also treated with antibiotics, antifungal agents and immunoglobulin, together with ongoing internal support provided intravenously.

Grave condition. On 25 December, Hannah told a social worker at the hospital that her husband had conducted a 'muscle test'[32] the previous evening and concluded the baby would be fully recovered in two weeks. Hannah's husband said he believed that an energy balancing technique, with which he had been treating his daughter, would contribute to her healing. The coroner believed that at this stage the parents still did not appreciate their baby's grave condition. The baby died on 26 December.

Manslaughter. The parents were charged with manslaughter. A magistrate at the committal hearing (to determine whether there was sufficient evidence to support the charge) found there was insufficient evidence on which a jury could find them guilty of gross negligence to warrant criminal sanctions:

There was too much disparate advice accepted at face value by the parents with ill-founded confidence.[33]

Findings

The coroner found that Hannah and her husband did cause the death of their daughter :

In breach of a fundamental duty of care they failed to ensure their infant child was adequately nourished resulting in severe protein energy malnutrition a deficiency resulting in disseminated candidiasis.[34]

The other basis upon which, in combination, the parents were in breach of their duty to the baby was the inordinate delay in seeking appropriate medical attention after it became, or should have become clear, that due to her perilous condition, the baby required specialist treatment.

The baby's death represents, from any perspective, a tragedy beyond comprehension.[35]

The coroner found that the rice milk product did contain a warning against feeding a child exclusively on the product and concluded by endorsing the magistrate's comment at the committal hearing :

I also hope the publicity surrounding this case will alert parents, and all health professionals, to the dangers of feeding alternative substances to infants without the supervision or advice of a qualified paediatrician or expert in the field of infant nutrition.[36]

....

In the first of the last two cases in this chapter, an English judge had to decide if a baby should be tested for its HIV status against the parents' wishes. A second issue was whether breast milk from the HIV-positive mother could endanger the baby. In addressing that problem, the judge posed the question whether 'the law should come between the breast and the baby.'[37]

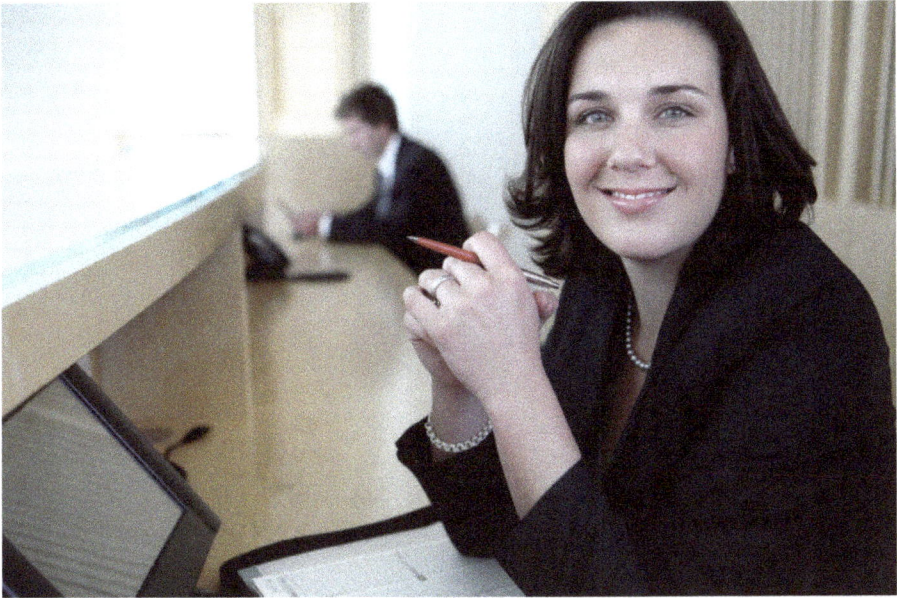

In Re C (a child) (HIV test) [UK, 1999][38]

The facts

Paula, aged 23, was devastated when her partner revealed that he was HIV-positive and she then tested positive. Their relationship finished. Paula remained in good health and read widely about HIV/AIDS. She rejected mainstream medical treatment, concentrating instead on a healthy diet and keeping fit. In 1997, Paula formed a relationship with Leon, who tested negative for HIV. Leon, who practiced in the holistic health area, also rejected conventional testing and treatment for HIV/AIDS.

Contrary to accepted opinion. The following year Paula became pregnant. Contrary to medical advice, she did not take recommended medication late in the pregnancy, nor did she have a caesarean section. Instead, and contrary to accepted opinion, she had a water birth at home (attended by a midwife) and breast-fed her baby.

Medical record. Paula's medical record had been transferred to a new GP, who had not read it prior to examining the baby during a routine developmental check. On later discovering Paula's HIV status, the GP contacted her and expressed grave concern about Paula continuing to breast-feed. The GP also wanted the baby tested for HIV.

Resistance. Paula and Leon remained resistant to all medical advice on HIV, including the administration of prophylactic antibiotics. The health authority then sought a court order that the baby be tested to determine its HIV status.

The hearing

The health authority argued that the result of a test, whether positive or negative, would enable doctors to provide advice to the parents as to whether their baby remained asymptomatic or would develop symptoms of the disease.

Parental autonomy. Paula and Leon argued that they were devoted parents who knew a great deal about HIV/AIDS and saw the court proceedings as an affront to their parental autonomy. In their view, all available tests had a degree of inaccuracy and, in any event, the results would not alter their stance. They did not believe the 'so-called virus'[39] was transmissible by breast-feeding.

Parental rights. The judge acknowledged that a court must move with extreme caution in the area of parental rights. The views of parents, looked at widely and generously, were an important factor in decision-making. To over-rule their wishes was to risk causing emotional distress to a degree that could affect their ability to care for their baby and so, indirectly, affect the baby's emotional stability. In this case, the parents (who were far from alone in their dissent from mainstream opinion) 'clung to their theories with the intensity of the shipwrecked mariner who clings to the plank of wood.'[40]

Proposed treatment. But having heard detailed medical evidence about the nature of tests and treatment for HIV/ AIDS, the judge concluded that if the baby was not tested and developed an illness, a treating doctor who knew of the possibility of infection would have to cater for that possibility. If the baby was uninfected, proposed treatment could be unduly aggressive.

The baby's rights. On the other hand, if a doctor did not know of the possibility and the baby was infected, the treatment could be dangerously slight. The case, at its heart, was not about the rights of parents. The rights of a tiny baby were not subsumed within the rights of parents. The baby had rights of its own acknowledged by the Children's Act 1989 and internationally under the U.N. Convention on the Rights of the Child 1989.

The order

Testing. The judge concluded that the case for testing the baby was overwhelming and made an order to that effect. The Court of Appeal refused the parents permission to appeal.

Breastfeeding. The judge then turned to the issue of Paula continuing to breast-feed the baby. Both Paula and Leon believed there was no risk of transmission of the 'so-called virus' [41] through breast-feeding. Paula said she would continue to breast-feed until it felt right not to do so.

Advantages/disadvantages of breast-feeding. The judge acknowledged the advantages of breast-feeding and said that if the baby was already infected the breast-feeding should probably continue. But unanimous medical opinion was convincing. If the baby was not infected, breast-feeding should cease. On the evidence, there was a 20 and 25 per cent chance that the baby was already infected.

The health authority made it clear that the court was not being asked to order the mother not to breast-feed her baby, however misguided her stance.

The judge concluded that there would be no point in doing so:

My belief is that the law cannot come between the baby and the breast. Indeed, if she cannot be persuaded by rational argument that she must curb her natural instinct to feed, I doubt whether the mother would comply with a court order, which would be, in effect impossible to enforce.[42]

The judge concluded with the hope that the parents would respond better to the judgment when they realised that it had intellectual merit and the case was out of the spotlight.

....

Eight years later, in 2007, an Australian judge found the law could come between the breast and the baby. In this case, the Department of Community Services in New South Wales (the department) commenced urgent proceedings eleven days before a baby was due to be born, seeking orders that (a) the baby be separated from its HIV-infected mother immediately after birth, (b) that the baby be treated against her express wishes and (c) that the mother not be allowed to breastfeed. This application was made in the woman's absence (ex parte). Doctors feared that if she were aware of the orders, she would not come to the hospital (or any hospital) for the birth and necessary drugs would not be available to treat the baby. Instead, the mother would be notified of the orders shortly after giving birth.

While this case appeared in *Chapter 2 Consent*, it is included again in this chapter to facilitate discussion about how the lactation issues were resolved.

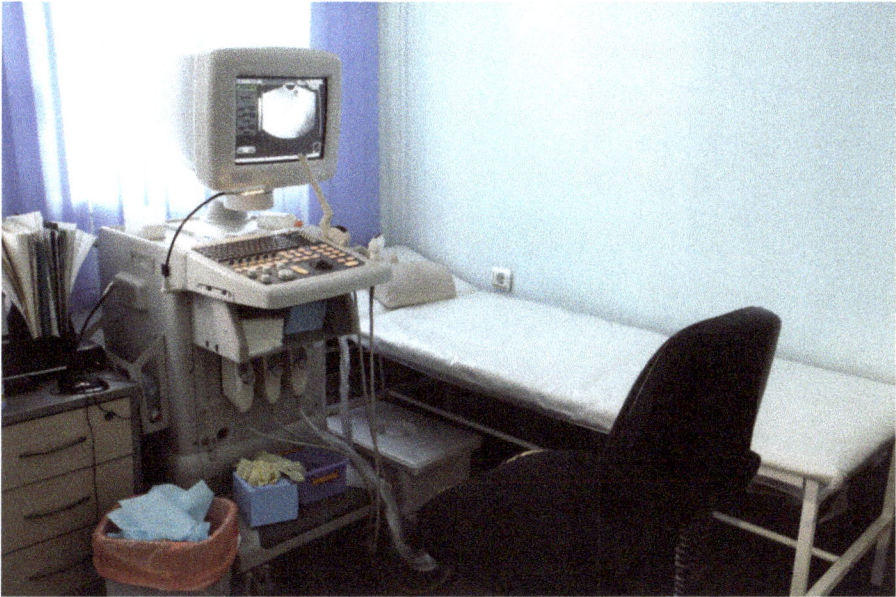

In Re Elm [2006] NSWSC 1137[43]

The facts

Illya arrived in Australia from a refugee camp in Africa in 2002. She later became pregnant, tested positive for HIV and was due to give birth on 22 September 2006. Illya initially agreed to take medication but ceased doing so in March, believing that God had cured her and would protect her child. An interview with officers of the department established that Illya did not know who the father of the baby was, appeared to have limited social networks, was on social security payments and had no family in Australia. It was also unlikely that she would be able to continue in the accommodation she shared with a male friend after the baby was born. (A decision on 1 September to appoint a public guardian for her under the Mental Health Act 1990 (NSW) was revoked on 4 September 2006.)

During a further interview with department officers on 5 September, Illya maintained that she would not agree to either herself or her baby taking anti-HIV medication, nor would she undergo a caesarean section. She did not believe that the baby would require on-going medical treatment and monitoring, and did not intend to breast-feed. She did not appear to have made arrangements about the baby's needs or alternative accommodation after the birth. Illya maintained that God had healed and would protect her.

Medical history. The judge found that Illya, despite her belief to the contrary, was still HIV positive. Her blood viral load had risen from a low 49 copies/ml on 6 March 2006 (shortly before she ceased taking medication) to more than 100,000 (the highest that can be reported) on 30 March. By 27 July she had a low CD4 count of about 270/ml, and a high viral load of about 83,900 copies/ml. Given her refusal to take anti-HIV medication or to permit her baby to do so, there was a serious risk that the baby would contract HIV from her at birth. This was a risk which would be reduced if she did not have a vaginal birth, and/or consented to the baby receiving anti-HIV medication at birth and for the following four weeks.

Risk element. Having regard for Illya's high viral load and low CD4 count, as well as her refusal to undergo an elective caesarean section, the risk to the baby of contracting HIV was about 50-70 per cent if no anti-HIV treatment was given at birth nor breast milk given. If anti-HIV treatment was commenced as soon as possible after the birth and maintained, the risk would fall to about 10-15 per cent. If the baby received breast milk from the infected mother, that risk would double, to about 20-30 per cent. Given that Illya intended to bottlefeed the baby, but refused to undergo a caesarean section (unless there were obstetric complications), there was the potential for a risk of HIV infection in the baby being reduced from as high as 70 per cent to as low as 10 per cent, if appropriate medical treatment was commenced promptly after birth.

Treatment of baby. The judge heard that the director of NICU at the hospital where Illya was to give birth had sought advice from an expert in the area of mother-to-child HIV transmission, and developed a protocol. The protocol provided for the baby to be washed thoroughly in the delivery suite, commenced on lamivudine syrup and nevirapine syrup, then admitted to NICU where an IV line would be introduced for a blood test, and the administration of zidovudine and vitamin K begun. The baby would then be transferred to the special care nursery and was not to receive breast milk. A second blood test would be performed 48 hours after birth. These steps were to begin as a matter of urgency as soon as possible after the birth, to reduce the risk of serious damage from HIV infection.

Common law rights

The judge found that as the right of a competent adult to refuse medical treatment (whether the reasons for doing so are rational or irrational, unknown or even non-existent')[44] is not diminished by pregnancy, an unborn baby's need for medical treatment does not prevail over the rights of the mother.[45] In these circumstances a court could not order Illya to undergo treatment necessary to save the life and health of the baby. However, the baby, once born, was a separate entity and entitled to the full protection of the law.

Protection of the baby. In order to protect the baby's rights, the department sought a number of orders including :

1. that the baby could be treated from birth by a doctor (the director of neonatal intensive care) against the mother's wishes – or, alternatively,
2. that the director of the department could assume care responsibility of the baby from birth (thereby having authority to consent to medical treatment recommended, notwithstanding the mother's refusal) and
3. an injunction prohibiting the mother breastfeeding from birth or removing the baby from the hospital without written approval.

Statutory authority. The judge found sections of the Children and Young Persons Care and Protection Act 1998 (NSW) were relevant in that they:

- authorized a doctor to carry out necessary and urgent medical treatment on a child without parental consent in order to save that child's life or prevent serious damage.
- authorized the director general of the department to (a) assume the care and responsibility of a child at risk of serious harm and (b) consent to medical treatment on the advice of a medical practitioner (notwithstanding that any other person who may have parental responsibility for the child does not consent, or refuses to consent).

Orders. The judge authorized the director general of the department to assume the care responsibility of the baby, including the authority to consent to medical treatment on the advice of a doctor (the director of NICU). The treatment was urgent. It was to be instituted immediately after the birth and administered continually for the following four weeks.

The judge further ordered that after the birth of the baby, the mother be prohibited from (a) breastfeeding (directly or indirectly) or (b) removing the baby from the hospital or any other hospital in New South Wales where she gave birth, without the written approval of the director general.

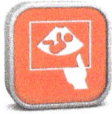

Discussion of Key Issues

Coronial investigation. (1) and *(2)* concern deaths of babies following hypoxic episodes during breastfeeding. Investigation *(3)* summarises the findings of investigations into four infant deaths – the majority relating to bed-sharing.

The mothers were variously described as 'very drowsy, 'extremely tired', 'extraordinarily tired', 'exhausted' and 'clearly exhausted.' If coroners acknowledge that midwives are the best judges of a mother's capacity to breastfeed:

- How do you assess a mother's 'tiredness'?
- How would you describe this process to a court?
- Do you agree that the 'general education' of mothers is not the responsibility of night staff?
- How often are midwives unaware of the nature and duration of a mother's labour because they have not had time to read the chart in detail? Do you see this as a risk?
- If so, how would you grade the risk?
- How would you reduce the risk?

The paediatrician compared the 'old practice' when mothers stayed in hospital for 4-5 days and nurseries were available to care for babies of tired mothers, with the 'new practice' of staying in hospital for 2.1 days. A midwife gave evidence that babies are the responsibility of the mother.

- As a generalization, which system best looks after the needs of new mothers/new babies?

- How would you support your views to a court?
- Give reasons – for and against – babies being counted as patients rather than grouped with the mother as one patient.
- Do your records have an 'easy to use' section in the care chart to record the time and physical location of the baby each time there is an observation/interaction with the mother?
- Would you add/subtract any factor from the risk list of mothers who should not breast-feed unsupervised?
- Are you surprised by the SIDS information (2008) that 30 to 33 per cent of midwives in two states incorrectly placed babies on their sides to sleep?

....

Coronial investigation. (4) There are many issues to discuss in this case concerning the early discharge of a baby who had lost weight in hospital, and was then not weighed for ten days.

For example, the court heard that the widely accepted guideline was 1800 − 2000 grams as minimum discharge weight, assuming a gestational age of 36 − 38 weeks, if the baby can:

1. maintain a normal temperature in an open cot,
2. feed satisfactorily and gain weight and
3. the mother (or parents) can care for the baby satisfactorily.

Expert medical opinion :

1. The paediatrician said it was rare to discharge a baby below 2000 grams. The hospital did not set a fixed minimum weight on post-conceptional age for discharge.
2. In one medical expert's opinion, the timing of discharge is not related to the baby's weight but more to its general condition and feeding capacity. Two reasons for delaying discharge would be the baby's failure to maintain body temperature and its failure to thrive.
3. Another medical expert believed weight gain is a very important factor in the discharge. Weight gain not only proves that the infant is maintaining its own integrity and getting adequate feeding, it also proves the general well-being of the infant.

4. The paediatrician explained that it is important that weight gain is steady and adequate in the week or so around discharge.
5. A medical expert said he would expect a baby to have a positive weight gain leading up to the day of discharge, to be feeding well from the breast every three-four hours, and that the mother was confident in handling the baby and keen to take it home.
   - Discuss the merits of each medical opinion.
   - Note (and discuss the possible reasons for) the lack of expert opinion from lactation consultants.

....

Coronial investigation. (5) Rice milk and dietary substances resulted in a baby's severe malnutrition, then death.

- What concerns (if any) have you had about a mother's proposed alternatives to breast milk or of planned dietary substances to be added to milk?
- Would your documentation demonstrate that you have discussed the matter of milk substitutes with the mother in hospital?
- How are your concerns communicated to M&CH nurses? Is this documented?

....

In *In Re C* and In *In Re Elm,* judges queried whether the law has any place 'between the breast and the baby.'

- How would you explain to a court the reasons for/against a HIV-positive mother continuing to breast- feed. When/why did a change of professional opinion occur?

Consider also what substances a breast-feeding mother might ingest.

- In what circumstances (if any) would you recommend that she stop breast-feeding?

The following concerns and answers about lactation issues were raised at midwifery and neonatal workshops I have facilitated.

- A mother being given the wrong baby to feed or a baby receiving the wrong stored milk.

Allegations of mix-ups and negligence have reached the media, if not the courtroom. Damage would lie in the transmission of infection (involving issues of causation), or the development of a phobic fear that a serious infection could occur. Hospitals must be able to demonstrate that checking procedures are in place, together with convincing evidence that they are followed.

- Have you known 'mix-ups' or 'near mix-ups' to occur? Discuss the circumstances.

Can you rely on the mother to recognise her baby?
    Apparently not! One midwife said she took a baby boy into a mother who fed, changed and cuddled the baby before handing him back. The mother had given birth to a girl. Or who would anticipate the father who, when walking his crying baby up and down the hospital corridors to allow his tired wife to sleep, was confronted by a woman in a dressing-gown who said: 'For heaven's sake give me the baby and I'll shut it up.' The father dutifully handed the baby over and it was promptly breast-fed in the corridor. (Presumably everyone settled down.)

....

Being accused of assault or battery after manually assisting with breast-feeding.
This is unlikely to succeed if the midwife has explained to the mother what is involved in that process (including possible discomfort) and the mother agrees. The mother is then verbally consenting to being touched in that way. A care plan could stipulate that such an explanation be given. Midwives may be unlikely to know if a mother has a history of sexual assault and sensitivity to being touched.

The mother signing a consent form for a complementary feed.
Mothers should be informed of current clinical concerns about 'breast to complementary' feeding and the fact that this information has been given can be documented. Whether a consent form adds anything to that process is debatable. Information on the dangers of 'breast to comp' given (and documented as having been given) during the antenatal period, and again in

hospital, should be sufficient to enable a mother to make an educated or 'informed' choice. You will recall that Chapter 2 included Lord Donaldson's caution to hospitals about producing forms for patients to sign that are in fact disclaimers of liability (to protect the hospital) rather than documents to inform patients about risk.

A signed consent form means little or nothing unless a balanced discussion about risk has first taken place. Midwives have commented that the purpose of the consent form can be to dissuade other midwives from giving the complementary feed without the mother's knowledge because it is quicker and allows a tired mother to sleep.

Pressure to breast-feed

M&CH nurses say new mothers have contacted them (having bought a bottle and formula on the way home from hospital) for advice about formula feeding. They explain they have no idea what to do and breast-fed in hospital 'to keep everyone happy.'

- However well-intentioned, do you think 'persuasion' can edge towards 'coercion' on this issue?

NOTES

1. *Inquest into Death,* No. COR 2145/05(7) (Brisbane).
2. *Record of Investigation into Death,* No. 1082/90 (Victoria).
3. Ibid., p.2.
4. No. COR 2145/05(7), p.12.
5. No. COR 2145/05(7).
6. Ibid., p.8.
7. Ibid.
8. Ibid.
9. Ibid.
10. Ibid., p.9.
11. Ibid.
12. Ibid.
13. Ibid., p.17.
14. Ibid., p.16.
15. Ibid., p.20.
16. Ibid., p.18.

17. *Record of Investigation into Deaths of Four Infants* www.magistratescourt.tas. gov.au/decisions/coronial_finding s.

18. *Record of Investigation into Death,* No. 1616/99 (Victoria, 2002).

19. Ibid., p.31.

20. Ibid., p.35.

21. Ibid.

22. Ibid.

23. Ibid., p.38.

24. Ibid., p.48.

25. Ibid.

26. Ibid., p.53.

27. Ibid.

28. Ibid.

29. *Record of Investigation into Death,* No. 4197/00 (Victoria, 2003) at p.8.

30. *Coronial Investigation Case,* No. 4197/00.

31. Ibid., p.3.

32. Ibid., p.5.

33. Ibid., p.8.

34. Ibid., p.8.

35. Ibid.

36. Ibid., p.9.

37. *In Re C (a child) (HIV Test),* 50 BMLR 383 Family Division.

38. *In Re C (a child).*

39. Ibid., p.286.

40. Ibid. p.293.

41. Ibid.

42. Ibid., p.294.

43. *In Re Elm,* NSWSC 1137 (2006).

44. *In Re T (adult:refusal of medical treatment)* 4 All ER 649 (1992) at 664.

45. *St George NHS Trust v S,* 3 All ER 673 (1998) at 691.

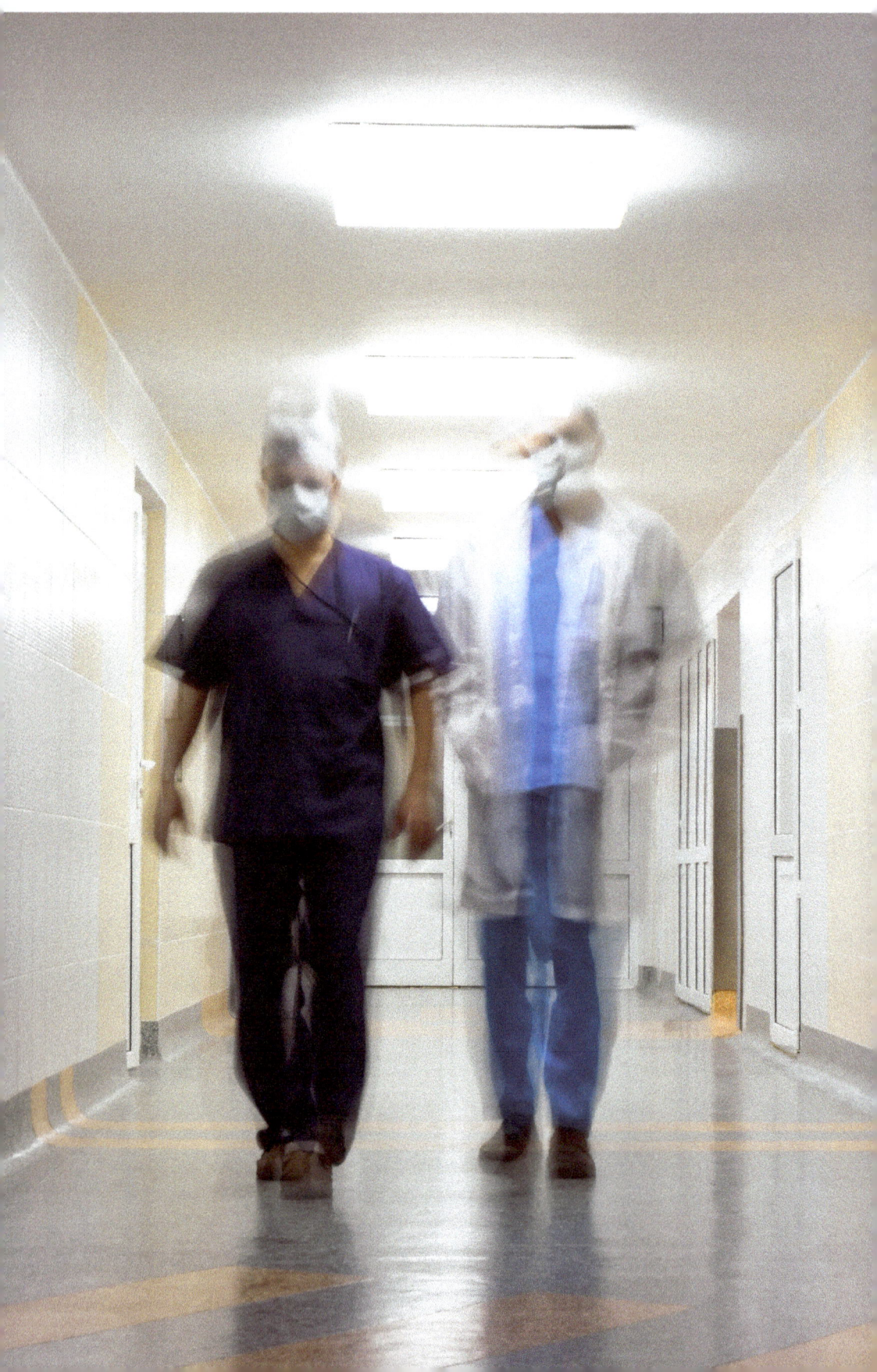

CHAPTER 13

Resuscitation and withdrawal of treatment

'We're in an environment where at 23 weeks, many of us do not believe that the aggressive treatment of babies with neonatal intensive care is necessarily in the baby's best interests.'

— Dr. Michael Stewart

Introduction

Amillia Taylor, an IVF baby born in the United States at 21 weeks and six days' gestation and weighing 280 grams, is reported to be the world's most premature baby to actually survive.[1] A newspaper report on Amillia Taylor's birth refers to the ethical dilemmas arising from the treatment of such a baby and cites a consensus statement based on a NSW and ACT workshop published in the *Medical Journal of Australia.* [2] This statement describes perinatal care at the borderlines of viability as demanding a delicate balance between parents' wishes and autonomy, biological feasibility, clinicians' responsibilities and expectations, and the prospects of an acceptable long-term outcome – coupled with a tolerable margin of uncertainty.

The statement indicates that in an otherwise normal infant born before 23 weeks, the prospect of survival is minimal and the risk of major morbidity so high that initiation of resuscitation is not appropriate.

Babies born between 23 weeks and 25 weeks and six days are described to be in a 'grey zone', where there is an increasing obligation to treat but it is acceptable medical practice not to initiate intensive care if that is the parents' wish. At 26 weeks and beyond, treatment should be initiated unless there are exceptional circumstances. Poor condition at birth and the presence of serious congenital anomalies have an important influence on any decision not to initiate intensive care within the grey zone.

Professor Lex Doyle of the Royal Women's Hospital in Melbourne, who has conducted wide-ranging research into the outcomes of premature babies at the hospital, is reported as saying:

If you have a baby born on time, you've got a 4 or 5 per cent chance that the child is going to have substantial problems. If you are at 23 weeks it's roughly half of them, at 24 weeks it's a third.[3]

The medical director of Victoria's Newborn Emergency Transport Service, Michael Stewart, was reported as being equally cautious:

We're in an environment where at 23 weeks, many of us do not believe that the aggressive treatment of babies with neonatal intensive care is necessarily in the baby's best interests.[4]

Nevertheless, Amillia's birth has prompted some doctors to say that there cannot be firm rules on the subject, just guidelines, and that these decisions must always be made with parents.

Loane Skene, Professor of Health Law at the University of Melbourne, writes that when assuming responsibility for the care of a patient, a doctor's duty is not to do everything possible to preserve life, but to act in accordance with good medical practice. That is, to take such steps as other reasonable doctors would have taken to save or prolong the patient's life in similar circumstances. Failure to treat, where there is a duty to treat, may be criminally negligent. It would appear that treatment may be lawfully withheld if it is futile to continue it, or if the burden imposed by the treatment exceeds the likely benefit; it is not then in the patient's best interests. Difficulties occur in relation to very young babies in determining what is 'futile' or 'burdensome', or when doctors and parents disagree about treatment or the withdrawal of treatment.[5]

Resuscitation and the decision whether to commence or withdraw treatment can therefore pose a number of difficulties, as explained in the *CCH Medical Health & Law Reporter*:[6]

- Scientific and medical advances have created a situation where many infants with congenital defects, immature organs or gross malformations (myelomeningocele, anencephaly and hydrocephaly) now survive birth for indeterminate periods.
- The policies of Australian hospitals vary as to the use of resuscitative efforts on malformed and very premature infants. Some are prepared to resuscitate all infants (except where gross malformations are present) over 23 weeks' gestation (weighing about 500g). Others will only attempt resuscitation in the case of infants weighing 700g or more. A variety of factors influence these policy decisions, not least the cost of care and availability of resources.

Survival after termination. The need for staff to have directions for the care of infants who survive terminations was noted by an Australian coroner during an investigation into the death of a baby in the Northern Territory.[7] The coroner found a protocol was lacking after a baby was unexpectedly born alive, having being induced at between 21 and 22 weeks' gestation.

According to a newspaper report at the time,[8] the midwife telephoned a doctor in charge of obstetric services at the hospital who, she said, gave no specific directions for care.[9] The midwife did what she could to care for the neonate, checking it every 10 to 15 minutes. After an hour, the heartbeat and breathing slowed. The baby died 80 minutes later.

The report noted that the coroner found the cause of death to be premature delivery, but that a 'responsibility vacuum'[10] had followed the birth. Despite the lack of medical direction, the midwife had acted humanely and was commended for this. It was recommended that hospitals put protocols in place to ensure that babies who survive terminations are immediately assessed for age and likelihood of survival. The coroner reiterated the principle that any baby born alive is entitled to value, respect, care and the protection of the law.

England

English paediatrician and medico-legal writer Professor Campbell writes that in the UK, any infant who is alive at birth has the full protection of the law.[11]

In Campbell's opinion, with very few exceptions infants of any gestational age, weight or apparent abnormality should be resuscitated if signs of life are present. Subsequent decisions about the wisdom of continuing life support should be the responsibility of the consultant, after discussion with the parents and other specialist colleagues, if indicated. Exceptions will include certain infants with gross abnormality of the CNS, such as anencephaly.

These problems have often been picked up in the antenatal period and discussions with parents should have included the appropriate care at birth. In such circumstances, there is then usually no justification for aggressive methods of resuscitation. The baby should receive all normal nursing attention with relief of apparent distress or discomfort until death.[12]

In 1990, an appeal court judge in England spoke of the checks and balances to be considered in coming to treatment decisions.

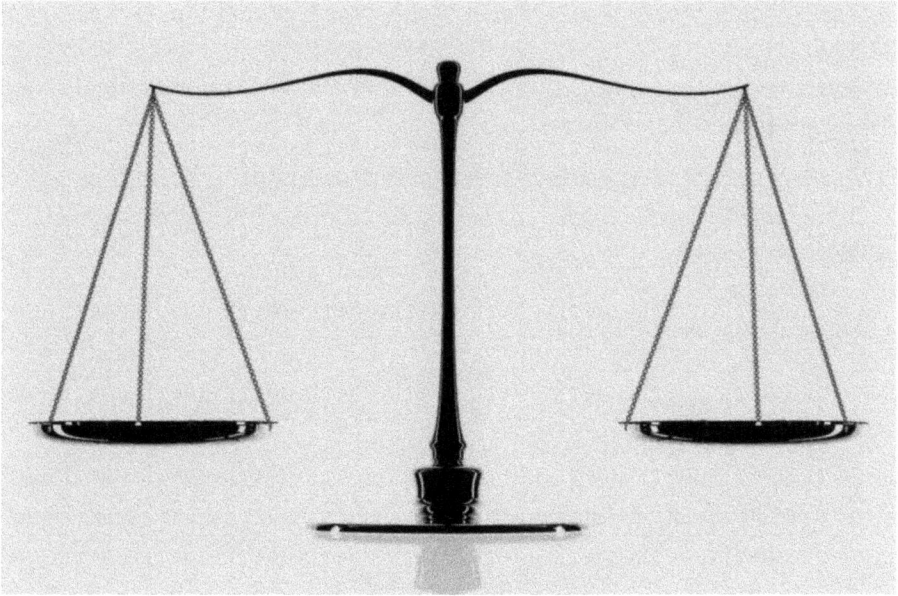

In Re J [UK, 1990][13]

The facts

Baby J was born 12 weeks premature in May 1990, weighing 1136g. He was not breathing and was severely brain damaged. The baby was placed on a ventilator, received antibiotics and remained oxygen-dependent until August, when he went home. Baby J was readmitted when he became cyanosed after choking.

Abysmally low baseline. During September, Baby J collapsed a number of times. He was resuscitated and put back on a ventilator. In late September, he began breathing independently. His condition slightly improved, but, as later described by a judge, 'from a baseline that could only be described as abysmally low.'[14] An ultrasound showed a large area of fluid-filled cavities where there ought to have been brain tissue.

Shortened life span. The court heard medical evidence that Baby J was likely to develop serious spastic quadriplegia, appeared to be blind, was likely to be deaf, might make some mood-reflecting sounds, but was unlikely to be able to speak or develop even limited intellectual abilities. He might be able to smile or cry, and it was likely he would feel pain in a normal way. His life expectancy, at most, was the late teens. Further ventilation in itself would involve the risk of deterioration. The treatment was described as 'invasive, unpleasant and distressing.'[15]

The first order. Baby J had been made a ward of the court. The judge, standing in place of the parents, then made an order in October authorizing medical treatment.

On appeal the court held that:

1. The doctors owed a duty to Baby J to care for him in accordance with good medical practice.
2. Because Baby J was a ward of the court, the choice of treatment was a joint decision of the doctors and the court instead of the parents and the doctor.
3. The right to choose a course of action which would fail to avert the death of a baby who is a ward of the court is that of the court. It is a choice which must be made solely on behalf of the baby and in what the court conscientiously believes to be his best interests, which are paramount.
4. The court and doctors had to decide whether, in the best interests of the baby, a particular decision as to treatment should be taken which, as a side effect, would render death more or less likely.
5. The court could never, even in the case of the most horrendous disability (that is, on a baby's inherent quality of life), sanction steps to terminate life and accelerate death; the court was only concerned with the circumstances in which steps should not be taken to prolong life.
6. Account had to be taken of the pain and suffering and quality of life which the baby would experience if life was prolonged; account also had to be taken of the pain and suffering involved in the proposed treatment itself. The correct approach was for the court to judge, in all the circumstances, whether the child's life would be so afflicted as to be intolerable for that child.

In Baby J's case:

Mechanical ventilation is in itself an invasive procedure which, together with its essential accompaniments, such as the introduction of a nasogastric tube, drips which have to be re-sited and constant blood sampling, would cause the child distress. Furthermore the procedures involve taking active measures which carry their own hazards, not only to life but in terms of causing even greater brain damage. This has to be balanced against what could possibly be achieved by the adoption of such active treatment.[16]

The three judges unanimously decided that it was in the best interests of the child that authority be withheld for reventilation if he stopped breathing. The court was not, in other words, authorising the withdrawal of treatment, but saying that if Baby J stopped breathing, he need not be resuscitated.

United States

No discrimination. In the United States, federal regulations govern the treatment of severely handicapped infants. Their purpose is to ensure that infants born with physical or intellectual handicaps are not discriminated against in being denied access to medical services. They require that all new-borns receive all possible treatment to prolong life.

Exemptions. The only infants who are exempt are those who are chronically and irreversibly comatose, or where the administration of treatment would not in any way ameliorate or correct the infant's condition; or where treatment would merely prolong life and, in the circumstances, be inhumane.[17]

Ethics questioned. Commentators have questioned the ethics of this type of statutory regulation which forces doctors to actively treat infants born with gross deformities instead of keeping them comfortable, without excessive treatment, to enable them to die peacefully.

U.S legal commentator Frank Rierdon, for example, writes that sometimes doctors refuse, in the face of a family's insistence, to treat, recognizing that their first and ultimate duty is to the patient's best interests.[18] Rierdon cites the case of Anthony MacDonald, which highlights this issue.

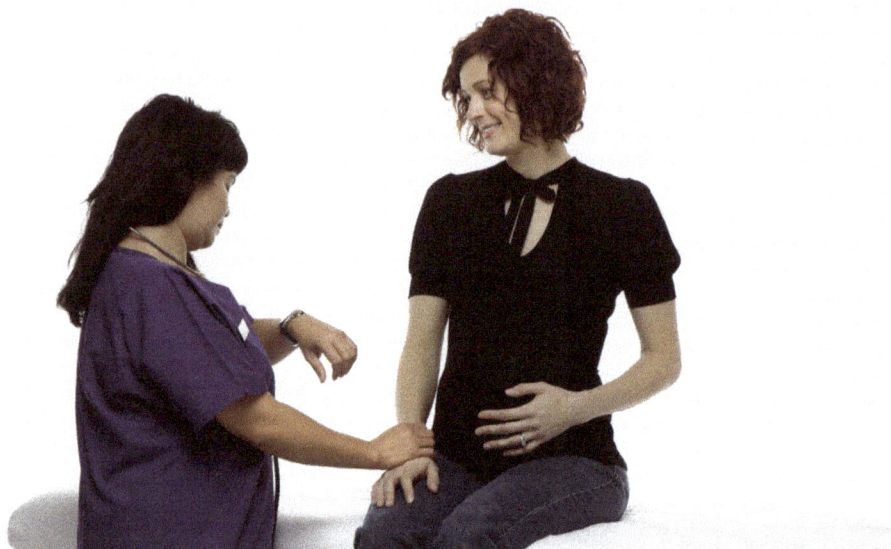

Anthony MacDonald, et al. v St Joseph's Hospital [US, 1989][19]

The facts

In 1989, Anthony's mother was rushed from Great Lakes Naval Hospital to St Joseph's Hospital, where at twenty-three and one-half weeks' gestation, she gave birth to Anthony. The baby was described as 'being small enough to fit in the palm of your hand with skin like wet tissue paper.' [20] After approximately 17 minutes of resuscitation with 100 per cent oxygen, the obstetrician was unable to get the heart rate above 50 to 60 beats per minute.

Admission to ICU. The parents were taken to a room to be alone with their baby. They were told he was not expected to survive beyond the next minutes to hours. But after being in the room for some time, Anthony suddenly cried out. He was rushed to neonatal intensive care and survived. At the time of the trial, Anthony was a severely retarded eight-year-old.

Arguments and allegations

Failure to provide oxygen. The parents alleged that the obstetrician had acted inappropriately by not providing Anthony with oxygen in the minutes following his birth. They argued that this failure led to oxygen deprivation with resulting neurological damage.

Infant too premature. Medical experts for the obstetrician disagreed. They said that such efforts were not successful in infants as premature as Anthony. To seek the consent of the parents to discontinue resuscitative efforts was not standard practice under these circumstances.

Rierdon comments that although the jury agreed with the obstetrician in Anthony's case, there is no assurance that another jury would do the same. The case had not led to an appeal court decision to guide doctors.

....

Parents took the opposite view about the resuscitation of their baby in the next case. On 8 February 1994, dermatologist Dr Gregory Messenger removed his premature infant son from a ventilator in the NICU at Sparrow Hospital in the United States. Dr Messenger was later charged with manslaughter.[21]

The discussion which follows is based on a report of the Messenger case by theologian Father John Paris.[22] Neonatologist Ed Beaumont,[23] who gave expert evidence for the prosecution at the trial, then comments on Paris's analysis of the circumstances.

This case note identifies a number of risk management issues: the care of a mother in premature labour, discussions between parents and doctors about resuscitation, and the procedures adopted in relation to a baby delivered at 25 weeks.

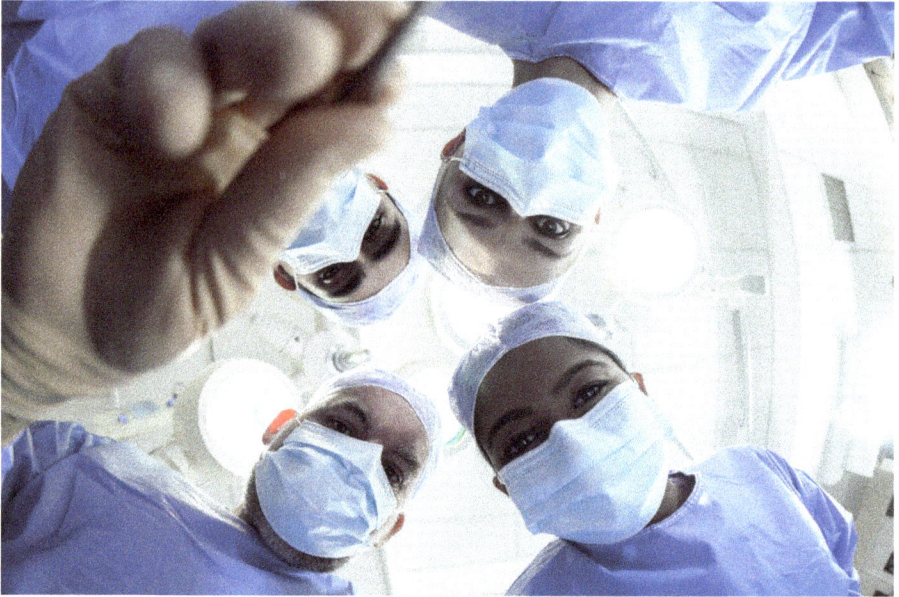

The People v Gregory Glenn Messenger [US, 1996][24]

The facts

Traci Messenger, a mother with high-risk factors in two previous caesarean section deliveries, was in the 25th week of a third pregnancy when she went into premature labour. An examination in hospital revealed the cervix dilated to 4-5 cm. Tocolytic therapy involving terbutaline and ultimately magnesium sulphate was instituted in an attempt to inhibit contractions.

Complications. This treatment led to hypotension, shortness of breath and the coughing up of bright red blood. Pulmonary oedema was diagnosed. Oxygen saturation levels were in the low 70s. The therapy was discontinued and Furosemide administered. On subsequent examination the cervix was found to be dilated to 8 cm and the patient in active labour.

The neonatologist. Before delivery and before the onset of pulmonary oedema, a consultation had occurred between Traci and her husband Gregory (who was a doctor) and Dr Padmani Karna, the neonatologist. Dr Karna told them that at 25 weeks' gestational age, and with the possibility of premature rupture of the membranes and sepsis, the baby had a 30 per cent to 50 per cent possibility of survival. If it did survive, there was a 20 per cent to 40 per cent chance of severe intracranial haemorrhage. The likelihood of substantial respiratory problems was also discussed.

No extraordinary efforts. Following this conference, the Messengers said they did not want any extraordinary efforts undertaken, nor any attempts at resuscitation. Dr Karna told them she preferred a 'wait and see'[25] approach for early gestational newborn. If, once intubated, the baby took a downward course, she would not hesitate to remove life support.

'Wait and see' approach. Dr Karna asked the parents to reconsider their treatment choice in the light of her suggested approach. She asked them to let her know of their decision. That was the only contact they had with the neonatologist before delivery. The meeting ended at 6.30 p.m.

'Vigorous or active.' Before leaving the hospital at about 8.30 pm. Dr Karna instructed her assistant that if the child was 'vigorous or active'[26] at birth and needed ventilation support, she was to intubate.

The obstetrician. In anticipation of an imminent delivery, an obstetrician also discussed the problems of a 25-week delivery with the Messengers, who indicated they did not want 'much or anything done.'[27] The obstetrician attempted vaginal delivery with the expectation of a stillbirth. After 40 minutes, when there was concern about a ruptured uterus, a caesarean section was performed.

The delivery. When the baby was delivered at 11.30 p.m, the obstetrician observed he was hypotonic and hypoxic with a 'black' head colour. The obstetric registrar described the baby as 'purple-blue in colour', 'floppy' and appearing 'lifeless.'[28] In the 15 to 20 seconds it took to place the baby on a warmer, a neonatal nurse detected a heartbeat in the umbilical cord of 80 to 90 beats/min. Dr Karna's assistant immediately intubated the baby, beginning manual respiration with a bag.

'Not vigorous.' Both the nurse and the assistant later testified the child was 'not vigorous'[29] at birth. The nurse said he was 'not active.'[30] The anaesthetist said the baby showed no movement and no change of colour in the delivery room. This led him to believe that either the baby's lungs were not developed enough to effect resuscitation, or the tube was not properly placed. He went to the NICU, where the baby had been taken, in order to speak with staff. The baby was then reintubated and given 100 per cent oxygen. The initial saturation level on 100 per cent oxygen was 14 per cent.

The NICU. Dr Messenger went to the NICU to ask why, despite his instructions, his son had been resuscitated. He requested that these efforts be terminated. Dr Karna's assistant told him she had no authority to stop the resuscitation. She said he was to wait until Dr Karna returned before a decision could be made to remove ventilator support.

At 12.15 am, Dr Karna examined the baby and ordered a blood analysis. She told the parents she wanted to do additional testing, as well as try surfactant to see how the baby responded, before terminating life support.

Removal from ventilator. The Messengers asked to be alone with their son. Dr Karna and the nurse left the room, closing the door. Gregory Messenger then removed his son from the ventilator, placing the baby in his mother's arms. When the monitoring equipment alarm sounded, Dr Messenger opened the door and asked a nurse if she would silence it. When she did so, the nurse saw that the baby, who was now 'pink', was off the ventilator. She ran for Dr Karna, who was standing in the hallway reading the blood gas results. (These indicated a pH of 7.19 and an elevated carbon dioxide value.) Dr Messenger closed the door.

When told of the situation, Dr Karna told the nurse it was 'okay'[31] and to let the parents be. She then instructed a paediatric resident to complete the notes. Dr Karna told the nurse to get a 'hoping packet' to contain photos of the baby, copies of its footprints and its identification bracelet as mementos for the family.

The autopsy. The pathologist found no congenital abnormalities. The infant was pneumonic and had a probable infection, and the placenta showed signs of fragmentation and infection. The pathologist found the infant's condition was not terminal. The cause of death was attributed to extreme prematurity and respiratory failure following removal of the ventilator. Based on his own understanding of the law, the pathologist concluded the manner of the death was homicide.

The trial and verdict

Manslaughter charges were brought against Dr Messenger, based on his failure to provide proper medical treatment for the baby, or gross negligence with regard to his child's care. A jury took less than three hours to return a verdict of not guilty.

In his discussion of the Messenger case, Father John Paris makes the following key points:

1. The consensus in the literature seems to be that for the never competent, such as the newborn, the 'best interest standard' should be used in the decision-making process. This rests solely on the protection of the patient's welfare and is particularly important for infants and children because they are now seen not merely as property of parents but as patients in their own right.

2. In the Messenger case, there was no certainty of a fatal outcome, nor was it certain that medical interventions would not help. However, there was certainty of the statistical probabilities of mortality and morbidity for this class of birth; the treating neonatologist had indicated these.

3. There was no question that if the Messengers had requested aggressive treatment, it would have been given to their son. The issue then became a matter of whether the information warranted a pre-delivery decision to withhold resuscitation and other aggressive medical interventions. Or (as Dr Karna had wanted) must the parents authorize resuscitation and aggressive life-sustaining measures until it became clear, if not certain, that the baby would not survive or, if he did, in such a devastated state as to justify removal of life-sustaining measures?

4. A statistical approach to determine which infants should be treated on the basis of objective criteria such as weight, gestational age and level of severity is widely used in European countries. Reliance on actuarial judgments consistently produces better overall results than does reliance on individual clinical judgments. While this might reduce the problem of profoundly compromised survivors, and that of parents who insist on treatments the doctor believes futile, it does not take into consideration the ability of an 'outlier' to survive and the willingness of some parents to cope with tragic circumstances.

5. In the United States, the response to uncertain outcomes in neonatal medicine is to give a chance to every infant who is potentially viable. Active treatment is then continued until it is nearly certain that the baby will either die or be so severely impaired that under any substantive standard, parents would legitimately opt for termination of treatment.

This 'wait-until-nearly-certain' approach was what Dr Karna proposed to the Messengers. While an appropriate approach when complete uncertainty is faced, it is one not well suited to moral situations in which there is data on which to base predictions.

6. This data was available. The statements of a 50 to 70 per cent death rate and a 20 to 40 per cent risk of severe bleeding in the brain, together with the probability of respiratory distress syndrome, were more than sufficient evidence of the disproportionate burden that awaited this child, and so justified the withholding of resuscitation. It was a decision well within the range of morally acceptable choices and in conformity with widely used medical standards, and should have been respected.

7. Had a neonatologist rather than an assistant been present at the birth, a judgment on the infant's medical status with regard to breathing, heart rate, colour, and activity, rather than a technical response to heartbeat alone, should have precluded resuscitation. The anaesthetist reported that at delivery the infant was 'practically dead and should have been reported dead.'[32] Had the parents' request for non-resuscitation been followed (a decision implemented in previous cases at the hospital), no one would have questioned the outcome.

8. Once the baby was put on a ventilator, the dynamics changed. Even though there is no moral or legal difference between withholding or withdrawing life-sustaining machinery, the Messenger case shows that 'psychologically and politically the gulf can be enormous.'[33] Both the pathologist and prosecution stated that if ventilatory support had not been initiated, they would have ruled the baby died of natural causes. Because the baby was in a stable condition, 'pink', and in no danger of imminent death, they held objective medical data of death or devastation was necessary before the ventilator could be removed. Dr Karna took a similar position and wanted to review the blood gas analysis, x-rays and a trial of surfactant.

9. What is missing in this reasoning is that the same justification for witholding medical treatment applies to its withdrawal. The baby should never have been placed on such support in the first place.

Neonatologist Dr Beaumont, who gave expert evidence for the prosecution at the *Messenger* trial, subsequently raised questions regarding the baby's care.[34] He was critical of Father Paris's analysis, arguing :

1. If the child was doomed, why was tocolysis begun?

2. There had been no mention in the chart of suspected uterine rupture.

3. Who asked the neonatal team to be present at the delivery? If the baby was not to be resuscitated, no call should have been placed and the team asked to leave. Someone in the delivery room must have felt differently at that point.

4. Who best knows how a 780g infant is doing? The colour and tone changes described, despite the observations of the anaesthetist and obstetrician, are quite common at this gestation. They are not indications to withhold resuscitation. Let the neonatal experts begin their initial treatment.

5. How did the baby respond to resuscitation? By 30 minutes of age the infant's Spo 2 was in the 90s. He was pink and his ABGs were good, given the amount of support he had been given up until that time. He gave no indication he was not a survivor.

6. At what percentage survival does the withholding of resuscitation become acceptable? The Messengers were told their son had up to a 50 per cent chance of survival.

Dr Beaumont comments:

I have never had a family refuse care given these odds. In fact, given much slimmer odds, most families opt for care. You have taken a 20 per cent to 40 per cent risk of haemorrhage and interpreted that to be a '20 per cent to 40 per cent risk of severe bleeding in the brain.' In fact most bleeds are small and of no long-term significance. Very few are severe and associated with brain damage. [35]

A hasty decision. Beaumont was also critical of the decision to use the baby's first ten minutes as a case for withdrawing treatment. He believed the child should have been given a chance and had been the victim of a hasty decision. Ventilator adjustments could have been made and surfactant given a try. If these had failed, then the situation could be reassessed.

Beaumont writes that in his NICU (De Vos Children's Hospital, Grand Rapids), parents are approached prior to birth to discuss difficult decisions. Ventilator support is removed if it is clear the child will not survive. As Beaumont explains: 'We are usually ready to make this move well before the parents are.'[36] In Beaumont's opinion, Dr Messenger's decision to take matters into his hands was most unusual and unjustified at this point in his son's life.

Absence of standard. Dr Messenger wrote:

A parent's worst nightmare is to lose a child. I can truly say a big piece of my heart died with my son that night on 8 February 1994. This tragedy was compounded by the absence of a clearly defined standard of care regarding removal of an infant from artificial life support. It was further compounded when I was prosecuted for manslaughter.[37]

To protect other parents who might find themselves in a similar situation, Dr Messenger drafted 'Compassion Care and Comfort Guidelines'. These adopt the 'best interest' and proportionate burden/benefit standards and were approved and adopted by the Michigan State Medical Society in May 1995.[38]

....

Withdrawal of treatment – further options

The next group of cases concern a further range of treatment options. Again, the central issue is 'the best interests of the child' as interpreted by parents, doctors and the courts. No legal generalisations should be drawn from the clinical circumstances. The legal certainty, as with resuscitation, lies in the principle that the welfare of the child is paramount.

But as one judge explained, the law's insistence that the welfare of the child is paramount is 'easily stated and universally applauded';[39] the difficulty lies in putting that principle into practice.

....

In the first case, legislation protects a baby's right to a blood transfusion.

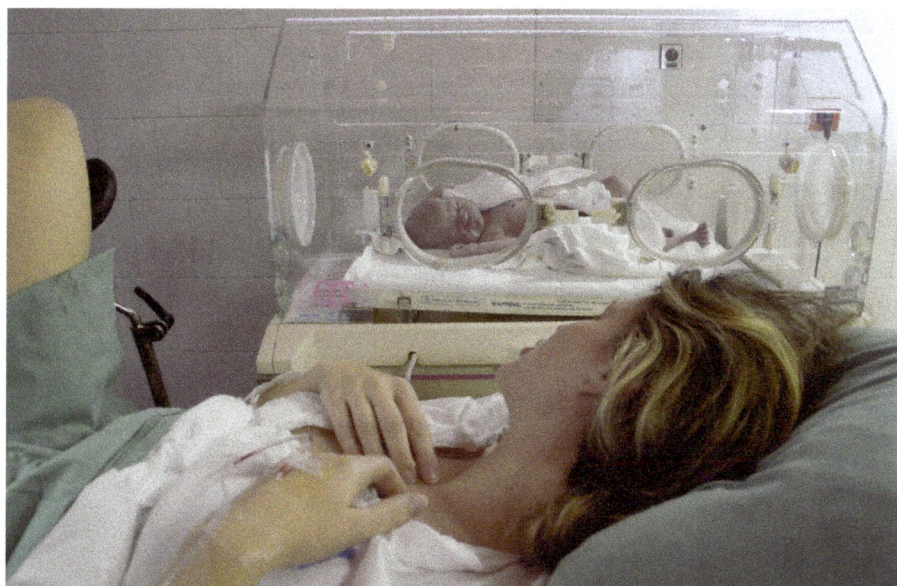

Birkett v Director General of Family & Community Services and Others [Aus, 1994][40]

The facts

When four-day old William developed gastro-intestinal bleeding, the paediatrician decided blood transfusions were necessary. The parents, who were Jehovah's Witnesses, refused on the basis of their religious beliefs. A care order was sought and blood was administered. The judge dismissed the parents' objections, holding that the transfusions were authorised under Care and Protection legislation. Such medical treatment could be given, despite parental objection, where a medical practitioner was of the opinion that it was necessary as a matter of urgency in order to save the child's life.

Similar legislation applies in all Australian States and Territories.

....

In the next case, the judge raised the possibility of criminal charges if the baby did not receive sustenance.

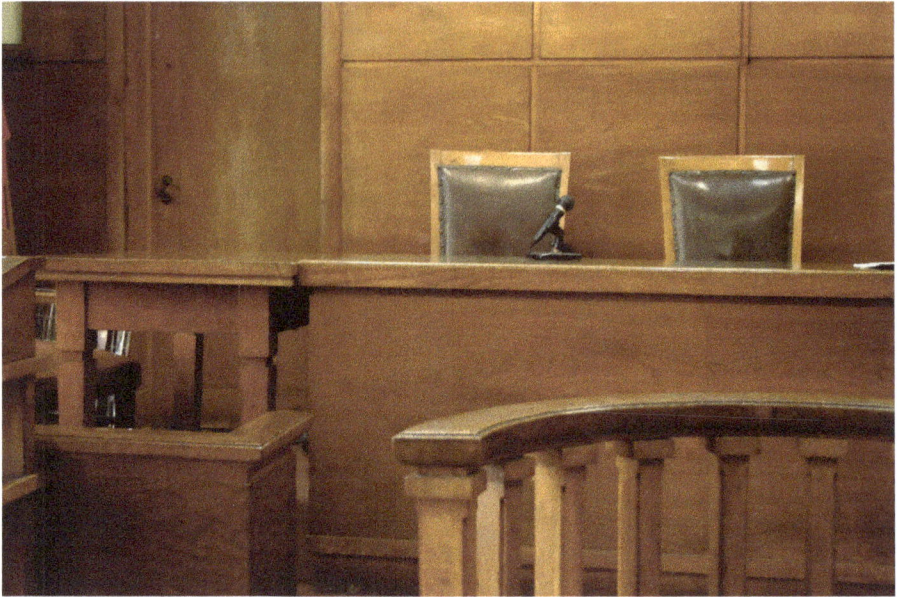

In Re F v F [Aus, 1986][41]

The facts

After Jacob was born with spina bifida, an application was made to the court at midnight by the grandfather. It was alleged that the baby was being starved by the hospital with the intention that it should die. The judge heard there was a risk of imminent death if no action was taken. When the grandfather requested that the hospital be ordered to provide sustenance, an interim order was made to that effect.

'*All necessary and relevant steps.*' The next day the judge made the baby a ward of the court and stated that he was confining his decision specifically to the present case and to the immediate issue of feeding:

No parent, no doctor, no court, has any power to determine that the life of any child, however disabled that child may be, will be deliberately taken from it ... [The law] does not permit decisions

to be made concerning the quality of life, nor does it enable any
assessment to be made as to the value of any human being.[42]

The judge added that any steps deliberately taken for this purpose would result in criminal charges 'of the most serious kind.'[43]

The hospital was then ordered to take all necessary and relevant steps, consistent with proper medical practice, to preserve the child's life. These measures included the provision of basic hydration and nourishment.

....

Six years prior to this caution from an Australian judge, criminal prosecution had become a reality for English paediatrician Dr Arthur.

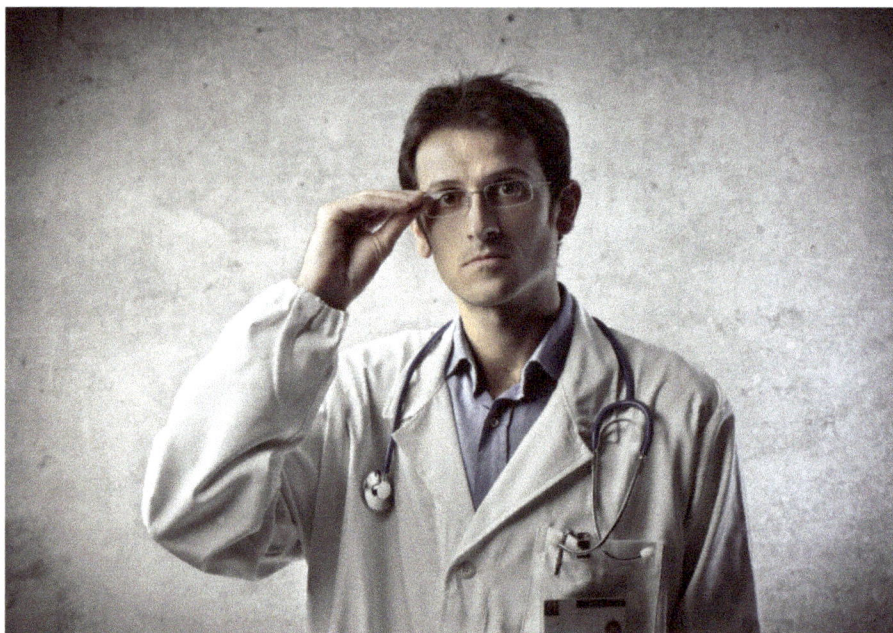

R v Arthur [UK, 1981]⁴⁴

The facts

In 1980, Dr Arthur examined a newborn baby suffering from Down's Syndrome, who had been rejected by his very distressed parents. Dr Arthur noted: 'Parents do not wish it to survive. Nursing care only.'⁴⁵ He prescribed DF 118, a morphine type drug (dihydrocodeine) to be given orally in 5mg doses, not more than four-hourly, to alleviate the baby's distress as and when it arose. The baby died four days later. The cause of death was given as broncho-pneumonia due to consequences of Down's Syndrome. The court heard evidence that 'nursing care only' involves dealing with the baby's bodily functions; the child must be kept warm, fed and cherished.⁴⁶

Police contacted. A nurse who was a member of the 'Life' organisation contacted police, alleging the baby had been drugged, starved and placed in a side ward to die. Inquiries were instituted and a postmortem performed. Dr Arthur was charged with murder eight months later. He pleaded not guilty.

The prosecution alleged:

1. The baby had died of lung stasis caused by the drug.
2. This had been the result of deliberate intent by Dr Arthur to kill the baby.
3. The baby had been deliberately deprived of food and medical treatment.

Most humane treatment. It was conceded that Dr Arthur's motives were of the highest order. He had adopted the course of treatment he considered the most humane for the baby and family.

Attempted murder. The prosecution case then largely collapsed when postmortem studies were found to be incomplete. The paediatric pathologist called for the defence found that the histology had shown calcification of the brain and fibro-elastosis of the heart, as well as congenital abnormalities of the lung. The charge of murder was withdrawn and a charge of attempted murder substituted.

Expert evidence for the defence

'A narrow distinction.' Dr Arthur did not give evidence, but after a number of paediatricians gave expert evidence on his behalf, it became clear to the court that the treatment had fallen within current norms of practice. Dr Dunn, for example, explained that intensive care would be given to any child, regardless of how severely handicapped, when it was the wish of the parents. But pressure would not be exerted on parents by a responsible paediatrician.

Dr Dunn said that reality had to be faced:

Sometimes children are born with such frightful handicaps it is reasonable or, at any rate we think it is, to accept the parents' decision that, in the interests of their own child, prolonging life is not in that child's interests. No paediatrician takes life, but we accept that allowing babies to die (and I know the distinction is narrow, but we feel it profoundly), is in the baby's interest at times.[47]

In summing up to the jury the judge acknowledged that interest:

Certainly in this country no individual is given sole power of life or death over another ... all must be alive to the danger of giving too much power to anyone, in the medical or any other profession, to exert influence over the life and health of the public at large ... Whatever ethics a profession might evolve, they could not stand on their own or survive if they were in conflict with the law. I imagine you will think long and hard before concluding that doctors of the eminence we have heard here, have evolved standards that amount to committing a crime.[48]

The judge then directed the jury to consider :

1. Whether the prosecution had convinced them that Dr Arthur had taken active steps to ensure the baby would die with the intention of bringing that event about.
2. If so, had they been convinced that such steps amounted to an attempt to murder the child?

After deliberating for two hours, the jury acquitted Dr Arthur.

English lawyers then questioned whether the criminal law, as written and administered, were two different things. Had it evolved to the point where doctors would be protected, while a parent in similar circumstances would be convicted of murder?

English legal writer David Meyers took a different view:

Hypocritical as the results of such cases are, few would find them unfair or ill-advised, even among those most firmly opposed to euthanasia. In other words, such verdicts bring about a just result in a particular case, but leave the thrust of the law on the side of preserving all life, regardless of its quality to the individual concerned or to society.[49]

The next four cases illustrate how English courts struggle to reach 'best interest decisions.' In the first, a court rejected the parents' wishes, and held that the baby was entitled to the normal life-span of a handicapped child.

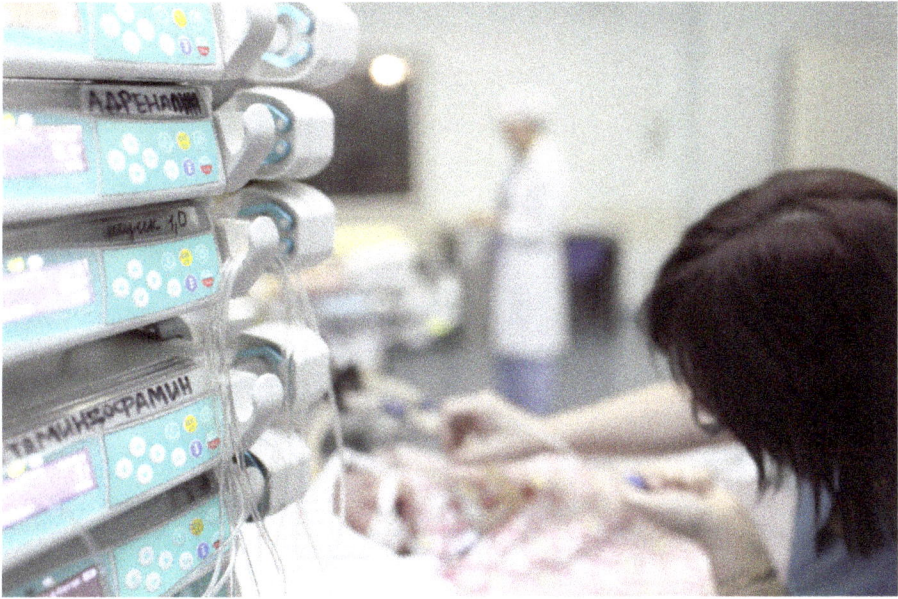

In Re B [UK, 1981][51]

The facts

A baby who was born suffering from Down's Syndrome also had an intestinal obstruction. Doctors believed surgery had a good chance of success, but without it the condition would quickly prove fatal. The parents felt that surgery was not in their daughter's best interests and that she should be allowed to die. The hospital then applied to the court for an order that it would be lawful to surgically remove the obstruction. The court heard that if surgery was successful, the baby was likely to have a life expectancy of 20 to 30 years.

The decision

Normal span. In examining the child's best interests, the wishes of the parents in these circumstances were considered irrelevant. If successful, the baby could go on to live the normal span of a child suffering from Down's Syndrome, with the defects and handicaps of that condition. The court held it was not for the court to say that life of that description ought to be extin-

*lustrates, poignantly and dramatically, the difficulties that are en-
countered when trying to put it into practice.*[56]

Treatment to make comfortable. The court held that the baby's best
interests required approval of recommendations designed to ease her suffering and permit her life to come to an end peacefully, with dignity, rather than
seek to prolong her life. It was better to give treatment, such as antibiotic
therapy for pneumonia or intravenous fluids for dehydration, in addition to
basic nursing care, rather than let the infant suffer.

This was the first time an English court had acknowledged the lawfulness
of managing some neonates towards their deaths. This lay in giving treatment to make them comfortable, rather than striving to save them at all costs.

....

In the last case in this chapter, an Australian coroner found the doctors and
parents 'entirely reasonable and appropriate' [57] in their decisions about a
baby's treatment.

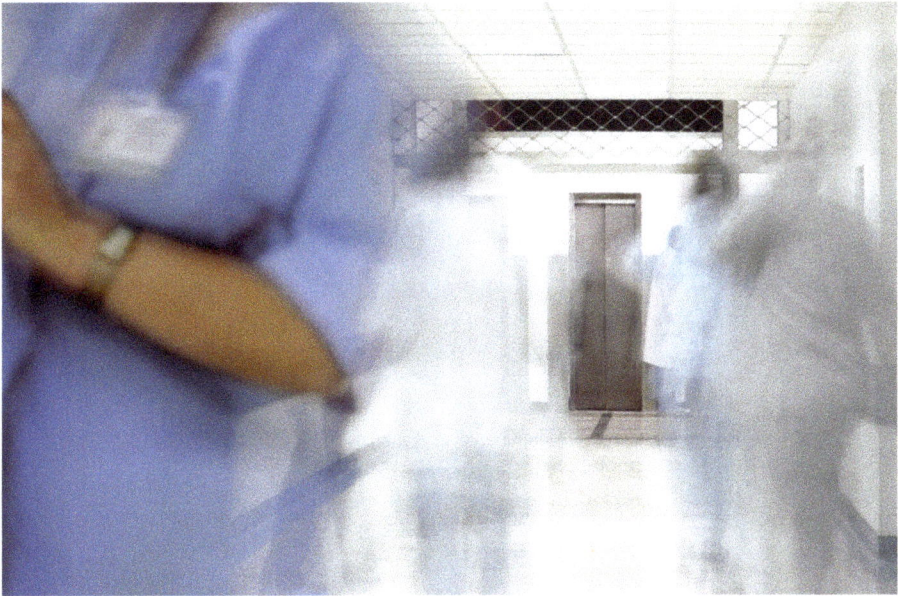

Baby M, No: 3149/89 [Aus, 1991]⁵⁸

[Note. The following discussion is based on a review of this case by Professor Loane Skene.⁵⁹]

The facts

Baby M was born with severe abnormalities, described by the coroner as: a severe form of spina bifida overta; large lumbar myelomeningocele (L1 or L2 level); hydrocephalus; Arnold-Chiari malformation of the brain stem; bilateral vocal cord paresis; severe leg deformities, including dislocated hips; dislocated knees; and talipes equinovarus. Baby M had severe wasting of muscles in all areas below the waist, would always be doubly incontinent and would have no sexual function. Her hips were in a constant position over her chest. Her knees were deformed and could not be bent in the correct direction. She had a severe degree of club feet. She had an 80 per cent chance of developing kyphoscoliosis (curvature of the spine), which might ultimately have prevented her from sitting in a wheelchair and might have restricted her lungs, causing respiratory failure and death.

Shortened life span. If she survived, Baby M would need numerous painful operations to straighten her bones. She had little spontaneous movement and little response to simple stimuli. She had shallow breathing and difficulty in swallowing and sucking. The latter suggested a severe form of Arnold- Chiari malformation and a significantly shortened life span. If she did survive, her quality of life was likely to be so poor that one might question whether she would want to live such a life.

The treatment. The doctors, in consultation with Baby M's parents and their Roman Catholic spiritual advisers, decided against surgery or other invasive life-saving treatment. Conservative treatment was instituted: an open cot, food by mouth on demand, and pain killers and sedatives to alleviate her pain and distress. Baby M died after 12 days.

The findings

1. The coroner found the baby died from natural causes (bronchopneumonia, hypoxia secondary to vocal cord paralysis in a baby with spina bifida and associated with upper airway obstruction in the presence of phenobarbitone and morphine at toxic level.)
2. No person was found to have contributed to Baby M's death. Although the amount of phenobarbitone and morphine were present in her blood at autopsy in quantities that might have caused death, the coroner found they were administered for the purpose of relieving pain and distress, and in the interests of the baby. They were not given to bring about or hasten her death: 'Rather the risk of death being hastened in such a manner was weighed against the need to prevent distress and pain.'[60]
3. The coroner found the decision not to operate in order to insert a shunt or to close the spina bifida sac was justified. The hydrocephalis was not progressive and the sac had not ruptured: 'She would be no worse off untreated if she lived, than if she had been treated.'[61]
4. The coroner commented that historically governments have been reluctant to intervene in private decision-making between doctors, family and patient, and that this principle should not be disturbed without good reason. Mature communities should have confidence in the medical profession, parents and their advisers, guided by the best available information, experience, good judgement, sincerity and common sense to reach the right decision in a particular case.

5. The coroner concluded that appropriate steps had been taken to ensure the decisions about Baby M were legally, ethically and morally sound, and were entirely reasonable and appropriate.

Coronial decisions. Professor Skene comments that while this is a strong statement supporting the doctor's role in making treatment decisions about critically ill newborn infants, coronial decisions do not bind courts, nor other coroners faced with a similar case. Coronial investigations focus on facts, determining cause of death and identity of the person. Their investigations are not concerned with fault.

English decisions. Though 'compassionate and just,'[62] the coroner's decision in the Baby M case seems at odds with some of the English Court of Appeal decisions. These sanction the withholding of treatment in only the most extreme case, and then only when the baby had stopped breathing. Skene concludes that in the absence of negligence, it is probable that another coroner or court would take a similar view.

The inherent legal principles in this case (as summarised by Professor Skene[63]) are discussed below.

In an emergency, where there is an imminent risk of death or serious injury, doctors may do whatever is necessary to treat a child.

- The parents of a child are legally entitled to decide what medical treatment their child will or will not have, provided they act in the child's best interests.
- Parents who have authority to consent are also entitled to refuse treatment that a doctor recommends, or choose an alternative, although this is subject to court intervention.
- If there is any doubt whether a decision meets the requirement of being in the child's best interests, then any person who is concerned may apply to a court for an order authorising appropriate treatment.
- A court's decision should be reached in a state of firm satisfaction upon convincing evidence.
- Applications to a court may also be made if the risk is serious but not life threatening. Again, the application can be made by anyone concerned about the child's welfare.
- The state's authority to act for children derives from its role as protector of children in society. The authority of this *parens patriae* jurisdic-

tion springs from the direct responsibility of the Crown to look after those who cannot look after themselves.

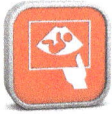

Discussion of Key Issues

It would appear that there is no legal duty to resuscitate patients or continue treatment that is futile and burdensome. However, disagreements occur as to what is 'futile' treatment for a very young baby.

- How strong is the midwifery voice in discussion about treatment?

In Professor Campbell's view, for example, with very few exceptions infants of any gestation age, weight or apparent abnormality should be resuscitated if signs of life are present. Exceptions include gross abnormality of the CNS.
Do you agree?

- List exceptions and discuss why.
- Are these legal or ethical reasons?
- What is the resuscitation policy in your unit?
- Discuss and justify any changes you would make.

Professor Campbell says that gross abnormalities have often been identified antenatally, and that discussions with parents would have included the appropriate care at birth. He believes there is usually no justification for aggressive methods of resuscitation and that a baby should receive all 'normal' nursing attention with relief of apparent distress or discomfort until death.

- Describe the antenatal midwifery role following such discussion between doctor and parents?
- How would you explain 'normal nursing attention' to a court?
- In your experience, is a baby's 'apparent distress or discomfort' adequately relieved in most cases?

- Would your documentation describe this distress and reflect its allevi-ation to a court?

A newspaper report[64] of a coronial investigation reported that a hospital did not have a protocol in relation to babies who survive abortion.

- Does your hospital have such a protocol?
- If so, how is it worded?

The Anthony MacDonald case. Rierdon comments that although the jury agreed with the obstetrician not providing oxygen within minutes following birth of a 23-week, 68g baby, 'there is no assurance another jury would do the same.'[65]

- What could you argue that might persuade a jury to reach a different conclusion?

....

In the *Messenger* case, the father (a doctor) was prosecuted unsuccessfully for manslaughter after he disconnected his newborn premature son from life support. Neonatologist Dr Beaumont, who gave expert evidence at the trial, took issue with a number of findings made by Father Paris and raised ques-tions regarding the baby's care.

- Review the findings and discuss the merits of the different clinical approaches.

Dr Messenger is reported as saying: 'I can truly say a big piece of my heart died with my son that night....'[66]

- Do you think staff have time to support (and if necessary, protect) shocked and vulnerable parents?

....

F v F: Note the judge flagged the possibility of criminal proceedings when he cautioned: 'No parent, no doctor, no court, has any power to determine that the life of any child, however disabled that child may be, will be deliberately taken from it.'[67]

....

In the *Arthur* case, expert witness Dr Dunn explained that some children are born so 'frightfully' handicapped that paediatricians think it reasonable to accept the parents' decision that prolonged or long life is not in their child's best interests. While no paediatrican takes life, allowing a baby to die (a narrow distinction but one felt profoundly) is in the baby's interest at times.

- Do you think that the difference between 'taking life' and 'allowing a baby to die' is a narrow distinction?
- Can you reconcile this view with the judge's warning in *F v F?*

....

In the case of In *In Re B,* parents of a baby born with Down's Syndrome refused to consent to surgery to remove a bowel obstruction.

- Compare the judge's rejection of the parent's wishes with Dr Dunn's view of the parental role (above) in the *Arthur* case.

In the case of *In re C* the Court of Appeal makes statements on easing suffering, and 'managing a neonate toward death.' The judge speaks of antibiotic treatment and IV fluids in addition to basic nursing care.

- Discuss the nature of medical orders in these situations. Have you disagreed at times? Why?
- Have you ever documented (objectively and subjectively) in a way that would make clear to a court that a baby was receiving treatment that was 'invasive, unpleasant and distressing'?

Professor Skene, in summarizing the issues in a coronial inquest which concerned the decision not to operate or resuscitate a baby born with severe disabilities, reports the coroner as saying that, historically, governments have been reluctant to intervene in the private decision-making between doctors, family and patient, and that this principle should not be disturbed without good reason.

- Do you agree?
- Do you believe there are adequate checks and balances at your hospital to protect the best interests of critically ill neonates?

NOTES

1. 'The Age', News p.3, (21 Feb. 2007).
2. MJA 2006; 185 (9): 495-500; perinatal care at the borderlines of viability: a consensus statement based on a NSW and ACT consensus workshop.
3. 'The Age.'
4. Ibid.
5. L.Skene, Law and Medical Practice. Butterworths, Sydney, 1998, p.2.
6. 2002 CCH Medical Health & Medical Law Reporter, Neonatal Care. Paras. 21–350.
7. 'Daily Telegraph' (April 11, 2000) at p.9, reporting on an inquest in Darwin.
8. Ibid.
9. Ibid.
10. Ibid.
11. Powers & Harris, Medical Negligence, Butterworths, London, (1994), p.702.
12. Ibid.
13. In Re J (a minor), 2 Med LR 67 (1990).
14. Ibid., p.69.
15. Ibid., p.76.
16. Ibid., p.73
17. 2002 CCH Medical Health & Medical Law Reporter, Neonatal Care, paras. 21-350.
18. February 1998, Legal Report: Disagreements on End-of- Life Care www.rmf .harvard.edu/publications/resource/legal-report s/feb1998/index.html
19. Ibid.
20. Ibid.
21. The People v Gregory Glenn Messenger, Ingham County (Michigan) Circuit, File No. 94-67694-FH (1995).
22. John J.Paris, Journal of Perinatology, Vol. 16, No. 1 (1996). Manslaughter or a Legitimate Parental Decision? The Messenger Case.

23. Journal of Perinatology, Vol. 16, No. 4 (1996). Letters to the Editor, Ed. Beaumont. Neonatologist, p.321.
24. Ibid.
25. Journal of Perinatology, Vol. 16, No. 4 at p.60.
26. Ibid., p.60.
27. Ibid.
28. Ibid.
29. Ibid.
30. Ibid.
31. Ibid., p.61.
32. Ibid., p.62.
33. Ibid, p.63.
34. Journal of Perinatology, Vol. 16, No. 4, Letters to the Editor (E. Beaumont.) at p.321.
35. Ibid.
36. Ibid.
37. Journal of Perinatology, Vol. 16, No. 1 (1996). Gregory G.Messenger, M.D. *Compassionate Care and Comfort- Guidelines,* p.65. (Approved and adopted as the standard of care by Michigan State Medical Society (May 6, 1995).
38. Ibid., pp.65–66.
39. *In Re C, 1 Med LR 46* (1989).
40. *Birkett v Director General of Family and Community Services and Others,* 5 Med LR 411 (1994).
41. CCH Australian Health and Medical Law Reporter Para 21–350, *In Re F v F, Unreported judgment of the Supreme Court of Victoria* (2 July 1986).
42. Ibid.
43. Ibid.
44. *R v Arthur,* 12 BMLR 1 (1981).
45. Ibid., p.8.
46. Ibid., p.9.
47. Ibid., p.18.
48. Ibid., p.22.
49. D. Meyers, The Human Body and the Law, Edinburgh University Press (1990).
50. *In Re B,* 1 WLR 1421 (1981) at p.1424.
51. Ibid.
52. Ibid.
53. *In Re C (a minor) (No.1),* 1 Med LR 46 (1989) at p.52.
54. *In Re C (a Minor).*
55. Ibid., p.47.

56. Ibid.
57. *Coronial Inquest,* No. 3149/89, reported in L. Skene, Law and Medical Practice, Butterworths, Sydney (1998) pp.254–255.
58. *Baby M, Record of Investigation into Death Case,* No. 3149/89 (1991).
59. Ibid., p.254.
60. Ibid.
61. Ibid, p.255.
62. Ibid.
63. Ibid.
64. *Daily Telegraph* (April 11, 2000), p.9, reporting on an inquest in Darwin.
65. Legal Report, *Disagreements on End-of-Life Care* (February 1998). www.rmf. harvard.edu/publications/resource/legal reports/feb1998/index.html
66. Journal of Perinatology, Vol. 16, No. 1, 1996. Gregory G. Messenger, p.65. *Compassionate Care and Comfort Guidelines.*
67. CCH Australian Health and Medical Law Reporter Para 21–350 *F v F.*

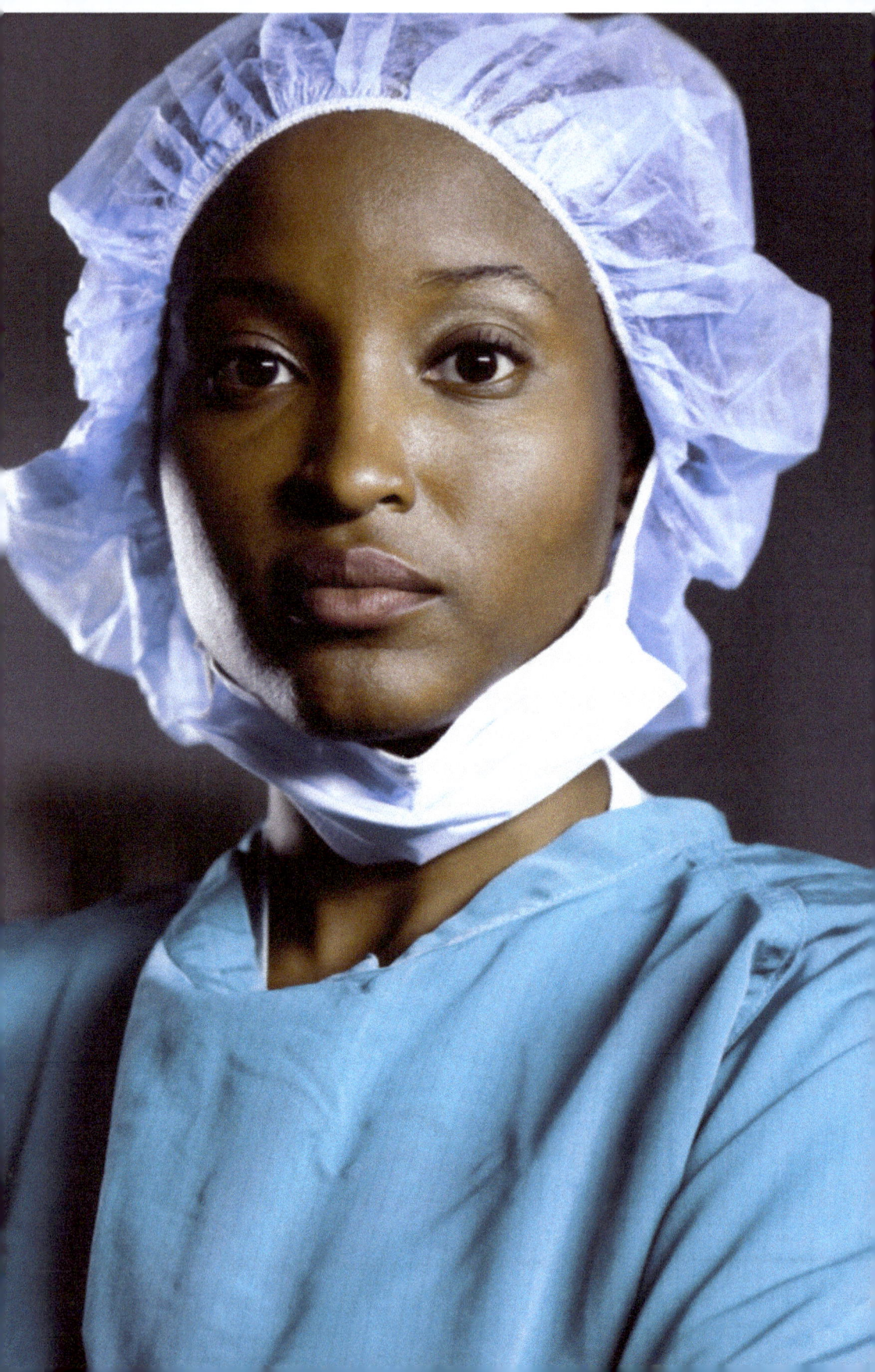

CHAPTER 14

The Neonatal Unit-staff/ equipment/ monitoring

'While most parents, even in the depths of their despair, will recognise that babies may be born abnormal or damaged and that nobody is to blame, some may recall certain incidents during pregnancy, labour or delivery which will cause them to question their care, and seek explanations.'

— Professor Campbell

Introduction

English paediatrician and medico-legal writer, Professor Campbell,[1] explains that while most parents, even in the depths of their despair, will recognise that babies may be born abnormal or damaged and that nobody is to blame, some may recall certain incidents which will cause them to question their care, and seek explanations. Rightly or wrongly, some blame nurses or doctors and legal action may follow, though not for many years until the full extent of disability becomes apparent. 'Blanket' allegations may be made against obstetricians, midwives, paediatricians and neonatal staff who have been involved in the whole perinatal and neonatal period.

Whatever the nature of the complaint, the baby's record will be critical to a court's understanding of the care given. Professor Campbell advises that nursing and medical notes should describe the clinical problems as they present, reflecting careful attention to the baby's needs. They should contain sufficient detail of the baby's condition and the actions taken or not taken to justify each action or inaction, for example, intubation:

It is also helpful to record the main points of any discussion with the parents. A summary of what they have been told about the infant's condition and prognosis should be part of any 'hand-over' note, a particularly important aid to continuity of care where there are frequent rotations of staff.[2]

This chapter examines three cases where inexperienced staff misused equipment in neonatal nurseries; a fourth case is concerned with the monitoring of a premature baby.

The duty to provide adequate numbers of competent staff

Hospitals offering specialised neonatal care have a duty to offer the particular level of care a vulnerable newborn requires. One aspect of a hospital's duty of care is to provide adequate numbers of competent staff to work with equipment.

The following three cases provide a strong disincentive to hospitals against placing inexperienced staff in NICUs without adequate supervision. While the first case concerns doctors, there is no reason why the court's reasoning would not apply to nursing staff.

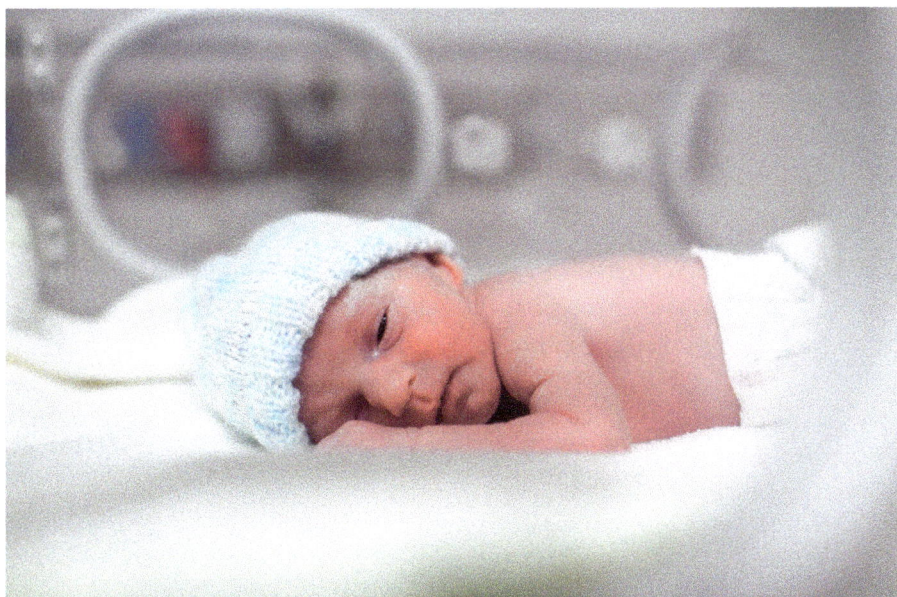

Wilsher v Essex Area Health Authority [UK, 1986][3]

The facts

Martin Wilsher was born three months prematurely and admitted to a NICU in December 1978. Due to a mistake by a junior doctor, an arterial catheter to measure his PO2 levels was inserted into a vein. The junior doctor asked a senior registrar to check the placement, but the registrar failed to see the mistake on the X-ray. Several hours later the registrar made exactly the same mistake himself. Consequently, mistaken readings of PO2 in the arterial blood led to excessive administration of oxygen in an attempt to raise the level. The true PO2 level, which remained excessively high for a substantial period, was alleged to have caused Martin's retrolental fibroplasia (RLF).

The negligence case that followed was appealed to the House of Lords eight years after Martin's birth. The decision provides an important guide to hospitals offering specialist units.

The decision

Inexperience. Inexperience was rejected as a defence. The court held that if a highly specialised standard of care is offered by a special care unit, then all those working in it will be expected to reach standards applicable to the positions they occupy.

Duty of care tailored to acts performed. The duty of care therefore ought to be tailored to the acts that the doctor elected to perform, not by the more limited skills the doctor brought to the task. One judge contended that an inexperienced doctor who was called on to exercise a specialist skill and who made a mistake, nevertheless satisfied the standard of care if he had sought the advice and help of his superior when necessary. (This will depend on the circumstances of each case.)

Consultation. The House of Lords found that in this instance, the junior doctor had satisfied the relevant standard of care by consulting the registrar. The registrar, on the other hand, had been negligent. He had the greater experience and had failed to notice that the catheter had been mistakenly placed in a vein rather than an artery.

Causation not proven. A re-trial was ordered on the basis that causation had not been proved. Medical experts explained that there are many causes of RLF, for example, prematurity. Martin's condition was too complex to ascribe simply to too much oxygen. Eventually the health authority negotiated a settlement with the family.

....

In the second case, a nurse was 'floated' to a neonatal unit, apparently unfamiliar with the way feeding tubes are attached.

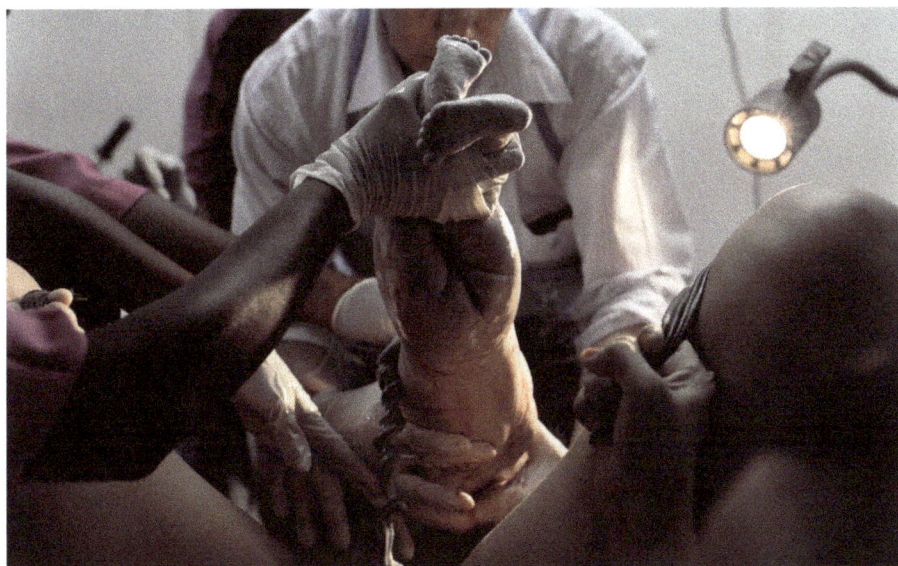

Anonymous v Anonymous Hospital [US, 1999]⁴

The facts

Annie was born in April 1996 (Apgars 7 and 9), but unable to suck or swallow. The results of a cranial ultrasound and head CTs were described as 'unremarkable' but Annie continued to have no suck or swallow reflexes.

Feeding tube. After a feeding tube placed through the abdominal wall failed to provide significant nutrition, a central line was placed in the right jugular vein (a week later) to allow for additional supplementation. This nutritional supplement had to be sterile because it went directly into the blood stream.

Re-attachment of feeding tube. When Annie improved, the central line was discontinued. Full nutritional support was supplied through the feeding tube in the abdomen. On the day Annie was to be discharged (two weeks after birth), the parents were allowed to take their daughter for a walk outside the hospital. The feeding tube was taken out and a button placed to close the tube. When they returned, the baby's primary paediatric nurse was on a lunch break. A temporary float nurse re-attached the feeding tube, re-implementing breast milk feeding.

Attachment to central line. The breast milk adaptor, however, was attached to the central line, which placed breast milk directly into the internal jugular vein. When the primary nurse returned, she immediately stopped the infusion.

Injury. The infused breast milk had gone to the brain, causing milk emboli to block the blood supply to numerous portions of the brain. Annie developed seizures, and went into a coma. A bacterial infection developed. CT scans confirmed a devastating injury, with some paraplegia.

Some recovery. Although Annie slowly began to recover, she still had a significant inability to suck and swallow on discharge from the hospital. At the trial three years later there was some further improvement but still cognitive deficit present. She was able to stand with assistance.

Settlement reached.

....

In the third case, a coroner explained that amendments to the Coroners Act in 1999 in Victoria have shifted the emphasis away from individual blame and, where appropriate, now focus more on systemic problems. In this case, a baby died after a nurse, unfamiliar with the way an ETT aspirate was obtained, mistakenly attached the suction tube to the oxygen instead of to the wall suction. The coroner also investigated the chain of events that followed.

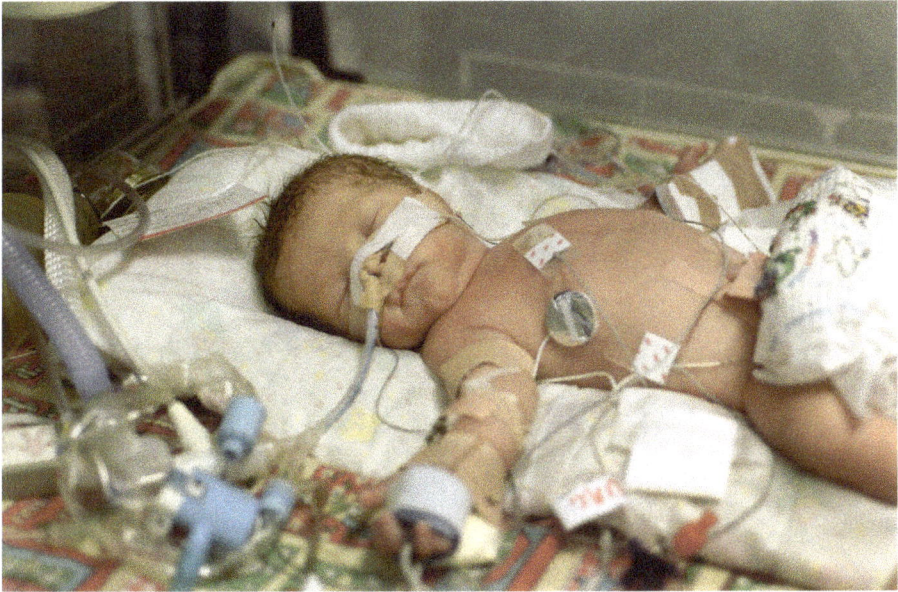

Coronial Investigation [Aus, 2002][5]

The facts

Justin, second of twins, was born at 26 weeks' gestation and weighed 810 g. He was in good condition but did require intubation due to hyaline membrane disease. Justin was extubated the following day, then placed on nasal intermittent positive air pressure. He developed intermittent bradycardia and apnoea.

A paediatrician later stated in an independent report prepared for the State Coroner that this is a typical complication of prematurity, which may occur many times during a day. If each episode is short and recovery complete after each apnoea, no harm is caused. If prolonged, or recovery incomplete, the baby may have to be put back on mechanical ventilation and intubated with an endo-tracheal tube. This was occurring to Justin in the NICU five days after his birth.

Nursing staff. Five nurses were managing eight babies in the bay. Nurse D, who was caring for Justin, called a trainee neonatal fellow (the doctor) at approximately 11.30 pm to see the baby, who had a prolonged episode of apnoea, with inadequate recovery. The doctor re-intubated the baby. He then asked nurse D to obtain an ETT aspirate (a sample of mucous for microbiological culture).

The ETT aspirate. Nurse D asked generally how this was done, but nobody volunteered an answer. She then asked one of the nurses directly, who told her to suction the ETT in the normal way and to use the oxygen tube from the wall unit to blow the contents of the tube into a specimen pot.

The incident report. Nurse D did not give evidence about what then occurred, but according to her Incident Report:

Took ETT aspirate for culture by suctioning ETT and then attached suction catheter to oxygen tubing to blow sample into specimen pot. Forgot to re-attach catheter to suction and returned catheter to ETT to further suction tube. While still attached to oxygen tubing. Baby collapsed with bilateral pneumothoraces.[6]

Calculations. The coroner heard evidence that calculations showed that 14 litres per minute of oxygen would have been the rate of flow, which equates to 233 ml per second. The paediatrician giving the independent report said that Justin's mechanical ventilator would have been delivering oxygen at 5 mls] per half second at a pressure of 20 cm H2O. Air embolism is a risk when ventilators are adjusted to deliver pressures of 40-50 cm H2O. The pressure from the wall unit would have been 4200 cm H2O until the catheter was withdrawn, two or three times the pressure used in most car tyres.

The paediatrician explained:

It is almost impossible to imagine that air embolism and extreme pneumothoraces would not occur under these conditions.[7]

The paediatrician concluded that an air embolism occurring at the same time as the suction catheter with oxygen flow was inserted would have caused severe and irreversible brain damage within minutes. Justin's heart rate had slowed and he became rapidly de-saturated and cyanosed.

Lack of information. Nurse D was heard to be sobbing and crying: 'I killed the baby.'[8] The doctor and the associate charge nurse were called. Justin was found to be poorly defused and discoloured, with a distended abdomen. The doctor initially thought it was an abdominal problem. As there was little bilateral chest movement, he took the baby off the ventilator and ventilated him manually with bag and mask. When the heart rate did not improve, he proceeded to cardiac massage and re-intubation. The coroner found that nurse D had not told the doctor what had occurred with the suction catheter.

Equipment malfunction. The doctor wanted to check if the baby had developed pneumothoraces, but the transilluminator in the unit, which was battery powered, was not working. This was later discovered to be due to a blown bulb.

Brain damage. An urgent X-ray confirmed bilateral pneumothoraces, which the doctor proceeded to aspirate and drain with good effect. But brain damage had already occurred. Neurological investigations continued over the next weeks. Justin's parents then consented to withdrawal of life support.

Incident not recorded. The coroner concluded that it was hard to resist the conclusion that there had been 'cover-up' by some nursing staff, or at least a failure to properly investigate the matter. The incident was not reported until some weeks later. It was never recorded in the nursing notes by nurse D. Nevertheless, there had been rumours.

Cross-examination

Counsel for the family to one of the nurses in the NICU on that shift:

Q: I'm asking you, was it common knowledge on the shift that night, and over the subsequent days, that there'd been an incident involving (Baby Justin)?

A: Yes.

Q: It wasn't simply that the patient had gone flat or simply crashed, it was during the procedure that this had occurred ?

A: Yes.[9]

A neonatal registrar said that the doctor had told him that he had gathered from the nurses, and from the distraught state one nurse was in, that instead of attaching the suction tube to the wall suction, the nurse had 'inadvertently and by mistake' [10] attached a tube to the oxygen. The baby had immediately deteriorated.

Failure to investigate. The coroner agreed with the family's submission that fear of consequences should not operate to conceal material facts that the family was entitled to know. But nurse D had actually said she had 'killed the baby.' The coroner found that it was unfortunate that in the immediate aftermath nobody quizzed her about what she meant by this. While no post-incident management could have altered the outcome, even if the true facts had been known, it was not hard to imagine a case where such concealment might have a dramatic impact on the subsequent course of treatment and management.

Effort to calm. The coroner accepted that the nurse was apparently hysterical at the time. Nevertheless, an effort should have been made in such an emergency to calm her to the point where she could give some coherent history of what had happened.

Assumption about equipment. The coroner also found that nursing staff assumed that when the transilluminator failed to function, the other transilluminator machine in the unit was away being repaired. In fact, it had been repaired and cleaned but returned to the wrong place (the equipment room). Nobody was aware of this.

Hospital initiatives. Since the baby's death, the hospital had developed a series of initiatives. These included training, staff education, equipment failure and incident reporting, as well as the method of sputum collection. These initiatives were aimed at ensuring there would be no replication of the chain of events that had occurred.

Monitoring – are alarms turned on?

....

In the next case, a Health Service ombudsman, investigating a complaint at an English hospital,[11] was critical that a premature baby had been left alone with the alarm on a monitor turned off.

Though brief, this case note (no citation) contains a cascade of errors.

The facts

Elsa, pregnant with twins and known to be at a high risk of going into premature labour, went to hospital after suffering period-like pain and a discharge. A junior doctor at the maternity unit dismissed this as caused by an infection, and gave her antibiotics and medication for pain. Appropriate medication would have delayed the onset of labour.

Premature birth. Shortly afterwards, twins were delivered, who being very premature, needed to be quickly treated with a drug to help mature their lungs. There was a delay in setting this up.

Alarm turned off. The babies, a boy and a girl, were transferred to the special care nursery. Ten days later the charge nurse left them in the care of a nursery nurse. Nursery nurses working in neonatal units in England usually work under an RN and are responsible for the feeding, changing and comforting of newborn babies.[12]

During this time the baby girl's heart rate dropped below 100 beats per minute. This would normally trigger an alarm by the cot to alert staff; but as the alarm had been switched off, the problem was not noticed for some time.

Investigation. The baby girl, who had previously been doing well, had been taken off the ventilator. However, a blood test the night before showed an infection which should have meant the resumption of ventilation. This test was overlooked by another junior doctor. Resuscitation was unsuccessful and the baby died later that day.

The decision

Monitor switched off. The ombudsman found that the baby should not have been left alone at all, and certainly not with the monitor switched off. The hospital had, since the investigation, improved staffing levels in the maternity unit, replaced the monitors in NICU and redesigned the unit so it would be easier to 'keep an eye' on the babies.

....

In the final case in this chapter, again concerned with the monitoring of a premature baby, a judge asked a neonatal nurse to explain just what 'keeping an eye' on a baby meant.

The judge said that premature babies now survive because of the very complex care they receive, but acknowledged that nursing and medical staff also have extensive demands on their skills and time.

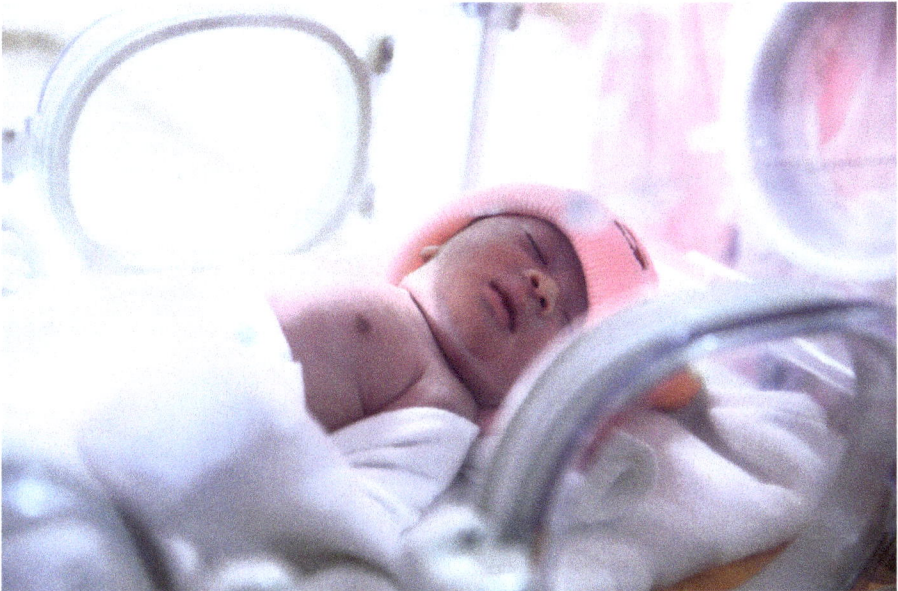

Nawoor v Barking Havering and Brentwood [UK, 1997][13]

The facts

On 10 April 1991, Surest was born at 28 weeks, weighing 566g. She suffered from a number of problems, including a heart condition. Surest received parenteral feeding: IV fluid consisting of a 10 per cent solution of glucose and amino acids. On 19 April, a leak from the IV line caused long-term scarring and deformity of the left foot and lower leg. Surest's mother alleged her daughter's injuries resulted from negligent nursing and medical care.

The trial

Management of leaking IV lines. The judge heard evidence that the skin of such fragile babies is very friable and that IV lines can leak even with careful management. Leaks occurring on 17 and 18 April had been adequately managed.

On 18 and 19 April, nurse Turner was on night duty. In the last hour before her final observations at 7.45 am, there had been some 6ml infused. At 7.45 am, she recorded the condition of the IV line, infusion site and cannula as satisfactory. Change-over occurred shortly before 8 am. Nurse Smith had first contact with Surest, noting:

8. am.   IV tissued, ankle of left foot noticed to be swollen. Skin broken in two places, appears bluish looking. Sister Parker (i.e. senior nurse) and another sister informed. Doctors informed re. Line removal.

8.30 am.   IV noticed to be tissued; tape and plaster removed. Ankle noticed to be bluish, two broken areas, necrotic areas around toes. Sister Parker and the other sister informed. Doctor informed re intravenous line removal.[14]

Removal of IV line. Sister Parker saw Surest shortly after 8 am, observing the condition to be more a matter of swelling than discolouration. She did not detect necrosis, nor did she find the swelling constituted an oedematous area. Sister Parker promptly arranged for the removal of the IV line. A burns unit was contacted at another hospital.

Sister Burke observed swelling, but did not notice any bluish marking or necrosis.

The treatment

Treatment from 19 April consisted of Jellonet dressing and bandaging of the wound. On 23 April, a consultant plastic surgeon advised: '3 x weekly cleaning with saline and the application of jellonet tulle. If pathogens are cultured the dressing should be changed to a single layer of bactigras tulle.'[15] Progress notes referred to many changes of dressings. On 22 May, light exercising of the foot and lower leg commenced. On 23 May, a splint was applied. Medical notes inferred that a consultant paediatrician in charge of Surest's care was pleased with her progress.

Contractures queried. A note on 25 May indicated the wound was healing well with granulation tissue well formed. It was also noted that Surest was keeping her leg in plantar flexed position. Contractures were queried. A plan indicated two-hour physiotherapy.

Injury. At the end of May, Surest was transferred to another hospital under the care of a second plastic surgeon.

This surgeon operated in January 1992, finding:

Most of the extensors and eventors of the left foot are enmeshed in scar tissue and destroyed. The planta flexion had been subsequently compounded by a caleaneal valgus whereby the foot, instead of being in the downward equine position of the plantor flexion, is splayed out in the valgus direction due to internal damage to tissues and tendons.[16]

The court heard this damage could be the result of:

1. The effect of added volume of liquid within the limb causing swelling and expansion.
2. A chemical reaction caused by the glucose and fluid on surrounding tissue having an osmotic effect, leading to scarring and potential destruction of deep tissue and muscle.

Evidence was given that a leak, if detected early, would not result in significant long-term damage.

Arguments and allegations

Conservative treatment. Surest's mother alleged that there was a failure on 19 April to promptly observe the leak, that the injury had continued to be caused by the leak over a considerable period and that medical treatment had been too conservative. Nursing staff told her they would continue to dress Surest's wound, reassuring her it would probably clear up within a few weeks. At worst, there would be a residual scar.

Not properly advised. The judge found Surest's mother to be a 'straightforward and reasonable witness'[17] whose evidence seemed to fit in with the actual experience of the unit at the time. Staff had never known such serious, long-term damage. Although not a basis for negligence, the judge found that the mother was never properly advised by any of the doctors as to what had occurred, nor what the future held for her daughter.

Monitoring

'Keeping an eye open.' Sister Smith could not be traced to give evidence. Sister Parker, an experienced neonatal nurse, described in detail how taping kept the cannula in place. Sister Parker agreed that the possibility of leaking and tissue damage in such babies was a high risk that merited frequent observations. She was not able to put a time on what was meant by 'frequent.'[18] One hour appeared to be normal, with one doctor preferring half an hour.

Sister Parker said nursing staff 'keep an eye open'[19] on the incubator to view the area of the foot around the infusion line. Her evidence was particularly important in describing the technique of observation. She explained that competent nurses needed to be alert to even a small amount of swelling or discolouration.

Touch. Nurse Turner explained her technique involved feeling by finger and thumb for swelling and warmth in order to determine any disturbance of the vascular supply. She would observe colour, and would also check the state of the cannula and attachment. She could not remember her observations at 7.45 am, explaining that Surest must have been satisfactory in order for her to make a note in that way. Nurse Turner's evidence was central to Surest's case. If she was right, there could not have been a leak occurring, so as to cause any significant damage at 7.40 am.

Another nurse, Sister Coates, told the court that on her examination of the child shortly after 8 am, she was more impressed by swelling and did not see any bluish or necrotic condition.

Expert medical evidence

Paediatricians

For the baby. A paediatrician, giving expert evidence on behalf of Surest, said he had never seen a child with such a severe injury. He admitted his experience with such small babies was very limited. The paediatrician concluded that at least 5ml must have leaked in order to cause such damage. It would have involved a 30 per cent increase in the transverse width of the leg. There would be a noticeable and very marked swelling. Even 2ml would have resulted in an 18 per cent expansion. This would be equally noticeable, if not as marked. His central thesis was based on the degree of injury, together with the length and quantity of the leak.

The paediatrician said that he would not have expected to see such effects as had occurred in a leak of less than an hour. On this view, it was contended that nurse Turner must have missed the swelling after a 'tiring, hard working night,'[20] her fourth consecutive night shift.

For the hospital. The paediatrician giving expert evidence for the hospital had significant experience in neonatal care, but saw such small babies 'irregularly.'[21] He had never seen such severe injuries. In his opinion, no more than 2ml of liquid could reasonably have accumulated. If it had, it would have occurred, at the rate of infusion, within 20 minutes. This was within the period between nurse Turner's observations and nurse Smith's discovery. The paediatrician said the effect of the liquid on surrounding tissue would inevitably have continued after nurse Smith's discovery, perhaps for up to an hour or more. It was this that had laid the foundation for what he thought was irreversible damage.

Plastic surgeons

For the baby. The plastic surgeon giving expert evidence for Surest had no real experience of neonates, but was experienced in extravasation injury. His 'strong view'[22] was that she should have received more active postoperative management. This would have involved assessment by a plastic surgeon, as well as an orthopaedic consultant. Light exercise and splinting would follow such assessment. These precautions would avoid the risk of contractures from scarred tissue and tendon damage.

For the hospital. The plastic surgeon giving expert evidence for the hospital did treat neonates. He said the plantar flexed position was probably the result of damage to the upper tendons. The foot drop was caused by the healthy lower tendons being able to pull down the foot, the upper damaged ones being unable to keep it in place. The calcaneal valgus was the result of scar tissue developing inevitably from the nature of the severe damage. This view was supported by the operative findings.

The condition of Surest's foot at 8. am. The absence of nurse Smith as a witness put everyone in difficulties as to what her note had meant. While the paediatrician giving expert evidence for the hospital had doubted the accuracy of her entry '? Necrotic',[23] the paediatrician on behalf of Surest had found it acceptable. The judge accepted the evidence of nurses Parker and Coates, both experienced neonatal nurses. They described a 'swollen and oedematous' area, but had not identified 'blueness or necrosis.'[24]

At what rate had the damage occurred? The judge said he had been concerned to understand and properly appreciate the type of injury process in such a small baby. He had been shown an injection capsule plus what constituted 2ml and concluded that it was a large amount of fluid in such a tiny limb. This was significant, given the lack of 'deep' experience in any of the medical witnesses in caring for such a child. They had all had to try to apply their minds to the likely volumes involved, together with the likely results, in terms of speed and effect, of fluid on surrounding tissue.

Foundation laid for severe injury. Expert evidence for the hospital was the more convincing. The probability was that the leak had started after nurse Turner made her 7. 40 am observations. It was likely to be well under way when nurse Smith discovered the problem at 8 a.m. This accorded with the rate of infusion, the likely size of the leg and the judge's assessment (from exhibits) of the amount of fluid going in. It was then probable that the damage progressed. In 1991, there had been no generally practiced system for the irrigation of fluid from the limb. The foundation had thus been laid for the severity of the injury.

Assertions of overload. Nurse Turner was described as 'an impressive witness.'[25] Her observations were accepted as accurate. This was so despite 'forceful' assertions that her workload and nearness to changeover may have contributed to her 'missing the obvious.' The judge noted that she had carefully observed and acted on matters earlier that evening. These actions had resulted in significant changes to Surest's condition. The first part of Surest's case therefore failed.

Postoperative management. The plastic surgeon (for Surest), contended that when such incidents occur, parents should be fully supported. Where feasible, they should be asked to participate in their child's care. In this instance, they could have assisted with light physiotherapy. This had not happened. The judge felt this probably represented 1997 thinking applied to 1991 circumstances. This thinking had coloured this plastic surgeon's view of the case.

Reasonable practice. The plastic surgeon (for the hospital), said that in 1991 such injuries were dealt with conservatively. The judge said times had changed. A different regime would be employed in 1997, with a likely 25 per cent reduction in damage. However, the practice followed had been reasonable in 1991. In any event, the treating doctors could not have known of the child's internal condition because in the first few weeks the scar was kept intact to avoid skin breakdown. The second part of Surest's case then failed.

The decision

Complex care. The judge acknowledged that not only do premature babies now survive because of the very complex care they receive, but that nursing and medical staff have extensive demands on their skills and time. In Surest's case, the hospital had given its best care. Her family would understandably feel such severe and long term injury could only be the consequence of negligence for which they should be compensated – but this was not the appropriate conclusion to what the judge described as a 'sad and difficult' case.

I regret to have reached the conclusion I have, because the child is clearly going to be affected in the longer term as a teenager and as an adult, but regret it though I do it is the conclusion I firmly reach.[26]

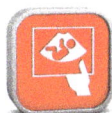

Discussion of Key Issues

Wilsher: The clear message for risk managers from this House of Lords decision (where both an inexperienced resident doctor and a registrar failed to pick up a misplaced in-dwelling catheter in a premature baby) is that staff in specialized areas will be expected to reach the specialized standard of care required by the position they occupy or the task they elect to perform. Because it is unlikely that inexperience will succeed as a defence, inexperienced staff must be supervised properly. (What excuses would you accept after being run into by a learner driver?)

This duty to supervise is only another version of a hospital's duty of care to provide adequate numbers of competent staff. The vulnerable and totally dependent newborn have a right to the standard of care their condition requires from a hospital offering specialist neonatal care.

- What are your concerns (if any) about the competency of staff in your nursery?

....

Anonymous: The reasoning in relation to medical staff in *Wilsher* can be translated to nursing staff in this case.

- What 'near misses' have you known when inexperienced medical/ nursing staff have been 'floated' to special care nurseries?
- Where do such problems originate?

Following a medication error (that would lead to a resident's death in a nursing home), the nurse involved said she was later 'crying in the day room – but no-one seemed to notice.'

- Do you think adequate counselling and care is given to staff (experienced/inexperienced) involved in serious incidents?

....

Coronial inquest: Victorian legislation has shifted the emphasis away from individual blame to a concentration on systemic problems, where appropriate. This inquest followed a baby's death after a nurse mistakenly attached a suction tube to the oxygen. Hospital initiatives then occurred in the areas of training and staff education, equipment failure and incident reporting, as well as the method of sputum collection.

The coroner agreed with the family's submission that fear of consequences in a hospital should not operate to conceal facts from a family.

- Have you known this to happen?

When examining the baby, the doctor was unaware a mistake had occurred.

- How would/do you manage staff in the highly charged atmosphere which surrounds an emergency, in order that doctors receive the best history possible?

....

Narwoor: The judge found that the mother was never properly advised by doctors about the leak in the IV, nor about what the future held for her daughter.

- Can you think of an instance when parents were not kept properly informed? Discuss your role.
- The nurses gave evidence that the risk of leaking and tissue damage in such premature babies was a high risk that merited 'frequent' observations. How would you define 'frequent' to a court?
- Discuss the nurses' explanations of what such observation meant – then give your own.
- Do you agree with the judge's decision? If not, give reasons.

NOTES

1.   Powers & Harris, *Medical Negligence,* Butterworths, London (1994), pp.696–697.
2.   Ibid.
3.   *Wilsher v Essex Area Health Authority,* 3 All ER (1986), 801 HL (1988), 1 All ER 87.1.
4.   *Anonymous v. Anonymous Hospital, King County (WA) Superior Court.* Nurse's Case of the Month, (Medical Malpractice Verdicts, Settlements & Experts) (Nov.1999). http://www. nso.com/case 0797.
5.   *Report of an Investigation into Death,* No. 1219/00, (Victoria, 2002). (Page references not available at the time of writing.)
6.   Ibid.
7.   Ibid.
8.   Ibid.
9.   Ibid.
10. Ibid.

11. BBC News, *The Health Service Ombudsman*. (27 October, 2000).

12. The NHS describes nursery nurses working in neonatal nurseries as usually working under an RN and being responsible for the feeding, changing and comforting of newborn babies.

13. *Nawoor v Barking Havering, QBD 313*.

14. Ibid., p.316.

15. Ibid., p.317.

16. Ibid., p.318.

17. Ibid., p.319.

18. Ibid.

19. Ibid.

20. Ibid., p.320.

21. Ibid.

22. Ibid., p.321.

23. Ibid.

24. Ibid.

25. Ibid., p.322.

26. Ibid., p.323.

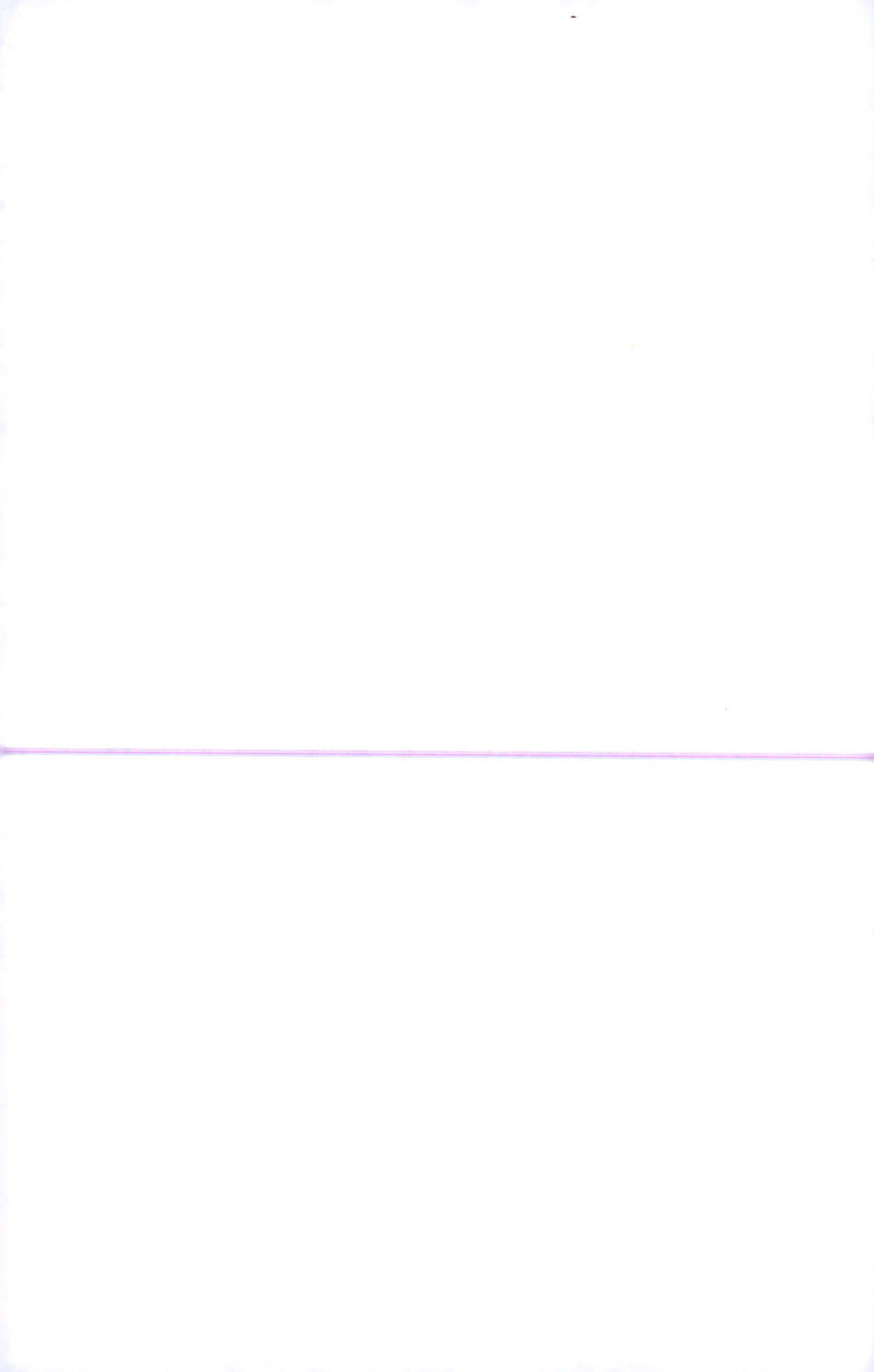

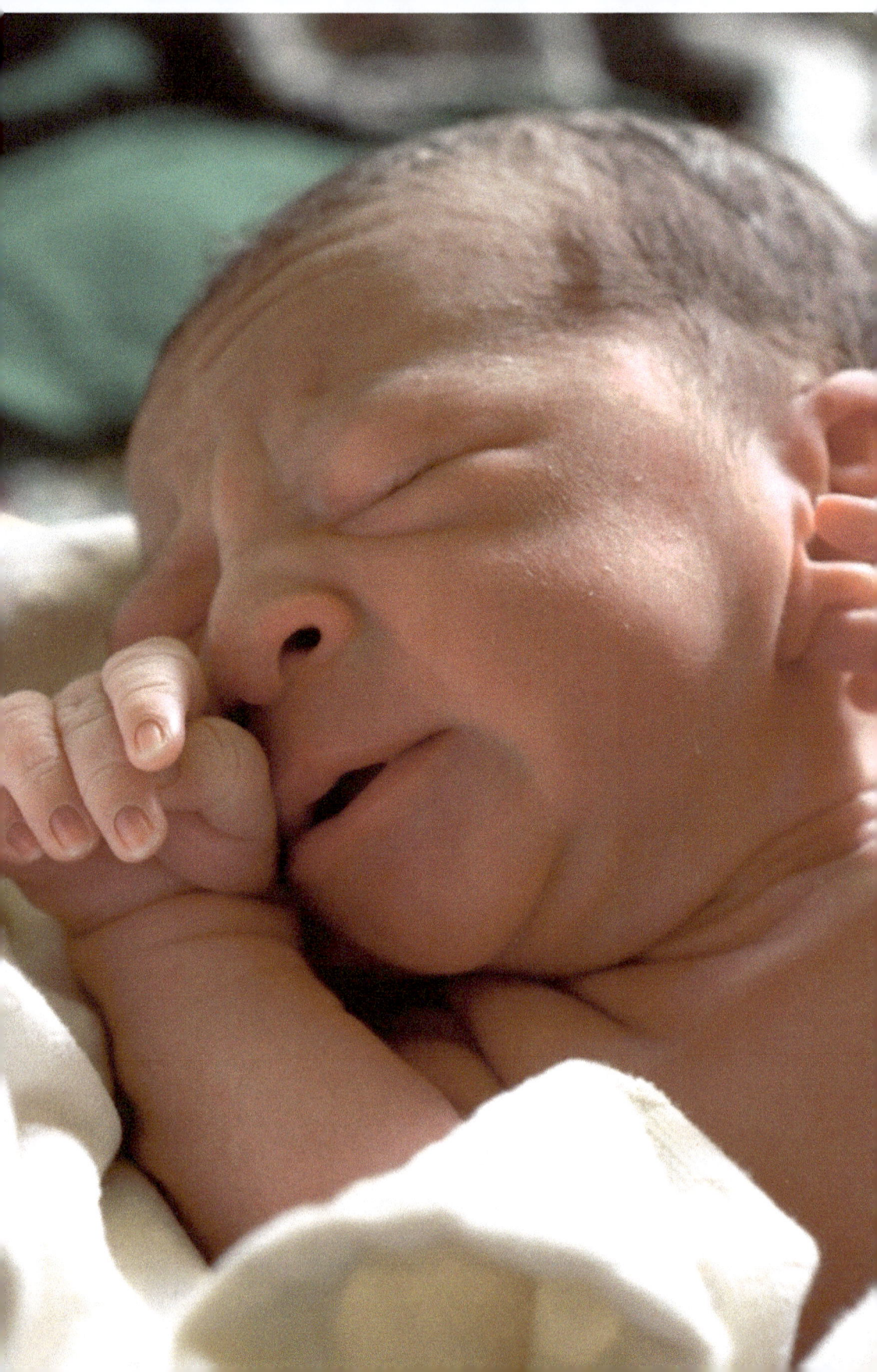

CHAPTER 15

The Neonatal Unit-times/ reporting problems

'Hospitals should have procedures for nurses to take patient care issues up the hospitals chain of command until they get appropriate results.'

—A lawyer

Introduction

In all four cases in this chapter, parents allege (with varying degrees of success) that nurses and doctors had not acted 'in a timely fashion' and that this delay was the cause of their baby's neurological injury.

In the first case, it was alleged that transfer to a NICU had been unreasonably delayed. What is 'reasonable' will depend on the circumstances of each individual case.

Blodgett v Kahn [US, 1996][1]

The facts

Mia, 26 weeks into her first pregnancy, went to an emergency department believing she was in labour. A doctor found her cervix was not dilated, but believed premature labour had started. As the hospital was not equipped to handle such a premature infant, the doctor arranged transfer to a hospital with appropriate facilities some 144 km away. An ambulance was called, arriving 50 minutes later. Mia was put on board 20 minutes after that. It then took approximately 30 minutes for the ambulance to leave with a nurse.

Re-direction of the ambulance. Halfway into the trip, Mia's waters broke. The nurse found the cervix dilated six centimeters and the baby's head visibly emerging. The nurse redirected the ambulance to the nearest hospital, where the baby was delivered. A neonatal transport team from the hospital that was the original destination, then arrived and took the baby the rest of the way. The baby was born blind and brain damaged.

The trial

In a negligence action against the first hospital, it was alleged that the nurse was negligent in delaying the original transfer. A neonatologist told the court the 50-minute delay from when the ambulance arrived until when it left was below the standard of care for the nurse.

The decision

No specific legal standard. Both the trial and appeal court dismissed the claim. The appeal court held there was no legal standard requiring a specific maximum number of minutes to effect a patient's transfer. Nurses and doctors are guided by their best professional judgment in all the circumstances.

....

In the second case, the central issue is whether a nurse notified a resuscitation team of an impending high-risk delivery 'in a timely fashion.'

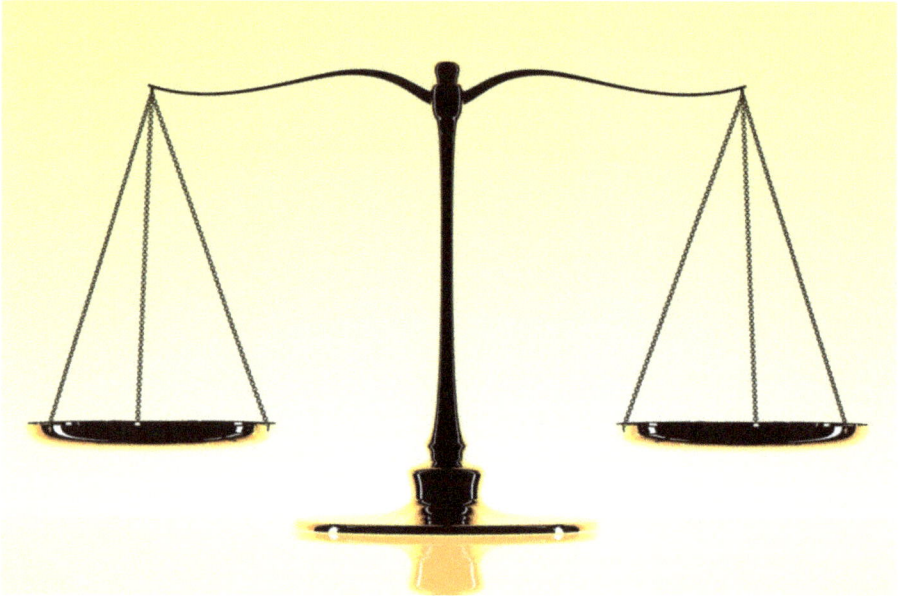

Salas v Wang [US, 1988][2]

The facts

Wendy was admitted to hospital in active labour. When the fetal monitor indicated distress, the obstetrician told a midwife to notify the charge nurse of the NICU of an impending highrisk delivery. The midwife called the charge nurse twice to update her on the situation. Twenty minutes prior to the birth she called the charge nurse again, telling her to send a resuscitation team to the delivery room immediately. The team did not arrive until several minutes after the birth. The baby sustained severe brain damage as a result of meconium aspiration syndrome.

The decision

The jury found the charge nurse of the NICU negligent. She had failed to notify the team in 'a timely fashion.' This delay had resulted in the resuscitation team's inability to arrive in time to assist the baby.

Re-admission

The third case is concerned with the re-admission of a baby to a NICU. The baby was discharged from the NICU but returned to the hospital via its emergency department. This case identifies the necessity for parents to have clear directions about the re-admission process. It also highlights the need to have nurses with paediatric training in emergency departments whenever possible in order to lessen the risk of miscommunication and delay. Courts hear evidence that babies and young children deteriorate quickly and that time can be critical.

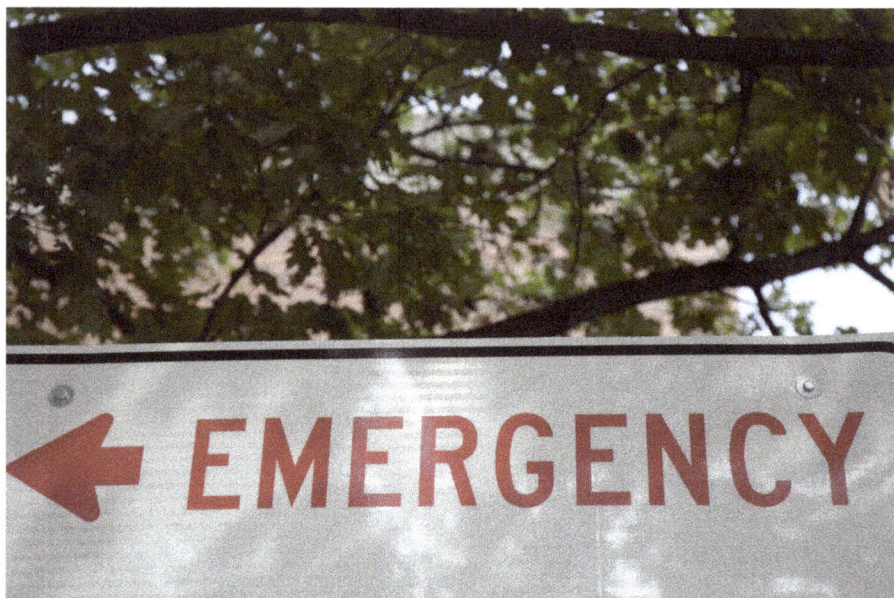

South Fulton Medical Centre v Poe [US, 1996][3]

The facts

When Sam was discharged from a hospital's NICU, his parents were told to bring him back to the hospital at once if he had even a slight fever, a change in feeding habits or a change in colour.

The parents brought Sam to the emergency department of the hospital the following day. They told the triage nurse that he had turned blue, had not had a bowel movement all day, appeared limp and that his eyes had rolled back.

Parents highly agitated. The parents were highly agitated, and wanted Sam to be seen immediately by a doctor. The triage nurse had insisted they fill out certain forms. She made a cursory examination of the baby, and repeatedly reassured the parents that he was fine, apparently in an attempt to stop their demanding behaviour.

Classification. The nurse then classified Sam as semi-urgent. This meant he would require medical intervention within eight hours, but did not have an immediate life threatening problem. The nurse told the parents to wait, as the doctor would be with them shortly. Based on these reassurances, the parents elected to leave. Sam died a few hours later.

Negligence was alleged against the hospital.

The trial

False reassurances. The court found the triage nurse negligent in that she had not taken a full history, nor assessed the gravity and immediacy of the baby's condition. Further, she had not brought his condition to the immediate attention of a doctor. In an apparent effort to control or defuse the situation, the nurse had falsely reassured the parents that Sam was alright. The court blamed the parents' decision to leave on those false reassurances, not for leaving against medical advice.

Damages awarded.

....

While a paediatrician bore the brunt of responsibility for the mismanagement of a jaundiced baby in the final case in this chapter, the court also found that nurses had delayed in bringing the jaundice to his attention and had not documented the progress of the jaundice. The court emphasized the need for a process to be in place that requires all medical and nursing staff to take problems that are not resolving up the hospital's 'chain of command' until the problem resolves.

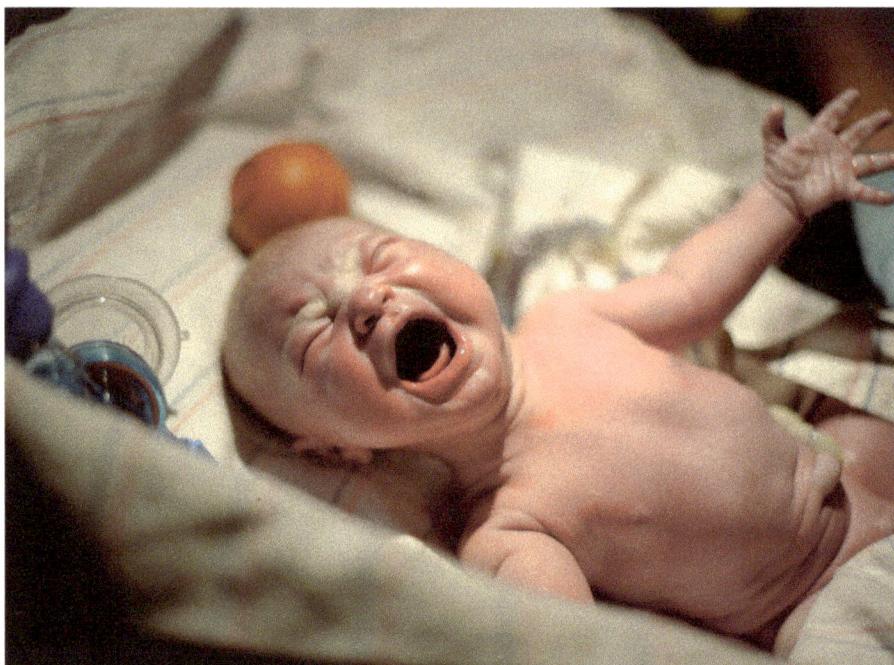

Sheridan v St Luke's Regional Medical Center [US, 2001][4]

The facts

Mark was born at 11.52 am on 23 March 1995. A paediatrician examined him approximately 10 hours later. Within 17 hours of Mark's birth, a nurse documented the presence of jaundice. The paediatrician was not notified. On the next shift, and within 24 hours of the birth, a nurse also noted jaundice. Again, the paediatrician was not notified.

Discharge. On 25 March, 33-34 hours after birth, the paediatrician examined Mark, performed a circumcision and arranged for his discharge. The medical chart noted that the baby 'has moderate icterus on head, mild icterus on body.'[5] The parents were given a handout on jaundice, but were not offered any special counselling about abnormal jaundice. Bilirubin levels were not measured.

Increased jaundice. The paediatrician next saw Mark, now five days old, on 28 March, approximately 78 hours after the hospital discharge. Mark's mother had contacted the paediatrician because Mark was not feeding as vigorously, seemed sleepy and lethargic, and was still yellow. The paediatrician noted the jaundice had increased and also discovered the baby had an ear infection in both ears. Oral antibiotics were ordered, but Mark was not hospitalized.

Admission to paediatric unit. On 29 March, Mark's mother telephoned the paediatrician again to say the baby was not improving and that the jaundice had increased. The paediatrician arranged for Mark's admission to the paediatric unit, where bilirubin levels were found to be 34.6/100 ml. The paediatrician arrived at the hospital at 6.30 pm and consulted with a neonatologist, who recommended a second bilirubin test. In the meantime, Mark was placed under a double bank of bili lights. When the results confirmed the high bilirubin level, phototherapy was continued. A blood exchange transfusion, which would have resulted in an immediate reduction in the bilirubin levels, was not performed.

Kernicterus. On 30 March, after Mark began exhibiting arching or hyperextension movements of the neck (opisthotonos) and had a sharp, high-pitched cry, an ear, nose and throat specialist ordered an MRI and other tests. Mark was discharged in April and ultimately diagnosed with kernicterus, a form of cerebral palsy associated with a neonatal history of elevated serum bilirubin and consequent jaundice.

Negligence was alleged.

The decision

The jury found in favour of the hospital and doctors. The judge then granted the parents a new trial on the grounds that there had been insufficient evidence to justify the jury's verdict and the hospital and doctors appealed.

The appeal court reviewed the evidence.

The diagnosis of kernicterus. The hospital argued that it had been an abuse of discretion for the trial judge, 'with no medical training or expertise, to presume to reach the sweeping conclusion that one side of this serious and complex medical debate was wrong'[6] and to discount the evidence presented for the defence.

Conflicting evidence addressed. The appeal court reiterated the principle that a trial judge (who sees and hears witnesses) is in a better position than an appeal court (where judges hear only legal argument) to weigh the demeanor, credibility and testimony of the witnesses, as well as the persuasiveness of all the evidence. In this case, the appeal court found the trial judge had specifically addressed the conflicting interpretations of the MRI studies, the evidence of one medical expert (who thought it was a virus), and two other doctors called for the defence who 'were only 49 per cent sure it was kernicterus.'[7]

The appeal court found the trial judge had 'clearly understood' [8] that the diagnosis of kernicterus was disputed, but was persuaded that this was what Mark was suffering from.

Causal link. The hospital also argued that a causal link had not been established between the alleged negligence of hospital staff and Mark's injuries. In other words, the hospital argued that even if there had been negligence, it was not the cause of the baby's injuries.

The appeal court reviewed the evidence the trial judge had considered on this point:

1. The hospital did not have in place any protocols or policies on jaundice. General policies and protocols required newborn nursery nurses to notify the paediatrician when any general abnormal symptoms or conditions were noted. None of the nurses had done so.

2. The nurses had instructed the mother only on the progress of normal jaundice. They had not warned her that Mark's jaundice might not be normal or that serious brain damage could occur if it worsened and was not treated.

3. The nurses also knew that no bilirubin tests had been conducted even though these tests were routine and readily available; nor did they suggest such tests to the paediatrician. The judge had heard that such suggestions were often made to doctors and usually acted upon. If not accepted or acted upon, there was a procedure within the hospital for a nurse to act as a patient's advocate and insist that the doctor's decision on treatment be reviewed. This had not occurred.

4. There was a failure to establish any policy with regard to the handling of cord blood retrieved at birth, particularly whether it was, or should have been, tested to reveal the possible blood incompatibility between Mark and his mother. The confusion in the chart led the doctors to assume the blood types were the same when they were not. The paediatrician said that if he had realized that Mark's blood was different from his mother's, he would have treated the hyperbilirubinemia more aggressively.

5. The two nurses who cared for Mark during his first 24 hours both noted the existence of jaundice, one at 17 hours and the other at 23 hours. Both testified they would be concerned if the jaundice progressed rapidly, and that it was the progress of the jaundice, rather than the mere presence of it, that would be of concern. However, neither nurse had documented any indicia from which progress could be ascertained by other members of staff. Nurses on later shifts made no inquiry of earlier nurses to ascertain the progress of the jaundice. The third nurse to care for Mark on the morning of his discharge noted that jaundice was present over his entire body - moderate on head, mild on trunk and extremities. The nurse had not considered this alarming.

6. While the paediatrician bore the brunt of responsibility for the mismanagement of the baby's care, some degree of fault had to be attributed to the failure of the nurses to be the 'physician's eyes and ears' at the outset of Mark's life. If the nurses had sounded the alarm upon the first observation of jaundice, and if they had pressed for bilirubin monitoring before he was discharged from hospital the first time, the catastrophe would have been averted.

The decision

'Chain of circumstances.' The appeal court concluded that although the hospital's actions were limited to the first 36 hours of Mark's life, and it was days later before the high bilirubin levels were measured, a jury could 'reasonably and naturally' [9] infer from the chain of circumstances that a breach in the standard of care in the first hospital stay was the proximate cause of Mark's brain damage. This decision was reached on the basis that:

1. Expert evidence had been presented that jaundice showing within the first 24 hours is pathological, requiring further evaluation such as a serum bilirubin measurement.

2. Evidence had also been presented that high bilirubin levels can be successfully treated by the use of bili lights and blood exchange transfusions. There had been no dispute that jaundice had appeared within 24 hours.
3. Nurses giving expert evidence said the hospital nurses had breached their standard of care by (a) not notifying the paediatrician when jaundice appeared; (b) not documenting the progression of the jaundice; (c) not noting the possible blood incompatibility problems of the mother and child; and (d) sending the parents home with information on physiologic or normal jaundice, but not warning them that Mark's jaundice was abnormal. Cerebral palsy associated with a neonatal history of elevated bilirubin, a symptom of which is jaundice, had resulted. Settlement reached.

Note the following comments from an American legal commentator on the Sheridan case.[10]

1. Hospitals should have procedures for nurses to take patient care issues up the hospital's chain of command until they get appropriate results.
2. Nurses must chart their observations. They must report to later nursing shifts in a way that allows those nurses to tell if the problem is resolving. None of the nurses on later shifts had talked to the earlier nurses to find out how jaundice was progressing. One nurse did not find it alarming that the jaundice had spread to Mark's entire body.
3. The court faulted the hospital for not having a protocol for incompatible maternal and umbilical cord blood types to be brought to a paediatrician's attention promptly. The court did not specifically state this was a nursing responsibility.
4. The nurses should have taken signs of jaundice more seriously. If a baby is not tested and bili lights not started (relatively easy and effective interactions), the condition can lead to a form of cerebral palsy (kernicterus).
5. If newborns are discharged with jaundice, parents must be taught what to look for. They must be impressed with the need to bring the baby back immediately if jaundice does not go away.

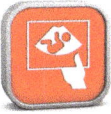

Discussion of Key Issues

In *Blodget,* there were allegations of delay in the intra-hospital transfer. The court found there was no standard in the U.S at that date requiring a specific time for transfer of neonates between hospitals. The matter was best left to the professional judgment of doctors and nurses. The important risk management point for hospitals and NETS is that delay was alleged and transfer times will have to be explained and justified.

Where transfer times are relevant, they will have to be explained and justified in the circumstances of that particular transfer. Hospital policy and protocols, professional standards and expert witnesses all inform a court of what would be considered reasonable in similar circumstances.

- Have you known any instances of 'unreasonable' delay? Discuss.
- Would your documentation support a 'timely transfer'?

....

Salas was concerned with intra-hospital delay. No explanation was given for the charge nurse's delay in organizing a resuscitation team to the delivery.

- Could you suggest to a court any circumstances in a NICU that would take priority over organizing a resuscitation team?
- Would documentation reflect these circumstances?

....

In *South Fulton,* the parents were trying to re-admit their baby to the NICU via the emergency department. Courts hear evidence that babies can deteriorate very rapidly.

- If parents are instructed by NICU staff to bring their baby back to the hospital 'at once' in the event of certain symptoms developing, how can quick access to appropriate care be ensured?

- Have you known unacceptable delays to occur when a baby is re-admitted through an emergency department ?
- Do you think that having nurses with paediatric training in emergency departments would alleviate delay?

....

In *Sheridan,* the paediatrician bore the brunt of responsibility for the mismanagement of the baby's care. The court also found some degree of fault could be attributed to the nurses, who were described as the 'eyes and ears' of the doctor. The following issues for discussion are drawn from the findings. No doubt you will find more. For example, would you have concerns about a doctor performing a circumcision on a jaundiced baby? What is the nursing/ midwifery role in this situation?

- Do you have a protocol requiring nurses to notify the paediatrician when abnormal symptoms or conditions (such as jaundice) are noted?
- Have you differed with a paediatrican as to what is 'abnormal'? What was the outcome? If you are a paediatrician, how would you see this issue?
- How are mothers educated about jaundice at discharge?
- Is there a risk (as occurred in this case) that on discharge a mother may be warned on the progress of 'normal' but not 'abnormal' jaundice?
- Are mothers made sufficiently aware of the risk of serious brain damage?
- Are mothers sufficiently impressed with the need to bring the baby back to hospital?
- Are they given clear instructions about quick access of care in the hospital?
- Whose responsibility is it to give advice on/before discharge? Are warnings in specific cases given in writing as well as verbally?
- Where are the possible breakdowns in communication with community or Maternal and Child Health nurses about a baby's jaundice?
- M&CH nurses say that mothers can be inappropriately relied upon by doctors as the historians of a baby's condition. What do you believe prevents a paediatrician communicating directly by phone and/or letter with M&CH?

- Is it a nursing responsibility to remind a paediatrican that routine tests have not been performed? Or to suggest other tests?
- Do you have a process requiring nurses and doctors to take a professional concern up the hospital's chain of command?
- In this case, there was no protocol for having incompatible maternal and umbilical cord blood types brought to the paediatrician's notice. The court did not specifically state this was a nursing responsibility. Do you have such a protocol? Whose responsibility is it?
- The court found that some nurses were not documenting information in a way that enabled nurses on later shifts to properly ascertain the progress of jaundice. Is there a risk that the 'existence' rather than the 'progress' of jaundice is documented?
- Do you agree with the court's description of nurses as 'the eyes and ears' of the doctors?

NOTES

1. *Blodgett v. Kahn,* 681 N.E. 2d 452 (Ohio App, 1996.) Note based on *Legal Eagle Eye Newsletter for the Nursing Profession* (5) 9 Sept. 1997.
2. *Salas v. Wang,* 846 F.2d 987 (1998).
3. *South Fulton Medical Center v. Poe,* 480 S.E 2d 40, Note based on *Legal Eye Newsletter for the Nursing Profession* (5) 4 April 1997.
4. *Sheridan v. St Luke's Regional Medical Center,* 25 P.3d 88 Idaho, (2001).
5. Ibid., p.4.
6. Ibid., p.6.
7. Ibid., p.7.
8   Ibid., p.6.
9. Ibid., p.10.
10. *Legal Eagle Eye Newsletter for the Nursing Profession,* Sept, 2001, p.7.

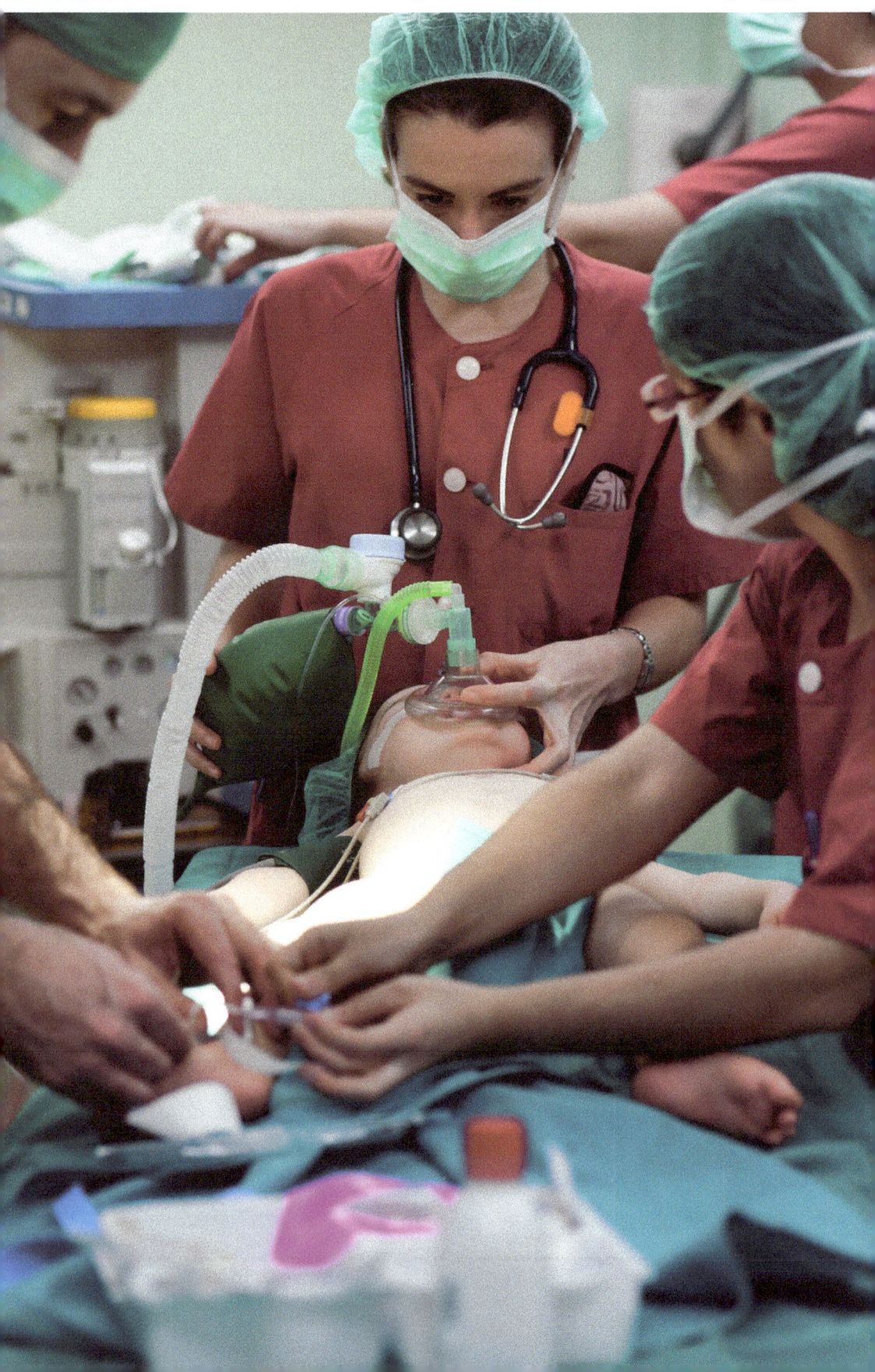

CHAPTER 16

The Neonatal Unit-medication

'The syringes were placed in a plastic bag and labelled with directions to administer 2.5 ml of the medication I.M. to equal a dose of 1,500,000 units (one full syringe and one quarter of the other). The correct dose should have been 150,000 units/0.25 ml.'

— A nurse

Introduction

Hospitals have a duty to put systems in place to ensure that medication is managed safely in neonatal units. The first case in this chapter, although set in a paediatric ward, is a cautionary note to risk managers that adverse outcomes can occur when staff come from adult wards to neonatal areas and administer medication. In this context note the warning of English paediatrician Professor Campbell (quoting William E Ladd) that: 'The adult may be safely treated as a child, the converse can lead to a disaster.'[1] Campbell explains that young infants are vulnerable to errors in the calculation of drug doses as the complex mechanisms involved in the absorption, distribution, metabolism and excretion of drugs may be relatively immature.[2] However, treat with caution the judge's statement in *Norton's* case that nurses are not held to the same degree of knowledge as doctors about the drugs they administer.[3] This was a judicial opinion in 1962. The contemporary view is that any person administering a drug has a duty to know the route, dosage, cause and effect of the drug they are administering.

That said, this case contains timeless lessons: to doctors to give clear, unambiguous medication orders; to nurses to be up-to-date in their knowledge of what they are administering; and to risk managers to ensure that not only is there a system in place in their hospitals whereby nurses can clarify an ambiguous order, but that the judge found that nurses have 'the duty and obligation of making themselves understood beyond the possibility or error' when clarifying such an order. Note how the doctors explained their role in the checking of another doctor's medication order.

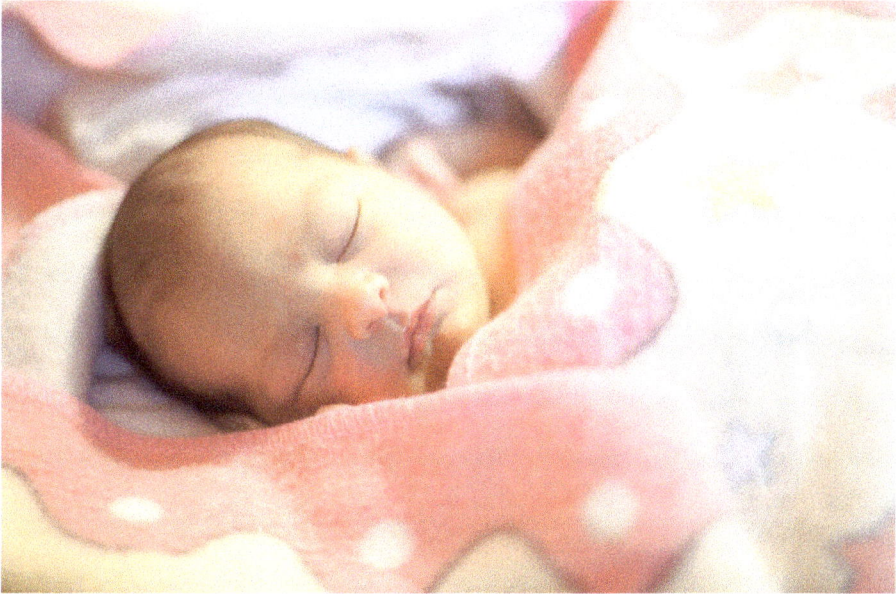

Norton v Argonaut Insurance Company [US, 1962][4]

The facts

When Elise was three months old, a paediatrician detected heart murmurs. After a cardiologist and a cardiac surgeon agreed that surgery was indicated, Elise was admitted to hospital for further examination and treatment. On admission, the cardiologist wrote orders for various drugs including: 'Elixir Paediatric Lanoxin 2.5 cc (0.125 mg) q6h x 3 then once daily.'[5] This order meant that the infant was to be administered 2.5 cc of Lanoxin every six hours for three doses and then once daily (a maintenance dose). The court heard that the function of Lanoxin, a derivative of digitalis, is to increase the efficiency or strength of the pumping action of the heart, while at the same time reducing the pulse, thereby minimizing strain on the heart. Evidence was given that Lanoxin is a potent drug that must be administered with caution and care.

Methods of administration. Lanoxin came in three forms: (1) elixir or in alcohol solution which was administered orally or by mouth by means of a calibrated medicine dropper; (2) pill or tablet form taken orally; and (3) in injectible liquid form which was contained in sealed ampoules containing two c.cs of the solution. (Note: The abbreviation 'c.cs' is the one used in the clinical documentation in this case.) Both the liquid and injectible forms of Lanoxin were measured in cubic centimeters.

Administration by mother. After Elise's mother became concerned that the nurses were not administering the drug on time, she was given permission by the cardiologist to administer the daily maintenance dose of 2.5 c.cs (from a calibrated medicine dropper) herself. Elise remained in hospital for two weeks, receiving Lanoxin from her mother as ordered.

Increased dose. Elise was then discharged home to await the scheduling of surgery, but 12 days later the paediatrician found her condition had deteriorated and readmitted her to the paediatric ward. Included with the paediatrician's admission orders was a statement that special medication was being given by the mother. This was in order to advise staff that some medication was being given by the mother other than that which he placed on the medication chart to be administered by nurses.

Three days later Elise was examined by the cardiologist, who concluded that an increase in the daily maintenance dose of Lanoxin was needed. He instructed the mother, who was in the room, to increase the dose to 3.c.cs instead of the usual 2.5 c.cs.

The cardiologist then noted the order on the medication chart as: 'Give 3.0 Lanoxin today for 1 dose only.'

A busy ward. The duties of the assistant director of nursing (ADON) at the hospital were primarily administrative and supervisory. However, hospital policy required that, when necessary, she was to assist nurses with routine nursing tasks. On the day on which Elise's medication order was changed, the hospital was understaffed and very busy. As the paediatric ward had only one RN and one SEN on duty, the ADON went there, accompanied by a senior student nurse. On checking patient records, she noticed the change of order for Elise's Lanoxin, noted that it had not been given and decided to administer it. Although an RN for many years, the ADON had been out of clinical nursing for some time, so was unaware that Lanoxin was now manufactured in elixir, as well as in injectible form.

Checking the order. Despite her limited knowledge of the drug, the ADON's training and 'womanly intuition'[6] warned her that 3 c.cs was a large dose to be given intramuscularly to a three-month-old infant. She discussed the matter briefly with the student nurse and asked the charge nurse whether Elise had previously received the drug. She then examined the hospital chart and found nothing which indicated the drug had been given. (This evidence was disputed.) Considering administration of the drug only by hyperdermic needle, the ADON, accompanied by the student nurse, then obtained two ampoules of Lanoxin each containing 2 c.cs of the drug in its injectible form.

While still pondering the advisability of administering such a large dose, the ADON saw Elise's surgeon, who was in the ward, and asked him. The surgeon advised that if the cardiologist had prescribed 3 c.cs., he meant 3 c.cs. Still not certain, the ADON discussed the matter with another doctor in the unit and was informed that although the dose was a maximum one, if the cardiologist had prescribed that amount, she could give it.

The overdose. The ADON obtained a syringe, drew up 3 c.cs of the drug from the two ampoules, injected one-half into each of the baby's buttocks and documented that she had administered the drug intramuscularly on the chart. A little over an hour later Elise, who had been upset after the injections, died. She had received five times the dose of digitalis than was prescribed.

Negligence was alleged against the cardiologist, who had written the increased order for Lanoxin, and the ADON.

The trial
The cardiologist

Failure to specify route. The ADON argued that the failure of the cardiologist to specify route was responsible for her injecting the Lanoxin because the order as written indicated the route to be intramuscularly by hypodermic.

The cardiologist argued that the order was written in accordance with common practice; this was contradicted by colleagues. The cardiologist also argued that in the event of any uncertainty, it was the duty of nurses to make sufficient inquiry to determine which type of administration was intended.

Misunderstandings. The ADON argued that she had checked with two doctors on the ward; both doctors said they were not made aware by the ADON of just what she intended to administer.

Double oral dose. The cardiologist conceded that he was in error for failing to note that on the morning in question the mother had already given (or was about to give) the 3 c.cs of Lanoxin. Without such explanation it was the duty of nurses to administer the dose. However he argued that at most, this error could have led to Elise receiving a double oral dose of the drug, which would have produced nausea but not been fatal.

A potent and highly specialized drug. The paediatrician explained to the court that because Lanoxin was such a potent and highly specialized drug, he at all times carried a pocket chart provided by the drug manufacturers and always consulted this before prescribing dosage rather than relying on memory.

The decision

The judge found the cardiologist negligent in failing to denote the intended route of administration and in failing to indicate that the medication prescribed had already been given or was to be given by the mother.

In dealing with modern drugs, especially of the type with which we are concerned, it is the duty of the prescribing doctor who knows that the prescribed medication will be administered by a nurse or a third party, to make certain as to the lines of communication between himself and the party whom he knows will ultimately execute his orders. Any failure in such communication which may prove fatal or injurious to the patient must be charged to the prescribing doctor, who has full knowledge of the drug and its effects on the human system.[7]

The duty of communication between doctor and nurse is more important when we consider that the nurse who administers the medication is not held to the same degree of knowledge as the doctor. It, therefore, becomes the duty of the doctor to make his intentions clear and unmistakable. If, as the record shows, the cardiologist had ordered Elixir Lanoxin, or specified the route to be oral, it would have clearly informed all nurses of his intention to administer the medication by mouth. Instead, he wrote his order in an uncertain, confusing manner considering the drug comes in oral as well as injectible form and in both forms dosage is prescribed in cubic centimetres.[8]

The ADON

Expert nursing evidence. The court heard that while some nurses consult any available doctor about an ambiguous order, the better practice, and the one they followed, was to consult with the prescribing doctor.

The student nurse. The student nurse who had accompanied the ADON to the paediatric ward gave evidence that the normal procedure at the hospital was to call the hospital pharmacy or the prescribing doctor when in doubt about a medication order.

Two doctors. Both the paediatrician and the second doctor consulted on the ward by the ADON said they were unaware of just what she intended to administer. The paediatrician said that he was under the impression she was referring to oral Lanoxin. The second doctor believed she intended only one cubic centimeter of the injectible drug. Both doctors told the court that in their experience, inquiries 'to any available doctor') are generally restricted to interpretation of the doctor's handwriting, and are not usually related to dosage or route.

The decision

Beyond the possibility of error. The judge found that the ADON had failed to meet the standard of care required of an RN when clarifying an order. Having elected to deviate from the general and better practice of consulting the doctor who ordered the medication, she was then 'under the duty and obligation of making herself understood beyond the possibility or error.'[10] It was reasonably clear that had the ADON consulted the cardiologist and advised him of her intention to administer the 3 cc of Lanoxin hypodermically, he would have warned her of the danger. The death would not have occurred.

Not only was she unfamiliar with the medication but she also violated what has been shown to be the rule generally practiced by the nursing profession – namely, the practice of calling the prescribing doctor when in doubt about an order.[11]

Damages awarded.

....

The next case concerns delay in diagnosing infection and administering antibiotics.

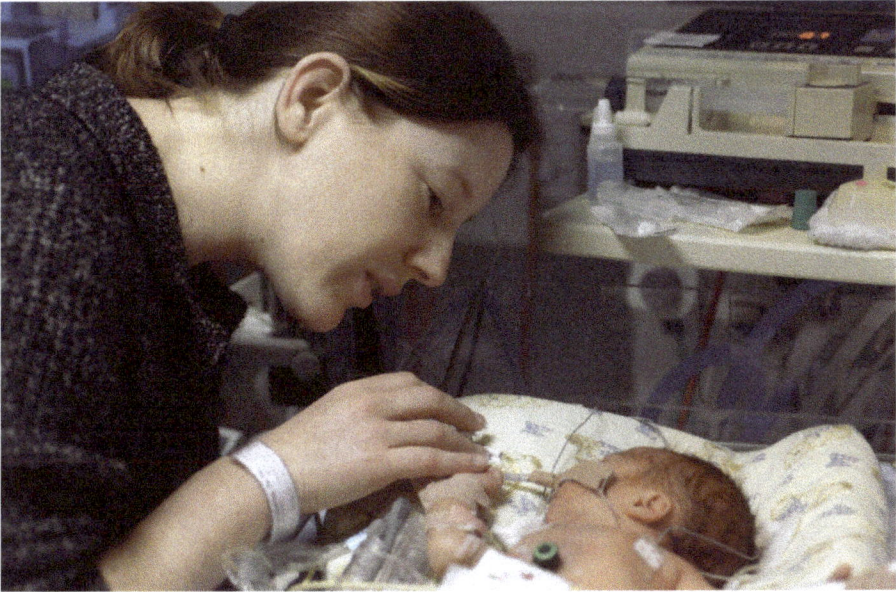

Wade v Tran [US, 1995][12]

The facts

The baby, one of twins, was born at 30 weeks, placed in a NICU and ventilated. After two weeks, inflammation developed in the left hand near an IV site. Approximately six hours later, breathing problems worsened, which required increased ventilator support.

Sepsis. That night, and early the next morning, the baby's condition deteriorated. After consultation with one of the two treating neonatologists, blood work was performed a few hours later. This showed increasing white blood cell and band cell counts. The second neonatologist then took over. The baby continued to deteriorate and a red streak was observed on his left arm later that afternoon. Antibiotics were administered, but sepsis had already developed. The baby was transferred to another hospital, but died 21 days later, survived by his twin brother.

The trial

The parents sued the two neonatologists, alleging failure to make a timely diagnosis and treat an infection. They claimed that in view of their baby's symptoms, staff should have ordered blood work sooner, tested for a suspected infection and initiated antibiotic therapy earlier. The jury agreed.

Damages awarded.

....

In the next case, the court had to determine whether pain relief administered to the mother during labour had an effect on the baby after birth and, if so, whether subsequent care in the nursery was appropriate.

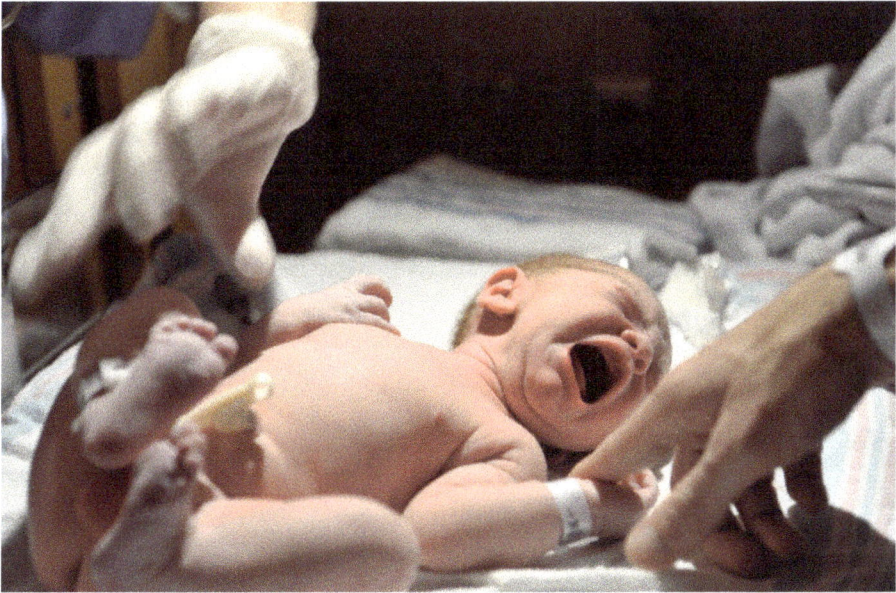

Chiricosta v Winthrop-Breon [US, 1994][13]

The facts

Rachel was given 25 mg of Demerol *(Pethidine Hydrochloride)* to relieve pain prior to giving birth to her son, Simon. There were no complications during delivery and the baby's condition remained stable for the first five minutes. However, after leaving the delivery room Simon had trouble breathing in the nursery. When his condition failed to improve, he was transferred to a second hospital.

Persistant fetal circulation. It was determined at the second hospital that Simon suffered from persistant fetal circulation of unknown etiology during the two and a half hours after delivery. What occurred during those two and a half hours became the subject of a trial after Simon was diagnosed with cerebral palsy.

Rachel alleged that:

1. The intravenous administration of Demerol to her approximately 30 minutes before delivery crossed the placental barrier, causing injury to the fetus.
2. The doctors and nursery staff at the first hospital were negligent in their treatment.
3. The package insert for Demerol was inadequate.

The jury found in favour of the hospital, doctors, nurses and the manufacturer of Demerol. Rachel appealed.

The Appeal Court reviewed the evidence.

The facts - reviewed

Rachel was admitted to hospital at 5.40 am on 22 March 1982 for the delivery of her third child. She was examined by the obstetrician who ordered 'Demerol, 25 milligrams I.V. p.r.n. for pain.'[14] Midwife Martin knew she was to give one dose when she thought appropriate and to contact the doctor if the patient requested more pain relief.

Demerol administered. At about 9.30 am, Rachel requested pain relief and midwife Martin administered a single dose of 25 mg of Demerol intravenously, taking between 50 seconds and one minute to give the injection. Before Rachel was taken to the delivery room, the fetal heart was checked eight times. It remained in the normal range of 120 to 160 beats per minute. Prior to the Demerol being administered at 9.30 am, the fetal heart tones had risen to 134-135. At 9.45 am, the heart rate returned to 120. No maternal depression was observed after the Demerol was administered.

The delivery. By 9.45 am, the cervix was fully dilated and at 10.07 am the obstetrician delivered Simon head first. There were no clinical signs of respiratory depression or reason to administer oxygen to the baby.

The Apgar scores. The one-minute and five-minute Apgar scores were made at 10.08 am and 10.12 am. Midwife Martin's scores were 8 at both the one-minute and five-minute scores, which she considered good. She gave Simon a score of 2 in the categories of heart rate, muscle tone and reflex irritability, and a score of 1 for respiration and skin colour.

(The court heard that a heart rate score of 2 would indicate a heart rate of 100 beats per minute at a minimum. A score of 2 for muscle tone indicated that the baby was moving spontaneously. Reflex irritation refers to whether the baby has a lusty cry and responds to external stimulation.) The nurse noted that the baby's throat had more mucous than normal.

Midwife Martin said the respiration score was because Simon was making a grunting or low congested sound after delivery. A score of 2 would indicate regular breathing at a rate of 35 to 50 breaths per minute. An 0 would indicate no spontaneous respiration. 1 is given for a slow breathing rate or some abnormal or irregular manner of breathing. She said the 1 for skin colour usually referred to a baby whose body is pink but whose extremities still have a bluish colouration.

The obstetrician gave a total Apgar score of 8 at the one-minute interval, with 1 for respiration and skin colour. At five minutes, 9 was given because he scored respiration at 2. The obstetrician believed that the grunting indicated the baby was making a good respiratory effort. (If Simon has been depressed from the Demerol after delivery, the obstetrician said he would not have expected to see scores of 2 for muscle tone and reflex irritability.)

Transfer to the nursery. Before his transfer to the nursery, Simon was held by both parents, who agreed that he 'looked fine.'[15] (midwife Martin said babies would not be given to parents to bond unless the babies were stable.) But as they approached the nursery, the father noticed his son's face turning blue.

The nursery. Nurse Long admitted Simon to the nursery at 10.30 am. Heart rate was within normal range, respiratory rate 36, temperature sub-normal, muscle tone fair, skin colour cyanotic. The nurse placed him in the special care section, deep suctioning for small amounts of mucous and fluids.

Heart rate was 134 and respiratory rate 34, with some retracting and pulling. Nurse Long said the baby was not going to sleep and did not appear narcotized. She placed him on an Ambu bag with a mask, which was set at 40 per cent oxygen. Simon showed some improvement in colour, which nurse Long described as 'very pale.'[16] He was still struggling to breathe. By 10.45 am, colour slightly improved to 'pale,'[17] but muscle tone was floppy. Heart rate decreased from 134 to 86.

Emergency calls. Simon was placed in an incubator and emergency calls were made to the obstetrician, a paediatrician and to a neonatologist.

The obstetrician. The obstetrician arrived first at 10.45 am, and remained in charge until the neonatologist arrived. The obstetrician had never resuscitated a baby in the nursery, but had experience in doing so in the delivery room. Simon was cyanotic, his heart rate down to 40 to 60 beats per minute. He appeared to be floppy and barely breathing. The obstetrician intubated him using the Ambu bag with 100 per cent oxygen, then suctioned. He periodically listened, observing to make sure the lungs were expanding on both sides.

No indication of respiratory depression. The obstetrician decided not to give Narcan. There had been no indication in the delivery room of narcotization or respiratory depression, or that the baby needed resuscitation. He thought the sudden change in condition was inconsistent with a diagnosis of narcotization. If Simon had been suffering from Demerol induced respiratory depression, he would have responded to the Ambu bag treatment by nurse Long or when he had reattached the bag with 100 per cent oxygen.

Tentative diagnoses. The obstetrician's tentative diagnoses were congenital heart disease and persistent fetal circulation secondary to pulmonary disease. The court heard that persistent fetal circulation means that the child's circulation system fails to make the transition from fetal circulation (where lungs are not used to oxygenate the blood) to post-fetal circulation (when the lungs are first used). The condition does not respond to oxygen therapy

In the obstetrician's opinion, Simon showed no signs of a typical case of respiratory depression due to medication. His condition had deteriorated over 30 minutes after delivery. Narcotized babies are slow to develop sustained, rhythmical breathing, usually do not cry and are sleepy. Simon, on the other hand, had Apgar scores of 8 at one-minute and five-minute intervals. Even if narcotization is delayed, it is usually apparent at the five-minute Apgar interval. This is because, after the adrenaline from the birth process decreases, the baby's respiration tends to drift off slowly between the one- and fiveminute scores.

Respiratory therapist. Shortly after 11 am, a respiratory therapist arrived and placed Simon on a ventilator, with 60 per cent oxygen and set pressure, inspiratory/expiratory ratio, rate and flow gauge as per the obstetrician's order. The flow was set to compensate for a minimal 'air leak' (the air returning from the lungs along the outside of the tube). This was desirable for a newborn. There was no improvement in colour. Adrenaline and Atropine were ordered. The heart rate increased to over 100. A chest X-ray was taken.

Paediatrician. At 11.02 am, a paediatrician arrived. Simon's colour had returned to cyanotic. Nail beds were dark. At 11.05 am, he was 'gaspy,'[18] making a respiratory effort separate and apart from the ventilator. Cardiac and respiratory monitors were attached. The heart rate was 107.

Neonatologist. At 11.10 am, a neonatologist arrived and took charge. He was aware the mother had received 25 mg of Demerol and knew from the package insert that :

1. Demerol, when used as an obstetrical analgesic, crosses the placental barrier. It can produce depression of respiratory and physiological functions in the newborn.
2. Demerol is a narcotic analgesic. Major hazards include respiratory depression and circulatory depression (to a lesser degree). Respiratory arrest, shock, and cardiac arrest have also been known to occur.
3. When used as an obstetrical analgesic, the usual dose is 50 to 100 mg, given intramuscularly or subcutaneously.
4. If given intravenously, Demerol should be given slowly and diluted, or given in a reduced dosage.

Primary treatment. The neonatologist also knew that the primary treatment for narcotic-induced respiratory depression is to re-establish an adequate respiratory exchange through a patent airway and assisted ventilation. He was aware the antagonist/antidote is Narcan and that an appropriate dose should be administered simultaneously with respiratory resuscitation.

Respiratory distress. When the neonatologist arrived in the nursery, Simon was suffering respiratory distress, serious shock and his colour was cyanotic. The neonatologist ordered 100 per cent oxygen from the ventilator, changing the inspiratory/expiratory rate from 1/1.5 to 1/1.1. He checked the position of the endotracheal tube, pulled it back a bit, then taped it in place. An X-ray confirmed that the tube and the arterial umbilical line were in place and the lungs were being filled with oxygen. By 11.30 am, respirator rate was 38, heart rate 168. Nurse Long noted the baby was warm.

The neonatologist did not think Simon was suffering from respiratory depression caused by Demerol. This opinion was based on the baby's history, the Apgar scores, appearance after delivery, the dosage of Demerol, and the fact that respiratory problems were not exhibited until after delivery. He saw no reason to administer Narcan.

Neonatal team. At 11.55 am, Simon's colour improved. He appeared more pink. The neonatologist continued to check the aeration. By 12.18 pm, colour was again cyanotic. Simon was removed from the respirator, then reconnected after an Ambu bag was used. The neonatologist continued to work with him until 1.00 pm, when the team from the second hospital arrived and assumed care.

Cerebral palsy. Simon remained at the second hospital for four weeks. The doctors determined that during the first few hours after his birth he had suffered from persistent fetal circulation of unknown etiology and, as a consequence, he suffered from cerebral palsy.

The decision

The manufacturer. The appeal court found the trial court had not acted unreasonably in accepting expert medical evidence that the package insert for Demerol was adequate in warning doctors of potential risk to mother, fetus and newborn child.

No delayed effect. A specialist in obstetrical anaesthetics told the court he had never read that 25 mg of Demerol given to the mother could cause respiratory depression in the newborn. The so-called 'delayed effect' of Demerol was not a delay at onset, but was a question of delay from the time of administration of the drug to the mother to the time of delivery. Where the drug is given one to four hours before the delivery, it accumulates in the baby's system. In some instances, this results in respiratory depression at birth. If the same dosage is given less than one hour before the delivery, it does not result in respiratory depression at birth.

The insert informed doctors that Demerol can and does cause respiratory depression, that resuscitation may be required and that an antidote may be necessary. The insert did not warn of a 'delayed effect' because such an effect did not exist.

Neonatologist. It was alleged that the neonatologist had been negligent in failing to re-intubate Simon (because the endotracheal tube was an inappropriate size) and for failing to give Narcan. Two experts called on behalf of the parents were critical that an inappropriately small endotracheal tube had been left in place. They agreed under cross-examination that if ventilation is being accomplished, the size of the tube is not important.

Lungs aerated. Evidence established that ventilation was being accomplished. The X-ray showed radiolucent lungs that were filled with air. The tube was working. It was also conceded that Narcan was not necessary because Simon was already on a ventilator when the neonatologist arrived. As long as the lungs were aerated, Narcan was not needed.

The trial court's verdict in the neonatologist's favour was upheld. Every step he had taken had helped the baby.

Paediatrician. The trial court found that in the eight minutes the paediatrician had been in the nursery, she had obtained a full history and examined the baby. The neonatologist had then arrived. It was reasonable that the paediatrician had not taken charge. The endotracheal tube was in, and drugs administered immediately before she had arrived. There was nothing about the care the baby was receiving in the nursery which would require her, as a paediatrician, to correct it.

The nurses

Time of administration. It was alleged midwife Martin's conduct had deviated from a reasonable standard of care in failing to have a specific order from the obstetrician to administer Demerol intravenously. Medical experts for the defence explained to the court that the p.r.n. (as required) order was a delegation of authority to administer the drug when the nurse deemed it necessary. Midwife Martin was the nurse during labour. She had complied with the standard of care, given the stage and level of labour, as well as the advancement the mother was making. The obstetrician said that had midwife Martin consulted him at the time he would have ordered the 9.30 am dose.

Hypothermic. It was also alleged midwife Martin had allowed Simon to become hypothermic. When Simon arrived in the nursery (about 30 minutes after delivery), his body temperature was 94.3°F (34.6 °C). A medical expert for the parents said that a newborn's body temperature will not drop if he is kept properly warm. midwife Martin had not complied with the standard of care by allowing him to become hypothermic.

The defence argued that this expert had not shown in what way the nurse's routine was incorrect. The decrease in temperature could be attributed to reasons other than nursing care.

Verbal/written communication. Finally, it was alleged midwife Martin had failed to verbally communicate to nursery staff that the mother had been given Demerol prior to delivery. The court heard that the fact Demerol had been administered was contained in the labour and delivery summary. This summary was viewed by all the medical and nursing staff treating Simon in the nursery. A medical expert explained to the court that the midwife was not required to verbally communicate this information because: 'The chart speaks for itself. It's very clear. It's distinct. There is no question about what went on in the delivery room.'[19]

Oxygen. It was alleged nurse Long deviated from the standard of care by improperly ausculating Simon's chest. Nurse Long had used 40 per cent rather than 100 per cent oxygen when Simon was admitted with observed signs of cyanosis and respiratory stress. Experts for both parties agreed that 40 per cent was within the standard of care. One doctor said that 40 per cent was proper as an initial treatment; that percentage could then be increased or decreased based on the baby's response.

Team responsibility. The court heard that it was not nurse Long's sole responsibility to auscultate the baby. The entire team was responsible for auscultating and placing the endotracheal tube. The respiratory therapist was also found to have met the appropriate standard of care. He had placed Simon on the ventilator at 11.00 am with 60 per cent oxygen, established the appropriate settings and auscultated the baby's chest to ensure proper placement of the tube.

The appeal court found there was ample evidence to support the jury verdict. The cerebral palsy suffered by Simon was not the result of negligence by medical, midwifery and nursing staff, nor by the manufacturers of Demerol.

....

In the final case in this chapter, nurses were the subjects of criminal prosecutions in Colorado. The case note is based on an article by Judy L Smetzer.[20] In criminal cases the prosecution has to prove its case 'beyond a reasonable doubt', not, as in civil cases (the majority in this book,) 'on a balance of probabilities' (more likely than not). Coroners have to be 'comfortably satisfied' on a balance of probabilities.

Smetzer writes that two types of failures can occur in an organization: latent and active.

Latent failures are weaknesses in an organization's structure, such as ineffective staff education. Inevitable in all organizations, latent failures lie dormant in the system.

Active failures are committed by individuals when they come in contact with those vulnerabilities in the system; that is when mistakes are made. Because system failures so frequently occur in the form of errors by staff, there is a need to move beyond blaming individuals and towards the strengthening of systems against chance combinations of latent and active failures.

Smetzer contends:

1. That the *Sanchez* case (discussed below) identifies many different system failures that allowed a medication error to develop, remain undetected and ultimately reach a baby.
2. That there is clear evidence that medication errors are almost never caused by the failure of a single element in the system or through the fault of a single practitioner.

If so, the *Sanchez* case will provide key lessons for risk managers. Smetzer's headings, which have been retained in the present discussion, will enable readers to systematically discuss whether similar circumstances could arise where they work. (Note: As the way the drug dosages were written is relevant to the misunderstandings that occurred in this case, the precise form of the abbreviations used in the clinical documentation relating to this case – i.e., 'I.V' and 'I.M' – have been retained.)

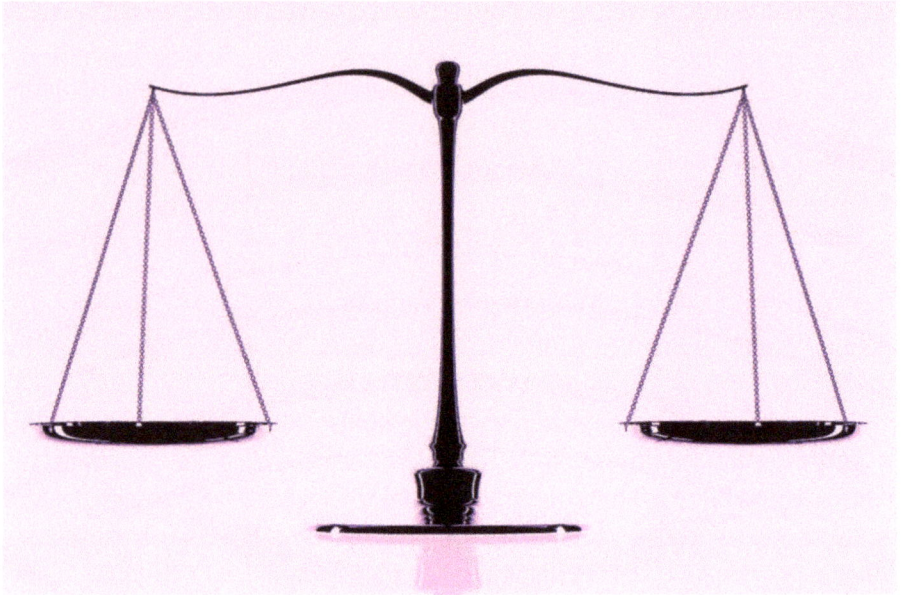

Circumstances surrounding the death of Miguel Sanchez [US, 1996][21]

The facts

A. Prescribing

1. Incomplete clinical information

Shortly after Miguel Sanchez, a healthy 3.2 kg baby boy was born, staff became aware his mother had a history of syphilis. A neonatologist was consulted. The parents spoke only Spanish, and although translators were available, staff could not easily determine whether the syphilis had been treated. A decision was made to investigate the possibility of congenital syphilis in the baby.

2. The language barrier

The language barrier also prevented staff from discussing treatment options. While there was no urgent clinical reason to treat Miguel before discharge, the neonatologist was not convinced the parents understood the need for follow-up and decided to treat the baby while he was still in hospital. This decision was made even though Miguel's test results would not be ready for several days.

3. Inconsistent procedure for communicating prenatal care
Years earlier, the mother had been diagnosed and treated for syphilis during her first pregnancy. Her first child (as well as two later children) was healthy and did not require treatment for congenital syphilis. After a series of tests, the obstetrician had chosen not to treat the mother because she was convinced the prior treatments were successful. This information was not clearly communicated to the hospital.

4. Staff inexperience and poor documentation
Staff at the hospital rarely treated babies with congenital syphilis. The neonatologist called an infectious disease specialist who recommended diagnostic studies, including a lumbar puncture. This consultant also recommended a single dose of penicillin G benzathine, I.M., at a dose of 50,000 units/kg.

Another staff member called a health department epidemiologist, who made the same recommendations. She then documented the recommendations directly onto the doctor's order form, in the right-hand column designated for progress notes. Her documentation was inaccurate. She noted the recommendation as 'penicillin G 50,000 units/kg.'[22] The health department recommendation had been for penicillin G benzathine. The route of administration was not recorded.

The neonatologist did not document the recommendation of the infectious disease specialist until the following day (after Miguel's death). The only order in place, therefore, was for penicillin G, with no reference to any administration route.

5. Non-standard method of writing the drug order
The day after Miguel was born, a different neonatologist (but from the same practice group), performed a lumbar puncture on the baby and wrote an order for one dose of 'Benzathine Pen G. 150,000 U I.M.'[23] But the doctor's method of writing the order was unusual. 'Benzathine' was capitalized and placed on a line above 'Pen G.' rather than after it on the same line. 'I.M.' appeared to be written over and looked somewhat like 'I.V.' The word 'units' was abbreviated as 'U.', which could be easily misread as one or two additional zeros.

Smetzer notes that up to this point the only recommended drug therapy was written directly across from the doctor's orders: 'penicillin G,' not 'penicillin G benzathine.' A possible explanation of the unusual way the order was written: the doctor could initially have written 'Pen G.I.V.,' and then added 'Benzathine' on the line above and changed the route to 'I.M.' after recalling that penicillin G benzathine was the recommended drug order.

B. Order processing

6. Insufficient drug information

The pharmacist was also unfamiliar with treatment for congenital syphilis and had limited knowledge about this rarely used non-formulary drug. There was no paediatric pharmacist on the staff, so she consulted the health department's recommendation and Drug Facts and Comparisons to determine the infant dosage for penicillin G benzathine. But she misread it in both sources as 500,000 units/kg instead of 50,000 units/ kg (the correct infant dose). The pharmacist also misread the drug order as 1,500,000 units instead of 150,000 units. Smetzer comments that with an infant dose on her mind, the pharmacist could easily have misinterpreted the 'U' as an extra zero, thus seeing 1,500,000.

7. No maximum dose warning

When the pharmacist entered this ten-fold overdose into the computer, the system did not issue any warnings about exceeding the maximum dose for a neonate. Consequently, she prepared the incorrect dose of 1,500,000 units.

C. Drug dispensing

8. Lack of a unit dose system

Because the nursery did not use a unit dose system, the pharmacist prepared two pre-filled syringes of penicillin G benzathine, 1.2 million units/2 ml each. She applied green stickers on the plungers reading 'Note dosage strength'[24] to indicate that the entire contents of the two syringes should not be administered.

The syringes were placed in a plastic bag and labelled with directions to administer 2.5 ml of the medication I.M. to equal a dose of 1,500,000 units (one full syringe and one-quarter of the other). The correct dose should have been 150,000 units/0.25 ml.

9. Insufficient information on infant injections

The pharmacist was unaware that a maximum volume of only 0.5 ml can be safely administered to an infant per I.M. injection. If this had been recognized, she would have detected that the ten-fold overdose she specified would require five separate injections.

10. Inconsistent independent double-check system

After preparing the drug, the pharmacist checked her own work and noticed that the medication in one of the pre-filled syringes had expired. After replacing the syringe, another pharmacist dispensed the drug without checking it against the original order. Once again, the ten-fold overdose was overlooked.

11. No staff education re the dispensing of nonformulary drugs

The hospital had no procedure in place to educate staff before they administered non-formulary drugs. Unfamiliar with this form of penicillin, neonatal unit nurses received the two syringes of penicillin G benzathine without adequate information from the pharmacy about the drug. No auxiliary warning labels were placed on the syringes or the pharmacy label to alert staff that penicillin G benzathine could be administered I.M. only. (Some other forms of penicillin G, such as penicillin G sodium or procaine, can be given I.V. or I.M.)

12. Insufficient drug information and inadequate drug references

After noting the order for penicillin G benzathine, Miguel's primary care nurse and a neonatal nurse practitioner (NNP) in the unit consulted the *1994 Red Book (Report of the Committee of Infectious Diseases)* to research the treatment of congenital syphilis. One drug recommended was penicillin G benzathine I.M. However, the text was not a specific drug reference and did not warn that the drug could be administered I.M. only.

Later, after glancing at the two syringes, the primary care nurse expressed concern to colleagues about the five injections that the baby would need. Anxious to prevent unnecessary pain to the baby, an advanced level nursery RN and the NNP decided to investigate administering the medication I.V. instead of I.M. Had the correct dose been dispensed, a single I.M. injection of only 0.25 ml (150,000 units) would have been needed.

The penicillin G monograph in *Neofax'95* (one of the medication resources the two nurses used to determine if penicillin G benzathine could be administered I.V.) did not specifically mention penicillin G benzathine. Instead, it noted that the treatment for congenital syphilis was aqueous crystalline penicillin G by slow I.V. push or penicillin G procaine I.M. Nowhere in the two-page monograph was penicillin G benzathine mentioned. Therefore, no warnings regarding "I.M. use only" were present (since corrected by the publishers). The NNP searched an additional medication resource, *NICU Medi-*

cation Administration, but penicillin G benzathine was not mentioned there either.

Unfamiliar with the various forms of penicillin G, the NNP believed that 'Benzathine' was a brand name for penicillin G. The doctor's unusual method of writing the drug order reinforced this misconception. In addition, the health department's recommendation was incomplete, recording only penicillin G and no route of administration.

Added to this was the fact that many texts use ambiguous synonyms when referring to various forms of penicillin. Penicillin G, for example, is frequently associated with the terms 'crystalline penicillin' and 'aqueous suspension'. Believing that 'aqueous crystalline penicillin G' and penicillin G benzathine were the same drug, the NNP concluded the drug could be safely administered I.V.

13. Unclear definition of non-physician prescriptive authority
Although hospital policies did not clearly define the prescriptive authority, nurse practitioners routinely prescribed medications within the scope of their practice. Routes of administration had been changed by nurse practitioners in the past. Also, the nurse practitioner assumed she was operating under a national protocol that allowed nurse practitioners to plan, direct, implement and change drug therapy. Consequently she decided to administer the drug I.V. Because Miguel's primary care nurse was not certified to administer I.V medications to neonates, his care was transferred to the nurse practitioner and advanced-level nursery RN.

14. Unclear manufacturer labelling
While preparing to give the drug, neither nurse noticed that the syringes were labelled by the manufacturer with the warning 'I.M. use only.' The warning was difficult to see as it was not prominently placed, and to view it the nurse had to rotate the syringe 180 degrees away from the drug name. In addition, once the pre-filled syringe was assembled for use, the orange plunger concealed part of the 'M' in 'I.M.,' making it possible to misread the warning as 'I.V. use only.'

15. The nurses also failed to detect the tenfold overdose
Both the pharmacy label and the manufacturer's labelling on the syringes expressed the drug's dose using multiple zeros, as in '1,200,000 units' and '1,500,000 units.' Had the dose been expressed as '1.2 million units' and '1.5

million units', as some manufacturers do, the nurses might have been less likely to have misread it.

16. Conflicting information on I.V. use of milky white substances
The nurses could see that the drug in the syringe was milky white. But their awareness that certain milky white substances, such as I.V. lipids and other lipid-based drug products, can safely be given I.V. conflicted with the widely recognized rule that only clear liquids can be injected I.V. Consequently, they did not recognize any problem with giving penicillin G benzathine I.V.

Believing that they were sparing Miguel unnecessary pain, the nurses began to administer the first syringe of the drug by slow I.V. push. After about 1.8 ml of the medication had been administered, the baby became unresponsive. Resuscitation was unsuccessful, and Miguel died.

The decision

In the criminal proceedings that followed, two nurses pleaded guilty in response to a plea bargain and the third nurse was acquitted by the jury.

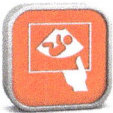 Discussion of Key Issues

Norton: In this case the RN, who had been working in administration for some years, was unfamiliar with the route of the drug. Her mistake (together with an ambiguous medication order) resulted in a baby's death.

Consider the following:

Hospitals have to be able to organize their staff when shortages occur. They also have a duty to provide adequate numbers of competent staff for the tasks staff undertake. Equally, midwives and nurses are advised by their professional bodies to stay within their field of competency. Vulnerable neonates, in turn, have a right to receive the care their condition requires.

Bearing this balancing exercise in mind (and you may think of more factors):

- Grade the risk (in terms of foreseeability) to a baby when, during a staff shortage, an RN is floated from an adult ward to a special care nursery, with the expectation that he or she could be involved in the administration of medication.
- Now advise the hospital, the RN and the charge nurse of the nursery on their responsibilities.

The ambiguous order:

Nurses advised the court that best practice requires an ambiguous order to be checked with the prescribing doctor.

- When this is not possible, what process (if any) does your hospital require nurses to follow?

The judge found that nurses have the duty and obligation of making themselves understood beyond the possibility of error when clarifying an ambiguous order.

- If the nurse is under such an obligation, is there a corresponding duty for the hospital to put a safe system in place to protect the patient?
- Could this process be formalized, for example, by a check-list?

The two doctors the ADON talked to about the order told the court that doctors usually see this role as checking 'handwriting,' not 'dosage or route.'

- Do you agree?

Note the risk of 'he said, she said' in this situation.

- Would your documentation demonstrate *what* you were checking and *with whom* in the ward or over the telephone?
- How do you inform yourself about the drugs a mother/ baby has received in another unit (e.g., the patient comes back from the OR and PACU)?

....

In *Chiricosta,* it was alleged that the midwife who had administered the p.r.n. dose of Pethidine during labour failed to communicate this 'verbally' to nursery staff. The court accepted expert medical evidence that the midwife was not required to communicate the information verbally because the 'the chart speaks for itself. It's very clear. It's distinct. There is no question about what went on in the delivery room.'[25]

- In your experience, have babies arrived in a NICU without a contemporaneous record from the labour and delivery area or the OR of drugs administered there?
- If nurses are floated to a NICU from adult areas, are they likely to know the cause and effect of drugs which may or may not have crossed the placental barrier?

....

The case of *Miguel Sanchez* identifies a considerable number of risks in chronological order.

- Could any of those risks pose a threat where you work? Either way, give reasons.

Judy Smetzer contends that medication errors are almost never caused by the failure of a single element in the system or the fault of a single practitioner.

- Do you agree? Either way, give reasons.

In workshops I facilitated, midwives and RNs identified a number of risks to the safe delivery of medication to neonates. Their comments and warnings provide an interesting postscript for risk managers:

0.1 mg Konakion (vitamin K) given IM where ampoule contains 0.2 mg, which is then given as an oral dose. A mistake could result in the baby receiving 0.2 mg IM.

....

The pharmacy delivered adult Kanakian instead of neonatal; i.e., 10 mg instead of 1 mg.

....

The birth suite midwife gave a second dose of Kanakian. The paediatrician had not written the order in the baby's chart but checked the ampoule with the midwife in the OR when mother went for an emergency LUSCS. The Kanakian order was written in the mother's history by the obstetric RMO.

....

Anti-D was given to a neonate by mistake.

....

In one neonatal unit, infusion pumps administer a dose with a decimal point. During a day shift, equipment was borrowed from an adult ward and a baby given 60 ml IV instead of 6 ml because the nurse failed to realize the adult pump had no decimal point.

NOTES

1. Powers & Harris, *Medical Negligence,* 2d ed., Butterworths, London, p.273.
2. Ibid.
3. *Norton v Argonaut Insurance Company*, 144 So.2d 249 (1962) at p.260.
4. Ibid.
5. Ibid., p.251.
6. Ibid., p.255.
7. Ibid., p.261.
8. Ibid.
9. Ibid.
10. Ibid., p.260.
11. Ibid.
12. *Wade v Tran,* Philadelphia County C.C.P. January, No. 3721 (1995).
13. *Chiricosta v Winthrop-Breon,* 263 Ill.App.3d 132. 635 N.E.2d 1019 (1994).
14. Ibid., p.1024.
15. Ibid., p.1025.
16. Ibid.
17. Ibid.

18. Ibid., p.1026.

19. Ibid., p.1030.

20. J.L. Smetzer, Nursing, *Beyond blaming individuals: lesson from Colorado* (May 1998).

21. Ibid.

22. Ibid., p.2.

23. Ibid.

24. Ibid., p.3.

25. *Chiricosta v Winthrop-Breon* at p.1030.

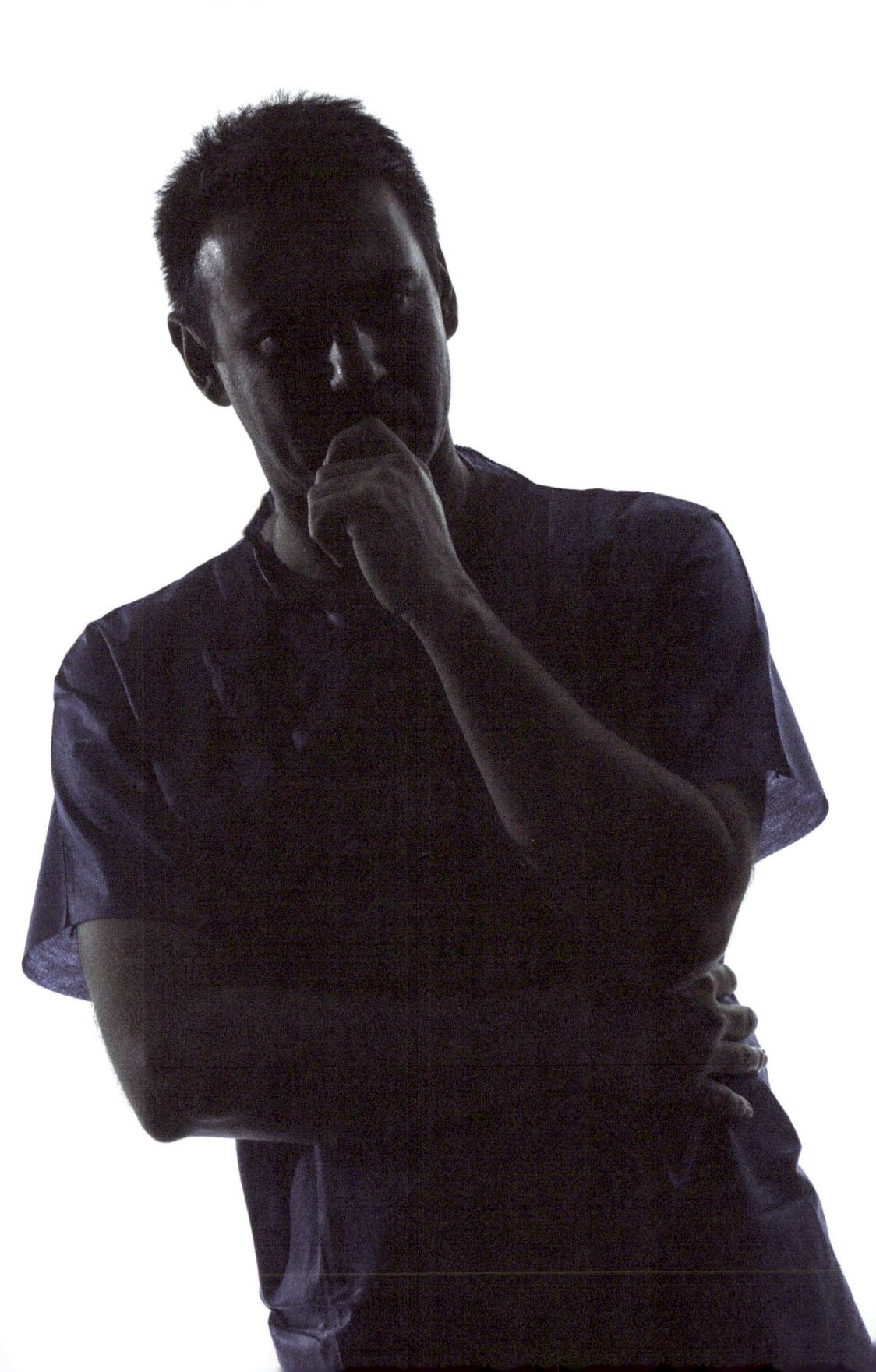

CHAPTER 17

The Neonatal Unit-intentional injury

'I don't know what is happening to me. I feel out of control. I can't even control my emotions.'

—A medical technician who later injured neonates

Introduction

The cases in this book have overwhelmingly dealt with instances of inadvertent harm. No one has set out deliberately to harm a baby or a mother. However, occasionally deliberate harm has occurred in neonatal care and hospitals should therefore have a properly functioning risk management/ quality assurance program in place to address and manage this risk. For example, how easily could someone come in off the street and take a baby from a nursery? Or, on some pretext, from a mother? Are signals being heeded that a member of staff or a parent could harm a baby?

While people are responsible for their own acts of intentional harm (subject to defences of diminished responsibility), it may also be alleged that the hospital failed to take reasonable steps to prevent foreseeable harm, for example, by a staff member.

....

Such were the allegations in the following case, where it was found that a medical technician working in a neonatal unit had deliberately harmed one mother as well as a number of babies. But as the judge observed, 'The case is not so much about what the technician did, as it is about what the hospital failed to do.'[1]

An expert witness, giving evidence on the function of a quality assurance supervisor, explained that what the hospital had failed to do was to implement a policy which ensured quality control, prevented foreseeable mishaps and managed risk, so that neonates did not continue to be injured. This case will enable risk managers and neonatal staff to compare the hospital policy and procedures put before the court with those prevailing at their own hospitals.

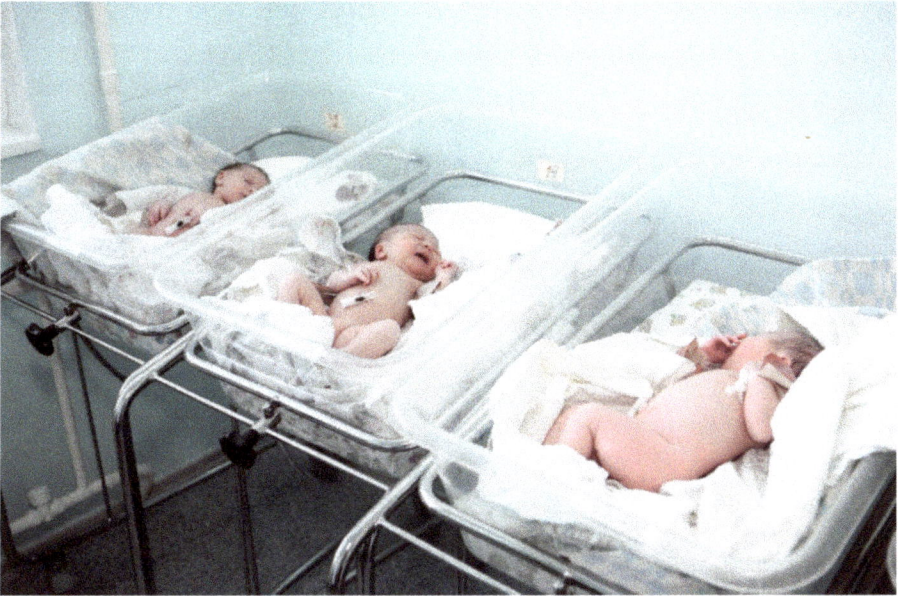

Gess v US [US, 1996][2]

Twelve of the thirteen patients in this case were newborn when they were deliberately injured. The judge commented:

> *Unfortunately newborn babies make poor witnesses; and only the adult plaintiff could directly testify about her experience. Nevertheless, the circumstantial evidence in this case obviates the need for the direct testimony of the infant plaintiffs.[3]*

The court then became primarily concerned with inferences drawn from circumstantial evidence rather than what was witnessed (direct evidence).

The judge explained to the jury how 'inferences' work as evidence:

> *If you go to sleep tonight and wake up in the morning and look out the window and see snow on the ground and rabbit tracks on the*

snow; you didn't see it snow, so it's not direct evidence; you didn't
see a rabbit walk across the snow after it snowed, so it's not direct
evidence; but you just know, because you may infer from what you
do see, that while you were asleep it must have snowed; and after it
snowed a rabbit must have walked across the snow.[4]

After hearing all the evidence, the judge concluded:

'This case is replete with rabbit tracks across the snow, all pointing
to the negligence of the defendant.'[5]

The facts

In February 1988, the first of what was to become a series of 'alarmingly similar'[6] emergencies arose in the obstetric ward of a United States Air Force Hospital. A newborn baby, seemingly in excellent health, suddenly stopped breathing and turned blue. Over the next sixteen months this emergency repeated itself in the case of one adult and twelve more babies. All of them, for no medically explainable reason, suddenly 'crashed from good health to the brink of death.'[7]

An investigation by the Air Force found that the symptoms displayed by the infants were not the result of infection or medical procedure; they were either caused accidentally or intentionally.

In 1993, the patients took their case to court alleging that they had been maliciously injected with toxic doses of lidocaine or a similar substance.

The court heard that several consistent, telling facts had emerged from the earlier investigation:

1. Each patient was under the exclusive care of the hospital when the life-threatening events occurred.
2. Anthony, a medical technician, was on duty and had some interaction with each of the patients shortly before the emergencies arose.
3. Anthony always seemed to be the first one on the scene; the one to 'discover' and come to the 'rescue' of the stricken patients.

4. Once the patients were transferred to a nearby medical centre, they experienced no more life-threatening events.
5. Once Anthony was removed from the obstetrics ward, the emergencies ceased.
6. Medical experts said the experiences of the patients were consistent with the injection of toxic doses of lidocaine or some similar drug.

A statistical analysis of events showed:

1. During 1988, more than six per cent of newborns at the hospital experienced a life-threatening event. The paediatric population as a whole experienced such events at the rate of 0.13 per cent.
2. Anthony was the only person on duty when each incident occurred. The chance of this being mere coincidence was one in ten million.

Anthony did not give evidence. The following extracts from the judgment relate to the one adult victim and two of the babies.

Louise

Louise, aged 24, was the only adult to be injured. Consequently, she was the only patient able to provide direct evidence.

On 1 November 1988, Louise delivered a baby at 8.39 am by caesarean section. At about 5.00 pm, Louise, now back in her room, complained of itching. Her doctor prescribed an intramuscular injection of Benadryl, which was administered by a nurse.

Respiratory arrest. At about 9.30 pm, the itching returned. Louise explained to Anthony, a medical technician in the unit, that she had been given Benadryl earlier. Anthony left the room, returned carrying a syringe, then began working with her IV apparatus. Louise said she immediately experienced a sharp burning sensation around the wrist. She also felt a strange feeling in her throat:

I complained to the technician who responded that this was 'normal.' The next thing I remember is violently coughing, at which time the technician told me to 'go with it.' I became unconscious and the next thing I recall is after the incident was over.[8]

The nurse who had earlier administered the Benadryl came into the room and called a Code Blue.

No medical cause. Subsequent examinations failed to disclose a medical or physiological cause for Louise's respiratory arrest. Duty rosters showed Anthony on duty at the time of the incident.

Missing record. Louise said she had tried on numerous occasions over the next two years to obtain her medical records. When she finally received them, there was no information about the injection of any drug in her IV by Anthony. The court noted the 'whole chapter' was missing from her record.

Emma

Emma was a full-term infant born without complications by vaginal delivery at 7.13 pm on 9 July 1988. She was stable until approximately 9.30 pm when she was found to have bradycardia and cyanosis.

Profound metabolic acidosis. A Code Blue was called. Emma responded to oxygen and stimulation. Later examination found she had suffered from profound metabolic acidosis.

Consistent with drug toxicity. The condition was characterised as consistent with lidocaine or bupivacaine toxicity but no medical cause could be found.

Emma's mother recalled handing her baby to Anthony shortly before the problems occurred. Duty rosters showed he was on the evening shift.

Bernadette

Bernadette was a full-term baby delivered vaginally at 12.38 am on 21 November, 1988. Meconium was present in the amniotic fluid; the fetal heart was decreased on delivery. Oxygen and Narcan were given to counteract the effects of the narcotic anaesthesia given to her mother. Oxygen was provided when she had tachypnoea.

Profound metabolic acidosis. At about 4.00 pm, Bernadette became mottled and started to grunt and gasp. She responded to stimulation. Respiration and colour improved until about 4.55 pm, when another period of mottling and decreased heart rate occurred. Bernadette was transferred to another hospital after failing to respond. She suffered profound metabolic acidosis.

Consistent with drug toxicity. The symptoms were later found to be consistent with lidocaine or bupivacaine toxicity. Lidocaine was found in the urine, but there was no record of the baby receiving that medication at either hospital. The mother had received an unknown quantity of one per cent licocaine as a local anaesthetic during delivery, but doctors concluded the amount present in the urine did not stem from this injection.

The mother identified Anthony as being present in the room shortly before the incident. It was Anthony who called a nurse to look at the baby at the time of the Code Blue. Duty rosters showed he was on duty at the time.

Very similar patterns emerged in respect to the other babies.

Anthony

Depression. The court heard that just prior to being inducted into the Air Force, Anthony spent six weeks in a psychiatric hospital, where he was treated for severe depression.

Mental instability. After induction, Anthony's mental instability appeared to have accelerated. He sought mental and physical medical attention some 50 times between induction and the injury to the last baby in 1988.

Outbursts. During 1988, Anthony's wife told his supervisor at the hospital that she was afraid of her husband's uncontrollable temper at home; he would hit her or the walls. She said she feared his outbursts over little things. Anthony was diagnosed as having an 'intermittent explosive disorder.'[9] He said during one group therapy session: 'I don't know what is happening to me. I feel out of control. I can't even control my emotions.'[10] Co-workers described Anthony as 'fishing for compliments, over-eager, under stress, nosey, craving attention, over-emotional and hyper.'[11]

The trial

The court found the case was not so much about what Anthony did, but what the hospital failed to do. Before reaching this conclusion, the court identified the duty of care and standard of care issues involved.

Duty of care

The hospital owed a duty to provide an environment where the health and safety needs of patients could be addressed. This 'broad, general duty'[12] included:

- Compliance with hospital administration standards.
- The existence of an adequate quality assurance program.
- Proper training and supervision of staff.

Third parties. The court also found the hospital owed a duty to protect patients from the foreseeable risks of deliberate harm from third parties. On this point the court referred to *Young v Huntsville 595 So.2d 1386* [1992], where a patient sued the hospital after being sexually assaulted by a trespasser. The court noted that in the absence of special relationships, hospitals have no duty to protect their patients from the criminal acts of third parties. But evidence indicated that the patient may have been sedated at the time of the attack. The court then applied a 'dependence test', holding the patient had a special relationship with the hospital: 'We can hardly imagine a situation in which a person is so dependent on another for basic bodily protection and care than the situation of an anaesthetised or sedated patient.'[13]

Utterly helpless and totally dependent. In *Gess,* the court found the need for protection of the babies from deliberate harm 'even more compelling' and observed that a newborn infant is 'utterly helpless and totally dependent on others for health, safety and protection.'[14]

Standard of care: quality assurance

Expert evidence

Mr Morris, who had worked in hospital administration for 34 years, gave expert evidence for the patients. He said accepted practice required the existence and function of a quality assurance supervisor. The supervisor's primary function was to ensure quality control, to prevent foreseeable mishaps and to manage risk so that similar medical problems do not recur.

Accepted practice

In the management of risk, accepted practice for a nursery included:

1. Direct, physical supervision by experienced nursery staff of staff with limited qualifications.
2. 24-hour skilled nursing cover throughout the hospital. This required the relaying of accurate, concise information between the administrative nurse on-call and the evening night supervisor.
3. Ensuring that staff relay all appropriate information to the chief of nursing services regarding incidents occurring on each shift.
4. The mandatory reporting and documenting of unusual incidents. The administrative nurse on-call must be contacted regarding any serious incident. Any evidence of child abuse, neglect or aggravated assault must be documented.
5. Hospital regulations ensuring medical technicians are adequately prepared to assume assigned responsibilities; new procedures performed in the presence of a qualified trainer.
6. Absolutely no prescribing/dispensing medications or performing surgical procedures by medical technicians.
7. Incident report documentations of any event inconsistent with routine care, such reports to be sent without delay to the risk manager for review and appropriate investigation.
8. A 24-hour report detailing any life-threatening or unusual incidents, specifically required to be completed by nursery staff.
9. Nursery staff required to identify, assess and resolve any problem area so as to eliminate any reasonable chance of recurrence during the current year.
10. All evidence bearing upon a fair adjudication of potential malpractice claims to be preserved.

Hospital standards. The court heard that relevant hospital accreditation standards as well as Air Force standards imposed a duty on the hospital to allow only competent staff with a commitment to the welfare of its patients to administer medical care to infants in a Level 1 nursery.

Potential danger. Contrary to this standard, the court found the hospital had been warned, both directly and indirectly, that Anthony was a potential danger and completely unsuitable for placement in the nursery.

Surgical unit. For example, prior to his assignment to the nursery, Anthony had worked in the surgical unit. The supervisor of that unit told the court that he communicated his 'firm belief'[15] that Anthony was capable of hurting a patient. A nurse who worked with Anthony in the unit said she had found him untrustworthy and told the staff member in charge that Anthony should not be transferred to the obstetrics ward.

Documentation missing. The supervisor remembered documenting his concerns about Anthony. The fact that this documentation, like other pieces of critical documentary evidence, had 'mysteriously disappeared'[16] was seen as significant by the court.

Foreseeability of injury

Frequency and similarity of injuries. As early as June 1988, the frequency and similarity of the injuries made further injury foreseeable. Mr Morris had highlighted to the court a 15-day period during which four babies experienced unexplained injuries.

Uncontrollable tempers. When Anthony's wife told his immediate supervisor that she was afraid of his uncontrollable tempers, the supervisor advised Anthony to seek mental health counselling, but kept these revelations to herself. She neither informed her supervisors nor documented the statements of Anthony's wife. She had not followed up on her referral. Ironically, she then gave Anthony the highest rating on his annual performance appraisal.

Frustrations. It was clear to the court that Anthony had been unable to segregate his mental and emotional problems from his work. He had also expressed frustration with his nursery assignment.

Breach of duty. Against this background, the court found 'overwhelming evidence'[17] that the hospital had breached its duty of care:

1. The hospital did not have a quality assurance program. If it did, it failed to adequately perform any important function. The patient's injuries were the unusual, severe, patterned type that a properly functioning quality assurance or risk management programme should have addressed. For example, Louise actually observed and identified Anthony tampering with her IV; this was not investigated.
2. Documentation was 'woefully deficient.'[18] Infant records did not contain significant information. Mandatory documentation was missing. The court found that if the hospital had followed reasonable docu-

mentation procedures, and adequately monitored this information, it would have known of the problems in the nursery and would have had an opportunity to prevent their recurrence.

3. The hospital had exhibited a 'pattern of neglect'[19] in not identifying and assessing medically significant information. There had been a failure to monitor, screen and investigate the infant crashes.

4. When problems occurred which had no medically explainable cause, the hospital had a duty to look for other causes. As an absolute minimum, drug screening should have been ordered.

5. A person of Anthony's history of psychological and emotional instability should never have been allowed to work in the nursery. This breach of duty was made worse by failing to ensure direct supervision. In addition, the physical layout of the nursery made such supervision difficult.

Damages awarded.

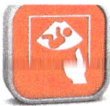

Discussion of Key Issues

Note that in *Gess* the court emphasised that a staff member is not necessarily incompetent to perform all tasks simply because of a mental health history. For example, the staff member may have received counselling or taken medication for such a condition. What the court did emphasise was that a hospital must consider a staff member's acts in the light of all relevant information. So Anthony's mental health history became relevant as the hospital learned or should have learned about his behaviour.

- Have you ever been concerned by the behaviour of a nurse, doctor or student in a nursery in terms of possible harm to a baby?
- Is there a process for taking your concerns further up the chain of command ?
- Has a mother/family member's behaviour in relation to their baby ever concerned you?

- Have you encountered Munchausen by Proxy? How was this resolved?
- Attempts have been made to steal babies from hospital nurseries. How difficult would it be for a member of the public to gain access to your neonatal area?

Expert witness Mr Morris stipulated 10 points for the management of risk in a nursery.

- Discuss and compare these with what is in place at your hospital.

NOTES

1. *Gess v U.S.,* 952 F. Supp. 1529 (1996) at p.1550.
2. *Gess.*
3. Ibid., p.1533.
4. Ibid. (citing the Hon. Frank Johnson's charge to a jury, some 50 years before.)
5. Ibid., p.1533.
6. Ibid.
7. Ibid.
8. Ibid., p.1539.
9. Ibid., p.1538.
10. Ibid.
11. Ibid.
12. Ibid., pp.1552,1553.
13. *Young v Huntsville,* 595 So.2d 1386 (1992) at p.1553 in *Gess.*
14. Ibid.
15. Ibid., p.1559.
16. Ibid.
17. Ibid., p.1560.
18. Ibid., p.1556.
19. Ibid.

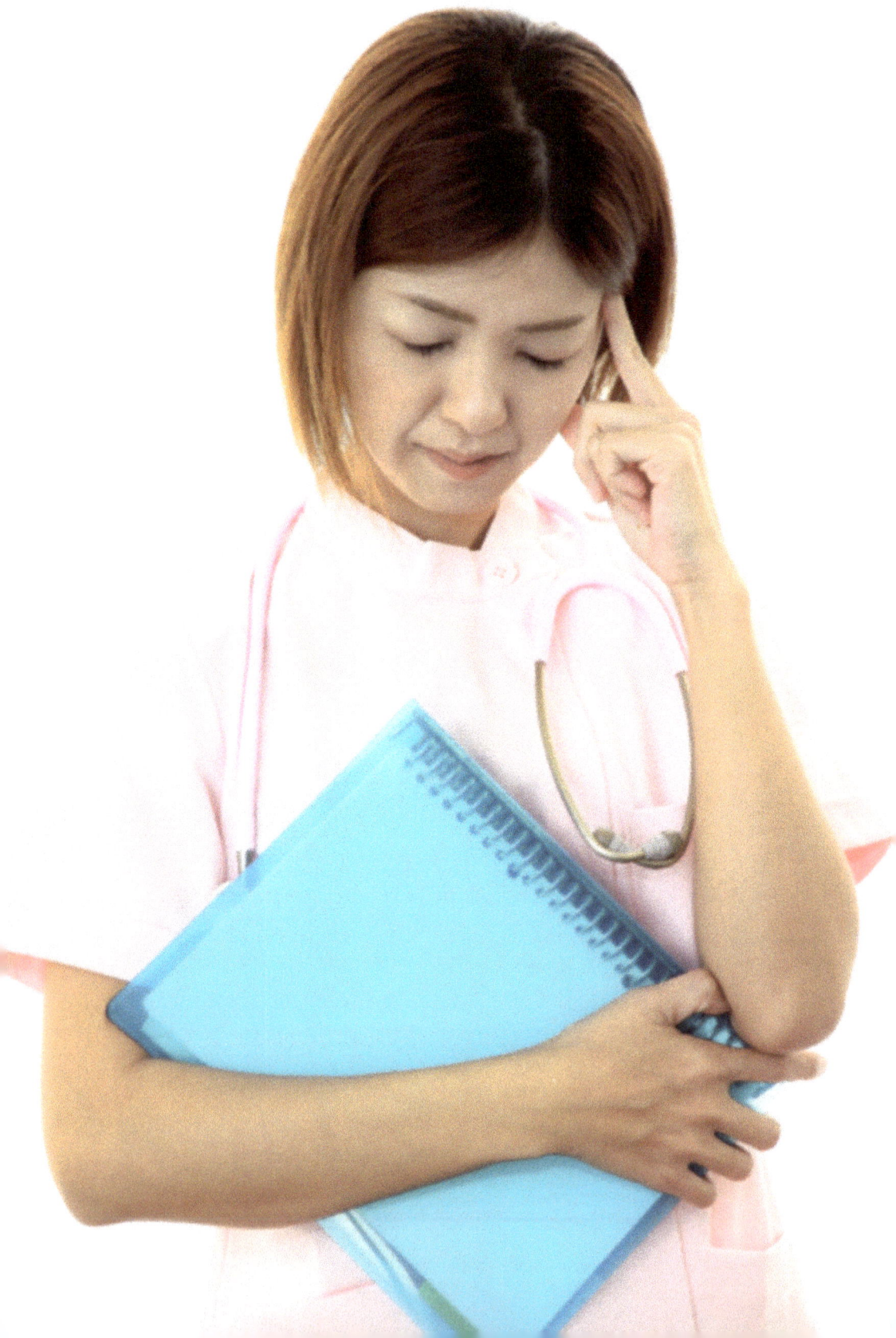

CHAPTER 18

Documentation

'It is appreciated that medical and nursing staff are often working under pressure, and in an emergency situation priority should correctly be given to providing the appropriate care. That said, when a critical incident occurs, the need to record accurately and while memories are fresh, is imperative.'

—A coroner

Introduction

Medical and midwifery records hold the story of the quality and quantity of the care mothers and babies receive in maternity services. The cases in this book will have left you in no doubt that the system of record keeping, and the way staff document events and processes, is critical if unsafe care is alleged or a 'consent' issue arises.

Hospitals have a duty of care to implement a system of record keeping that does not put the patient at foreseeable risk of harm. Effective risk management clearly requires that records of mothers and babies reflect the story of safe midwifery and obstetric care. Australian legal writer Pat Staunton[1] believes that, if kept accurately, contemporaneously and objectively, these records will:

- indicate a patient's progress or deterioration to staff on later shifts,
- provide a record of their treatment on discharge and
- provide a history for future consultation.

Lawyers are well aware that if a hospital and its staff become involved in a civil or criminal matter, documentation can 'make or break' the defence of a hospital.

For example, in *Gabaldoni v. Board of Physician Quality Assurance*[2] the court (finding the patient's death was avoidable), contrasted the doctor's negligent documenting with the competently kept nursing records. The court found the midwifery notes contained exact times when tests were ordered by the obstetrician, exact times when samples were taken and sent to the lab, exact times when results came back or when someone was sent to get them, and exact times when, and exactly how, the doctor was notified.

Hospital records are equally central to the coronial process, as one coroner explains:

An inquest that involves the examination of the circumstances of a death following admission and treatment in hospital will invariably result in the close examination and scrutiny of medical records. Regrettably in too many cases the documentation and attention to detail is deficient. It is appreciated that medical and nursing staff are often working under pressure, and in an emergency situa-

tion priority should correctly be given to providing the appropriate care. That said, when a critical incident occurs, the need to record accurately and while memories are fresh, is imperative.[3]

Judges and coroners decide what documents will be relevant to be put before the court as evidence.

Documents that could come under scrutiny include:[4]

- admission records sheet;
- antenatal information;
- in-patient medical, midwifery and nursing progress notes;
- CTG traces;
- partograms;
- clinical pathways;
- care plans;
- charts – temp, blood pressure, fluid balance, etc.
- test and investigation results;
- drug sheets;
- correspondence (other hospitals/doctors);
- physiotherapy, social work, psychological records;
- X-rays;
- anaesthetic records;
- consent forms;
- neonatal unit charts/records;
- incident reports;
- hospital policies & protocols; and
- in a fatal case, coronial notes and postmortem report.

In addition to other evidence of appropriate and contemporary standards, a hospital's policies, guidelines and protocols will establish the standard expected by that hospital from their maternity services unit. As such, these documents become important evidence. A hospital's requirements in relation to record keeping/documentation need to be achievable and not unrealistic in the face of staff/patient ratios and heavy workloads. Establishing 'state of the art' policies is a first step. Staff then need to be educated about policy requirements, and a process put in place to ensure compliance. How, for example, are policies disseminated where you work? How are new/ agency staff orientated to policy requirements? As cases come to court years after an incident, the relevant policies will be those at the time of the incident, not at the date of the court hearing. Copies should therefore be archived.

Guidelines

While there are no specific 'legal' rules for report writing, here are some basic guidelines from Patricia Staunton:[5]

1. Reports should be concise and clinically relevant to the next health professional reading them.
2. Reports should be accurate and complete. Unless you have actually witnessed the incident, what someone else says occurred is clearly hearsay evidence and must be reported as such. Always record that a patient has refused treatment or medication prescribed, or acts contrary to advice.
3. Reports should be legible. Incorrect interpretations lead to many mistakes. If unsure, check with the writer where possible.
4. Reports should be objective, definite statements of fact. Record what you see, not what you think you see. The word 'appears' suggests uncertainty. Only use it if that is the case.
5. Entries should be prefaced by the date and time, and the signature of the relevant health professional.
6. Abbreviations should not be used unless they are accepted hospital practice or are widely acknowledged medical abbreviations.
7. Draw a line through an incorrect entry and initial it before continuing. Total obliteration suggests something may be being hidden; writing over mistakes and inserting words is confusing. Liquid correction fluid should not be used (forensic tests quickly expose what is underneath).
8. Do not make an entry in a patient's record by an identifying room or bed number, or before checking the name on the record. The patient's name and identifying number should be on every sheet of their record before making an entry. Single sheets that are not properly identified can be filed in the wrong record.
9. Every time an entry is transcribed, a margin for error exists; the note can also end up in the wrong record.
10. No entry concerning a patient should be made in their record on behalf of someone else unless this is made clearly evident.

11. The destruction of records following an adverse incident will raise an inference of a cover-up.
12. 'Not documented – not done' is not a legal principle, but failure to document will raise an inference that something was not done. This allegation may be able to be rebutted by other evidence, for example, of 'usual practice.'
13. Record keeping must be designed so that it is practical and stream-lined. To achieve compliance, the system of record keeping must 'work on the floor' for staff. There is little use drafting state of the art policies and protocols for the instruction of staff if workloads and staffing levels mean they do not have time to read them.

It is therefore important that staff/patient ratios and workload enable:

14. Staff to keep contemporaneous records; memories fade and events may be overtaken by subsequent events, particularly if a patient's condition worsens and various treatments are commenced and tests undertaken.
15. Staff taking over a patient's care from other staff have *time* to read their patient's records thoroughly and regularly. Staunton observes that even though there is a strong oral tradition in nursing (and a stronger written culture in medicine) verbal reports at handover should be seen as an *addition* to the written report, not instead of it.

Guidelines for the keeping of essential health records in NSW also advise:

16. Documentation in the health care record is to occur at the time of, or as soon as practicable following, the provision of care, observation, assessment, diagnosis, management/ treatment, professional advice, or any other matter worthy of note.
17. Entries do not contain prejudicial, derogatory or irrelevant statements about the patient. (Nor should they contain criticism of other health professionals; perhaps written under stress, such opinions may be incorrect and reflect only one view of a complex situation.)

18. All entries in the health care record are integrated in chronological sequence, and, in the case of electronic records, are accessible and linked to the individual main record.

19. Records stored electronically shall be capable of being reproduced on paper and adequate back-ups kept.

20. All computerized and handwritten systems shall have the capacity to enable identification of individual health personnel. In a computerized system, this will require the use of an appropriate identification system, e.g., computer signatures.

Confidentiality

21. As both highly personal and sensitive material is contained in medical records, both statutory and common law recognize a duty of confidentiality to the patient.

Exceptions exist when the record/information about the patient is divulged:

- with the patient's consent;
- when there is mandatory reporting of child abuse and certain notifiable diseases;
- when records are required for the purposes of legal proceedings, e.g., pursuant to a court order/subpoena;
- when information is divulged (to the appropriate person/authority) in order that the safety of the patient or others is protected;
- subject to privacy requirements, the records can also be used for research and teaching purposes.

Privacy

22. The collection, use, protection, storage and disposal of health records require clear hospital policy directives in line with privacy legislation.[6]

Admission of patients' records

In *James v. Camberwell Health Authority* (discussed earlier in this text), the hospital argued that an apparent delay in responding to a trace showing the baby's heartbeat was slowing down, was in fact due to faulty CTG equipment. The clock had 'flipped', making an actual and acceptable nine-minute response time appear to be a negligent 69-minute delay. To support this argument the hospital was allowed to refer to the times and traces of patients upon whom the equipment had been used on the same shift.

The following case is a further reminder that the records of other patients (with appropriate measures taken to preserve confidentiality) can be admitted into evidence if relevant to an issue.

....

In *Deacon v McVicor [UK, 1984]*[7] the patient, who had a shirodkar suture in situ, was admitted to hospital for delivery of her first child. She claimed that labour room staff had failed to act quickly enough to remove the suture, with consequent damage to her cervix and risk to future pregnancies. The hospital acknowledged that no emergency existed, but argued that the ward was very busy that night and in that context, the patient had received appropriate care. At the hospital's request, the judge then directed that the notes of other patients (referred to by code names to protect their confidentiality) should be made available to the court to show what was going on in the labour ward at that time.

The judge closely examined all the ward records and found they indicated that the doctors were busy, but also established that the patient was not the only patient who presented problems. What they did not show was that there was anything to prevent the doctors performing a vaginal examination or removing the suture sooner than they did.

As you will see throughout this casebook, accurate concise and contemporaneous records documenting the continuing safe care of mothers and babies are critical to the effective defense of the hospital and its maternity services staff.

NOTES

1. P. Staunton & M. Chiarella, *Nursing and the Law,* 5th ed., Churchill Livingston, Ch.7 Report Writing (Sydney, 2006).
2. *Gabaldoni v Board of Physician Quality Assurance,* 785 A.2d 771 (2001). Note based on Legal Eagle Eye Newsletter for the Nursing Profession (March, 2002) p.7.

3. His Honour, Magistrate Carl Milovanovich, Deputy State- Coroner of NSW.
4. Powers & Harris, *Medical Negligence,* Butterworths, London (1994) p.177.
5. Staunton & Chiarella; refer to NSW, *Circular No. 98/59, 'Guidelines for Essential Documentation, Management,Storage and Disposal of Health Records.'*
6. For example, Health Privacy Principles introduced by *Principles Health Records Act 2001 (Vic).* These cover Collections, Use and Disclosure, Data Quality, Data Security and Data Retention, Openness, Access and Correction, Identifiers, Anonymity, Transborder Data Flows, Transfer or Closure of the Practice of Health Provider, and Making Information Available to another Health Provider.
7. *Deacon v McVicar,* QBD (7 Jan 1984).

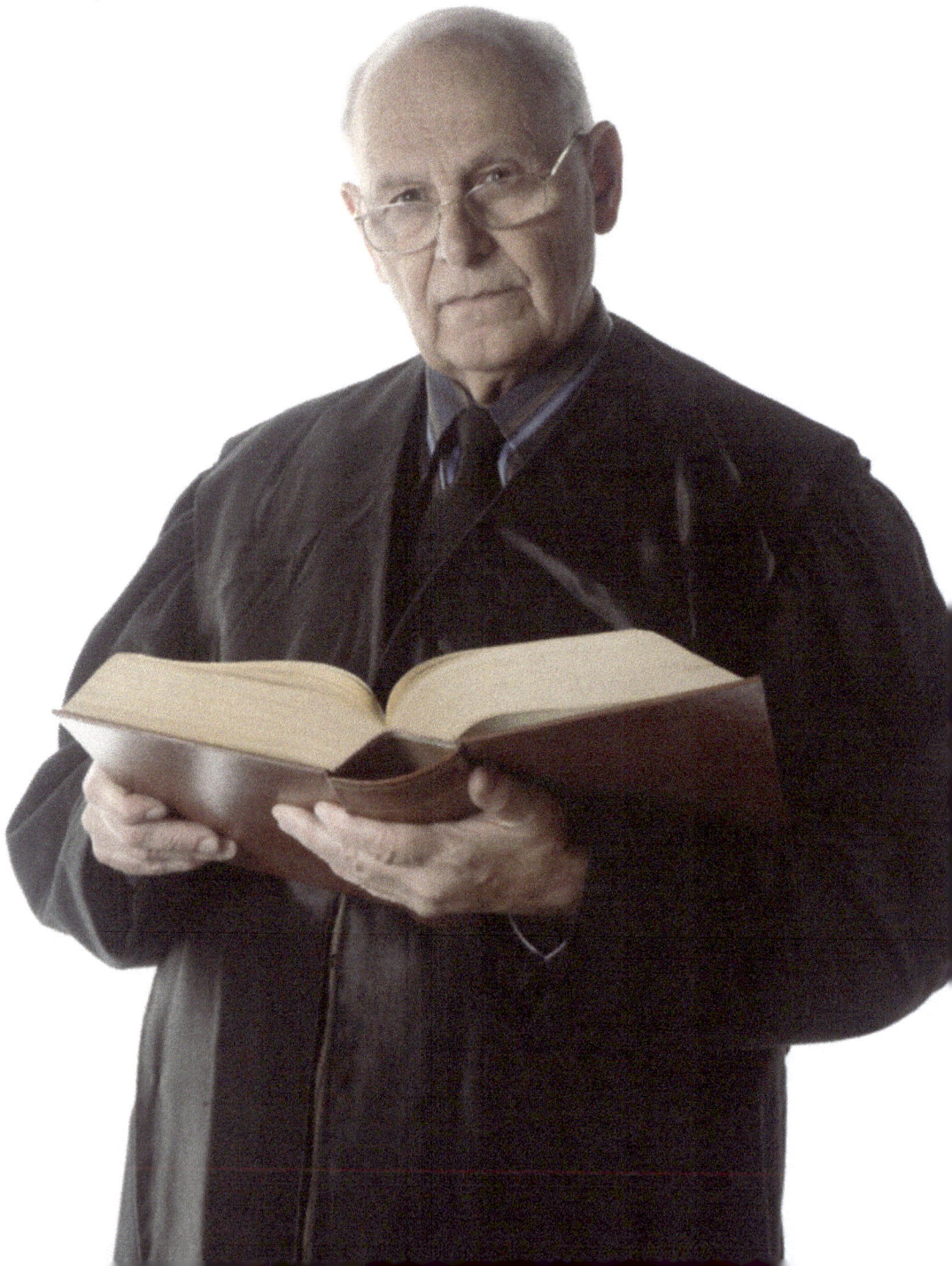

Conclusion

In his introduction to *Medical Negligence,*[1] Lord Nathan cautions that a study of past decisions will be unrewarding, if not misleading, unless it is recognised that the facts of each case and the decisions given in them are of value only as indicating in what manner the courts will apply the general rules of law to individual fact situations. The vital question in the majority of cases in this book has been whether the hospital and/or its medical, midwifery and neonatal/nursing staff exercised skill and care in the circumstances, and whether the circumstances have inevitably differed.

Nevertheless, it is hoped that the cases, while chronicling many sad and painful moments for both patients and staff, will contribute to safe care. Numerous risks and systemic issues in maternity services have been identified by judges and coroners. Judges, usually having heard expert evidence, have gone on to make considered statements on standards of practice. Coroners, in their comments and recommendations, have sought to lessen the risk of avoidable deaths in similar circumstances. Collectively, this not inconsiderable list of risks and strategies should assist in the development of policy and in the management of risk in hospitals.

Readers will have varying views on whether the judges and coroners have been sensitive to the pressures that occur on a daily basis in busy birthing suites and neonatal nurseries. However, Mr Justice Kay shall have the last word:

... in this area, even more than in many other areas of medical litigation, a great deal revolves around matters of judgment, that more than one view can co-exist within the range of the acceptable and that one must be careful before categorising something as negligent if it was simply an alternative but acceptable judgment which has only become unfortunate with the benefit of hindsight. I am also conscious of the need to make allowances for the pressures within which decisions have to be taken by clinicians.[2]

NOTES

1. Nathan, *Medical Negligence,* Butterworths, London 1st ed. (1957) p.4.
2. *Dowdie v Camberwell Health Authority,* 8 Med LR 368 (1997). At p. 375, Mr. Justice Maurice Kay, speaking of shoulder dystocia.

Table and summary of cases

Note on Citation Format:

The citation format in this table will include (with few exceptions): name of case, (date) or volume number, or both, abbreviated name of law report series, beginning page of reference and year of hearing. A reference to 'at page' is a reference to a particular page in the case report. For example, McCrystal v Trumbull Memorial Hospital. 115 Ohio App.3d 73, 684 N.E. 2d 721 (1996) at p.723. In the text, the full citation will be given and thereafter reference to the case will be to the first party; for example, McCrystal or McCrystal's case 'v', means 'versus'. 'Re' means 'in the matter of.' For a list of abbreviations of law reports/legal publications, see the Legal Glossary.

Coronial cases will include (where available) a case number, the year of hearing and the state or territory within Australia.

Chapter 1 Consent to treatment

Cohen v Smith 648 N.E 2d [1995] 329 (U.S)
Assurance by doctor that patient would not be seen unclothed by male nurse during caesarean section; nurse saw and touched patient during surgery; ignoring religious beliefs; insulting and offensive behaviour constituted battery.

In Re MB (CA) [1997] 8 Med LR 217 (U.K)

Baby in breech position; mother agreed to caesarean section; refused anaesthetic by needle; detailed examination of law; order that caesarean lawful, including needles for IV and anaesthetic.

In re T (Adult: Refusal of Treatment) WLR [1992] at 803 (UK)

Injured, pregnant and critically ill patient refused blood transfusion; refusal not effective because of mental and physical state; pressure by Jehovah Witness mother, misleading response to enquiry about alternatives to blood; Refusal of Consent form designed to 'protect hospital' rather than inform patient; refusal of consent did not extend to emergency that subsequently developed.

Davidson v Shirley, 616 F.2d 224 [1980] (US)

Consent to caesarean section, tubal ligation plus any procedure therapeutically necessary; tumour discovered and removed; life-threatening blood loss; hysterectomy; removal of tumour therapeutically necessary. No battery.

Re Elm NSWSC 1137 [2006] (Aus)

Woman (refugee and pregnant) HIV-positive with very limited networks; refused medication and consent to caesarean section or medical treatment for baby after birth; orders made in her absence for government department to assume responsibility for baby; director of NICU authorised to give baby necessary medical treatment immediately after birth; baby not to receive breast milk from mother or to be removed from hospital without authority.

Khalid v Barnet & Chase Farm Hospital NHS Trust [2007] (UK) 97 BMLR

Delay by midwife in calling registrar and misinterpretation of true contraction rate by registrar, both negligent; parents making decisions not to be overloaded with technical information but given simple explanation of whether to continue trial of labour or proceed to ceasearean section; wisdom of seeking consent from labouring woman queried. Negligence proved.

Chapter 2 Communication

McCrystal v Trumbull Memorial Hospital, 115 Ohio App. 3d 73, 684 N.E.2d 721 [1996] (US)

Patient cramping and bleeding; telephone calls, visits to hospitals; advised to stay home, relax; ruptured uterus; midwife and supervisor not listening to patient when exploring history of bleeding; negligence.

Coronial Investigation Case No. 2896/96 [1999] (Vic)

No vaginal examination after patient complained to midwife of 'something coming out'; management of high-risk patients examined; hospital's internal review process examined.

Nguyen v Tama, 688 A.2d 1103 [1997] (US)

Midwife and RMO observed, noted signs of pre-eclampsia; no medication orders by obstetrician; caesarean section; patient suffered stroke; management of pre-eclampsia examined; obstetrician negligent.

Lopez v Southwest Community Health Services, 833 F.2d 1183 [1992] (US)

Patient 28 weeks' pregnant; abdominal pain; disagreement between patient, nurse, paediatrician, obstetrician as to cause; induced labour; brain damaged premature baby; nurse's faulty assessment influenced obstetrician; obstetrician, nurse negligent.

Coronial Investigation Case No. 3480/92 [1993] (Vic)

Midwives concerned at GP's lack of response to CTG tracings, information to consultant over telephone; traces represented terminal tracing of heart beat; query whether midwives should have taken matter to the director of nursing.

Coronial Investigation (Aus 2000) Case no: N.A.

Communication error; forceps delivery; midwife unsure whether obstetrician attempting rotation, or, having successfully rotated, attempting traction; obstetrician responsible for directing midwife; ritualised checking and communicating to avoid human error recommended.

Chapter 3 Supervision of junior staff

Rouse v Pitt County Memorial Hospital., Inc., 116 N.C. App. 241, 447 S.E.2d 505 [1994], rev. granted 339 N.C. 615, 454 S.E.2d 257 [1995]

Delivery of high-risk patient by RMOs below standard; supervising doctors negligent; no record of having visited that day; supervision defined in various ways.

Director of Proceedings (Mrs V) v Dr Mc 447 S.E 2d 505 [2001] (NZ)

Registrar delegated management of labour to senior midwife and senior house surgeon; no personal assessment; supervising doctor needs to assess competence; delegation must not put patient at risk.

Mozingo v Pitt County Memorial Hospital, Inc., 331 N.C. 182, 415 S.E.2d 341 [1992]

Supervising doctor at home on-call; delivery by RMOs negligent; supervision negligent, responsibility to call hospital, ascertain continuing condition of new patients, formulate care plans.

Greater Southern Area Health Service v Angus NSWSC 1211 [2007]

Allegations of negligent care following administration of Syntocinon; case against health authority settled; health authority claimed contribution to damages from obstetrician on-call at time of incident; obstetrician (though present in labour ward area at the time) was held not to have been consulted by junior doctor about Syntocinon administration.

Coronial Investigation Case No: 0057/2007, (Darwin Aus 2009)

Delay in reporting neonatal death; primary midwives new to birthing suite teamed with inexperienced resident, misunderstanding as to responsibilities; high-risk labour managed by midwives rather than senior medical staff; documentation issues, request by patient not documented.

Grainger v Ottawa General Hospital 7 O.T.C 81 (Ont.Gen.Div) [1996]

Acting midwife failed to assess trace, alert doctor; supervising midwife failed to supervise properly; hospital breached duty to ensure minimum competency levels.

Chapter 4 Malfunctioning equipment

Anderson v Salvation Army Maternity Hospital N.S.J. No. 339 [1989] (Can)

Malfunctioning paging system; delay in reaching obstetrician; obstetrician held to be able to rely on hospital paging system; hospital liable.

James v Camberwell Health Authority 5 Med.LR 253 [1994]
Apparent delay of 69 minutes in recognising severe abnormality in fetal heart was in reality only nine minutes because of malfunction of CTG clock; propensity of clock to 'flip' common knowledge to staff but not communicated; no negligence.

Chapter 5 Neurological injury

Dissidomino v Newnham & Anor, Supreme Court of Western Australia, No.84, CCH Australian Health & Medical Law Reporter [1994](Aus)
Cerebral palsy allegedly caused by delay by GP in calling specialist when meconium noted; 'extraordinary' lapse of time between incident and trial; both doctor and midwife now elderly; mother's evidence effected by distortion of memory; early placental insufficiency likely; no negligence.

Ren v Mukerjee and Anor. ACT Supreme Court, No. SC 440 of 1989, 12 Dec. 1996
Confusion as to whether OR was needed for caesarean section following failed attempt at forceps delivery or for a trial by forceps with possible caesarean section; delay; negligence.

Allan v University Hospital's Board, A.J. No. 880 (Q.B) (Q.L), Alberta Court of Queens Bench [2000](Can)
10-30 minutes standard for high caesarean section appropriate; 45-50 minutes for this procedure in tertiary hospital substandard.

Bauer v Seager MJ. No. 356 (Q.B) (Q.L) [2000](Can)
Failure by nurses to notify doctors in timely manner of main cause of injury; RMO slow in involving obstetrician and moving mother for examination.

Whitehouse v Jordan, 1 All ER 267 [1981] (UK)
Neurological damage allegedly caused by registrar pulling 'too long and too hard' on forceps; no negligence; distinction drawn between 'error of judgment' and 'negligence.'

Chapter 6 Shoulder dystocia

Gaughan v Bedfordshire Health Authority, 8 Med LR 182 [1997] (UK)
Big baby; mother significantly overweight; midwife continued traction with more force and longer than necessary; brachial plexus and Erb's palsy of right arm; negligence.

Dowdie v Camberwell Health Authority, 8 Med LR 368 [1997]
Big baby; possibility of cephalopelvic disproportion; arrest of secondary labour; Syntocinon; negligent failure to abandon vaginal delivery at appropriate time; shoulder dystocia delivery managed appropriately; brachial plexus nerve injury of right arm; negligence.

Croft v Heart of England NHS Foundation Trust, WL 1933467 [2012]
Injury to nerves of neck; loss of function in right arm; allegations of negligence by midwife; diagnostic traction acceptable; need to demonstrate factual evidence of use of excessive force or inappropriate management, particularly from eyewitnesses to delivery; brachial plexus injury multifactorial; growing acceptance that propulsive forces of uterine contractions may contribute to injury; no negligence.

Chapter 7 Medication

Webster v Chapman, 155 D.L.R (4th) 83 [1998] (Can)
Fetus injured by prescribed drug; causation issues as to when damage occurred; GP should have sought specialist advice earlier and advised mother of dangers and treatment options; negligence.

Look, et al. v Hamel, Ont.Ct. (Gen.Div) [1991] (Can)
Prostin induced labour; failure to monitor; no link between nurses' actions/inactions and baby's injuries.

Coronial Investigation Case No. 1765/93 [2006] (Vic)
Patient (42 weeks plus two days' gestation) exercised choice to go home after administration of Prostin; re-presented in labour, perinatal asphyxia; continued admission after Prostin for induction of labour recommended.

Ritchie v Chichester Health Authority, 5 Med. LR 187 [1994] (UK)

Toxic drug administered to mother during epidural; circumstantial evidence: fatigue, failure to check top-up, 'rogue drug' in drug cupboard; negligence.

Coronial Investigation Case No. 2477/02 [2004] (Vic)

Syntometrine instead of Pethidine given prior to delivery; single checking of dangerous drug; preparation and placement of Syntometrine; difficulty in locating reversing agent; delay in seeking expert medical help; employment issues; incident reporting; individual and systems failure.

Chapter 8 Pain Relief

Ackers v Wigan, 2 Med. LR 232 [1991] (UK)

Awareness, pain, inability to communicate during anaesthetic for caesarean section; patient withdrawn and fearful; difficulty bonding with baby; fear of future surgery; second pregnancy required caesarean section; fear of a third pregnancy; sexual relations affected; negligence admitted; amount of damages disputed.

Taylor v Worcester v District Health Authority, 2 Med. LR 215 [1991] (UK)

Awareness, pain and discomfort experienced during reversal of anaesthetic, not during surgery as patient alleged; detailed clinical reasons for decision; no negligence.

Tucker v Hospital Corporation Australia Pty Ltd & Ors, NSW SC No. 12575/92 [1998](Aus)

Unacceptable level of pain experienced during epidural for caesarean section; emotional difficulties and personality changes; negligence.

Lunn v Giblin Supreme Court of the Northern Territory, 98008 [1998]

Placenta removed manually without anaesthetic soon after birth; complications; further surgery; severe trauma; negligence.

Chapter 9 Infection

Starkey v Connell, et al., Supreme Court Victoria No. 12477 [1996]
Pregnant patient very ill and vulnerable to infection; Hickman catheter inserted; septicaemia, gentamicin administered; deafness; allegations of sub-standard infection control not proved; nursing care plan decisive as to safe handling of Hickman catheter; no negligence.

Troxel v A1 Dupont Institute, 6675 A. 2d 314 [1996]
Mother and baby contracted CMV; pregnant friend handled baby; baby died after contracting CMV; doctors have duty to inform patient about infectious nature of CMV and how to prevent its spread; negligence.

Hughes v Sydney Day Nursery, NSWCA 11 [2002]
Pregnant child care worker in nursery contracted CMV; pattern of child's disabilities pointed to primary rather than reactivated infection early in pregnancy; failure to warn negligent.

Coronial Investigation Case No. 903/96 [1998] (Vic)
Mother pregnant with twins tested positive for Strep. B in public hospital; pathology results not transferred to private hospital where twins delivered by obstetrician who had attended mother in public hospital; one twin died after contracting Strep. B; coronial recommendations: steps should be taken to ensure test results reach interested parties.

Lindsay County Council v Marshall, 2 All ER 1076 A.C. 97 [1937]
Neither patient nor doctor warned of infection in hospital; patient infected; duty to warn doctors admitting patients of 'hidden dangers' so doctor can decide whether to admit a patient and, if so, what precautions against infection should be taken; negligence.

Inderbitizen v Lane Hospital, 124 Cal. App. 462, 12 P.2d 744 [1932], reh. denied, 124 Cal. App. 469, 13 p.2d 905 [1932]
Vaginal and rectal examinations performed; too many 'students' involved; torn uterus, infection; allegation that hands not washed.

Chapter 10 Postpartum

R v Inner London North Coroner, ex parte Touche,
[2001] 60 BMLR 170 [2001] (UK)
Twins delivered by caesarean section; headaches; failure to monitor mother's BP; left-sided hemiplegia; maternal death; coroner refused inquest; court found grounds for holding inquest.

Coronial Investigation Case No. 4210/91 [1994] (Vic)
Maternal death; trial of labour after previous caesarean section; response to postpartum bleed adequate; no cause found.

Le Page v Kingston and Richmond Health Authority,
8 Med LR 229 [1997] (UK)
Delivery of twins by caesarean section; uncontrolled postpartum haemorrhage; delay in transfusion; falling blood pressure; no routine palpation of fundus; failure to detect blood in uterus; shock; negligence.

Coronial Investigation Case No: 615/2007 [209] (NSW) [2009]
No policy of taking a full blood count, group and hold or cross/match prior to emergency caesarean section by hospital; failure by recovery room nurse to recognise internal bleeding in patient following a postpartum haemorrhage during a caesarean section; medical staff assumed recovery room nurse experienced and trained in this area; compartmentalizing of perceived areas of responsibility between disciplines.

Gregorie v Spencer, 300 A.P.R. 1 (Q.B) [1991]
Mother complained of pain in upper left quadrant day after delivery; delay in examination by doctor; ruptured diaphragm; negligence.

Prosser v Eagle, NSWCA 166 [1999]
Mother complained of severe pain in pelvic area following delivery; no immediate X-rays; physiotherapist reported diastasis of symphysis pubis; undiagnosed pelvic fracture.

Chapter 11 Nervous shock

Kralj v Mc Grath, 1 ALL ER 54 (Vic) [1986]
Internal rotation of second twin attempted without anaesthetic; mother in extreme pain; caesarean section; mother saw baby convulsing and unable to cry or swallow before death; nervous shock; negligence.

Tredget & Tredget v Bexley Health Authority, *5 Med LR 178 [1994] (Vic)*

Big baby; long labour; hospital admitted negligent delivery; parents saw baby in distressed state following birth; aggravated reaction to neonatal death examined; nervous shock (both parents); negligence.

Hunter Area Health Service v Marchlewski & Anor [2000] *NSWCA 294*

Asphyxia during shoulder dystocia delivery; baby removed from life support without parents' consent; no information about autopsy; aggravated and exemplary damages considered; nervous shock; negligence.

Bro v Glaser, 22 Cal. App.4th 1398, 27 Cal. Rptr. 2d 894 *[1994] (Vic)*

Baby's face 'nicked' during caesarean section; no permanent injury; claim 'bordering on frivolous'; no negligence.

Allin v City and Hackney HA, 7 Med LR 167 [1996]

Emergency delivery; mother incorrectly told that baby had died; post-traumatic stress disorder discussed; negligence.

Chapter 12 Lactation

Coronial Investigation Case No. 1082/90 [1993] (Vic)

Baby suffered hypoxic episode during unsupervised first breast feed, later died; mother very tired post caesarean section; Pethidine drip; recommendation that such feeds are supervised and probably assisted; documentation issues.

Coronial Investigation Case No: 2145/05 (7) [2006] (Qld)

Baby suffered severe hypoxic episode during unsupervised first breast feed, later died; mother exhausted after long labour; very busy shift, staffing issues; midwives unaware of policy re monitoring; recommendation that mother/baby be classed as two patients- not one.

Coronial Investigation Case No. 1616/99 [2002] (Vic)

Early discharge of premature baby who had lost weight in hospital; breakdown in communication between hospital and mother; hospital and community agency; baby not weighed for ten days; recommendations re roles of community agencies; communication between hospital and agencies; keeping records of telephone calls; need for adequate medical notes; recognition of medical emergency.

Coronial Investigation Case No.4197/00 [2003] (Vic)

Baby weaned from breast; deterioration when fed fortified rice milk; delay by parents in seeking medical assistance when baby critically ill.

In Re C (a child) (HIV test), 50 BMLR 383 Family Division (UK)

Mother HIV- positive; disagreed with proposed mainstream treatment; water birth at home, breast fed; court ordered HIV test for baby; query as to whether law should come between breast and baby.

In Re Elm NSWSC 1137 [2006] (Aus)

Woman (refugee and pregnant) HIV-positive and very limited networks; refused medication and consent to caesarean section or medical treatment for baby after birth; orders made (in her absence) for government department to assume responsibility for baby; director of NICU authorised to give baby necessary medical treatment immediately after birth; baby not to receive breast milk from mother.

Chapter 13 Resuscitation and withdrawal of treatment

Coronial Investigation, Daily Telegraph, April 11 2000 (Northern Territory)

Baby born alive after termination between 21 and 22 weeks; responsibilities unclear; recommendation for protocol to cover future contingencies.

In Re J (a Minor), 2 Med LR 67 [1990] (Vic)

Premature baby born severely brain damaged; readmitted when cyanosed; approval given to continuance of treatment; duty to act in accordance with good medical practice; pain, suffering and quality of life considered.

Anthony MacDonald, et al. v St Joseph's Hospital, Legal Report [1989] (US)

Baby born severely disabled at 23 and a half weeks, 68 g; not responsive to resuscitation; survived unexpectedly; obstetrician not negligent in failing to give oxygen immediately after birth.

The People v Gregory Glenn Messenger Ingham County, (Michigan) Circuit, File No. 94-67694 – FH [1995]

Father (a doctor) acquitted of manslaughter after removing baby (born at 25 weeks and appearing 'lifeless') from life support; opposing opinions from theologian and neonatologist.

Birkett v Director General of Family & Community Services, [1994] (NSW)

Baby developed gastro-intestinal bleeding, parents opposed blood transfusion; blood authorized under Children (Care and Protection Act); similar legislation in all states.

In Re F: F v F, Unreported Judgment of the Supreme Court of Victoria, [2 July 1986]

Baby born with spina bifida; hospital ordered to take all necessary steps consistent with proper medical practice (including hydration and nutrition) to preserve baby's life; comment on quality of life and criminal charges.

R v Arthur, 12 BMLR 1 [1981] (UK)

Baby born with Down's Syndrome; rejection by parents; nursing care only ordered, plus medication to relieve distress; baby died; doctor acquitted of attempted murder

In Re B, 1 WLR 1421 [1981] (UK)

Baby born with Down's Syndrome and intestinal obstruction; parents refused surgery; order that surgery to remove obstruction lawful; baby entitled to normal lifespan of a Down's Syndrome child.

In Re C (a Minor), 1 Med LR 46 [1989] (UK)

Baby born with severe and irreversible brain damage; best interests of baby required court to approve recommendations to relieve suffering and permit life to end peacefully.

Coronial Investigation Case No. 311149/89 [1991] (Vic)

Baby born with severe abnormalities; parents decided against surgery/life-saving treatments; drugs administered with intention to relieve distress; doctors' and parents' actions found reasonable and appropriate; comment re coronial role.

Chapter 14 The Neonatal Unit: staff/equipment/monitoring

Wilsher v Essex Area Health Authority, 3 All ER 801 HL, 1 ALL ER 871 [1988] (UK)

Junior doctor in NICU mistakenly inserted arterial catheter into vein; registrar failed to pick up misplacement on X-ray; premature baby (RLF); inexperience rejected as defence; registrar held to specialised standard of NICU.

Anonymous v Anonymous Hospital, [1999] (US)

Temporary float nurse re-attached feeding tube; breast milk adaptor attached to central line; milk directly into baby's jugular vein. Settled.

Coronial Investigation Case No. 1219/00 [2002] (Vic)

Nurse in NICU took ETT aspirate for culture by suctioning ETT; attached suction catheter to oxygen tubing to blow sample into specimen pot; returned catheter to further suction tube while still attached to oxygen tubing; baby suffered bilateral pneumothoraces; doctor not made aware of incident. Nurse should have been 'calmed'; assumptions about repair of equipment.

Nawoor v Barking Havering and Brentwood HA, QBD 313 [1997] (UK)

Baby received perenteral feeding; leakage; damaged foot; monitoring met reasonable standard; acknowledgement that premature babies survive because of very complex care. No negligence.

Chapter 15 The Neonatal Unit: times/reporting problems

Blodgett v Kahn, 681 N.E.2d 452 [1996] (US)

Patient in A&E in premature labour; transfer by ambulance to second hospital; birth started; brain damage; delay alleged; no specific legal standard re time to effect patient transfer.

Salas v Wang, 846 F.2d 987 [1996] (US)

Obstetrician told labour and delivery charge nurse to notify NICU of impending high-risk delivery; team arrived late; charge nurse negligent; failed to notify team in timely fashion.

South Fulton Medical Center v Poe, 480 S.E.2d 40,
224 Ga.App.107 [1996] (US)
Baby discharged from NICU with instructions about returning; baby brought back to hospital via A&E; gravity of condition not assessed by triage nurse; medical opinion not sought; delay; nurse negligent.

Sheridan v St Luke's Regional Medical Center,135 Idaho 775, 25
P.3d 88 [2001] (U.S)
Mismanagement of jaundice; nurses negligent; paediatrician not notified when jaundice appeared; possible blood incompatibility of mother and baby not noted; parents not given information at discharge on abnormal jaundice; nurses should document so that nurses on later shifts can tell if problems identified on earlier shift have been resolved; hospitals need procedures to take patient issues up hospital chain of command. Negligence, paediatrician bore brunt of responsibility.

Chapter 16 The Neonatal Unit: medication

Norton v Argonaut Insurance Company, 144 So.2d 249
[1962] (US)
Deputy DON went from administration to paediatric ward; failed to clarify ambiguous medication order; medication injected dose; meant for oral administration; doctor negligent, ambiguous order; nurse negligent, failure to check.

Wade v Tran, Pa; Philadelphia County C.C.P No. 3721
[1995] (US)
Baby in NICU; inflammation developed near IV site; severe infection; allegations that neonatologists failed to diagnose and delay in administering antibiotics; negligence.

Chiricosta v Winthrop-Breon, 263 III. App.3d 132, 635 N.E. 2d
1019 [1994] (US)
Baby, cerebral palsy; allegations that medication for pain relief crossed placental barrier; that manufacturer supplied inadequate information; that care in NICU below standard; no negligence.

Criminal proceedings : Death of Miguel Sanchez,
[1996] (US) Nursing, May 1998
Examination of chain of errors leading to baby's death by overdose.

Chapter 17 The Neonatal Unit: intentional injury

Gess v US, 952 F.Supp 1529 [1996] (US)
Medical technician deliberately harmed mother, babies in a neonatal unit; circumstantial evidence pointed to technician; not picked up; hospital negligent; lack of supervision; ignoring staff concerns; failing to monitor instability; failure to have quality control programme; poor documentation; recommendations for risk managers.

Chapter 18 Documentation

Gabaldoni v Board of Physician Quality Assurance,
785 A.2d 771 [2000] (US)
Doctor's negligent record keeping contrasted with accuracy of nursing notes.

James v Camberwell Health Authority, 5 Med.LR 253 [1994]
Apparent delay of 69 minutes in recognising severe abnormality in fetal heart in reality only nine minutes because of malfunction of CTG clock; propensity of clock to 'flip' common knowledge to staff but not documented/ communicated; no negligence.

Deacon v McVicor, [1984] (UK)
Patient claimed labour room staff should have removed shirodkar suture before cervix damaged and future pregnancies put at risk; hospital argued patient received appropriate care in context of very busy shift; notes of other patients (de-identified) viewed by court; demonstrated busy shift but did not explain why suture was not removed earlier.

Legal abbreviations

Abbreviations used in cases cited in text

Australia

AC	Appeal Cases
ALR	Australian Law Reports
ACT SC	Australian Capital Territory, Supreme Court
CLR	Commonwealth Law Reports
CCH	CCH Australian Health & Medical Law Reporter
NSWSC	New South Wales Supreme Court

England

All ER	All England Law Reports
BMLR	Butterworths Medical Law Reports
Fam	Family Division (UK)
Med LR	Medical Law Reports
QBD	Law Reports, Queens Bench Division
QB	Law Reports, Queens Bench
TLR	Times Law Reports
WLR	Weekly Law Reports

United States

A	Atlantic Reporter
A.2d	Atlantic Reporter (Second Series)
ATLA	American Trial Lawyers Association
F.2d	Federal Reporter (Second Series)
F. Supp	Federal Supplement
N.E.2d	North Eastern Reporter (Second Series)
P.2d	Pacific Reporter (Second Series)
S.E.2d	South Eastern Reporter (Second Series)
So.2d	Southern Reporter (Second Series)

Canada

DLR	Dominion Law Reports
OTC	Ontario General Division
(QB) (QL)	Alberta Court of Queens Bench

Other abbreviations used in text

In Re	In the matter of – somebody or something
Ex parte	On the application of one party
v	Versus

Glossary of legal terms and concepts

Note: Definitions are based on Concise Australian Legal Dictionary, 3rd ed, Butterworths, Australia, 2004.

Accident. Something that happens without intention or design.

Action. Any proceeding in a court.

Accusatorial/adversarial system. The common law system of trial which requires one party, usually the plaintiff or the prosecution, to collect evidence and present it to a judge to prove a cause of action against another party.

Admissible evidence. Evidence received, or capable of being received by a court or tribunal for the purpose of proving a fact in issue because it is relevant to the proceedings. The rules governing admissibility of evidence are found in legislation.

Adult. A person who is of or above the age of 18 years. At that age, a person is of full legal capacity subject only to the law relating to mental illness.

Advocacy. The art of conducting or presenting proceedings before a court. An advocate's work comprises argument or making speeches, questioning witnesses, and preparation and planning for these tasks.

Affidavit. A statement given under oath.

Aggravated damages. Substantial, general compensation awarded when the manner in which a tort is committed is particularly insulting and humiliating. A tort is a civil wrong, e.g., negligence or defamation (distinguished from other areas of law e.g. the law of contract, criminal law). The law of torts aims to restore the injured person to the position they were in before the tort was committed by awarding damages in compensation.

Appeal. An application to a higher court to reconsider the decision of a lower court, on the ground that there has been an error in the decision of the lower court. The term includes an application for a re-hearing.

Assault. An act that intentionally or recklessly causes another to apprehend immediate and unlawful personal violence.

Balance of probabilities. The weighing up and comparison of the likelihood of the existence of competing facts and conclusions. A fact is proved to be true on the balance of probabilities if its existence is more probable than not, or if it is established by a preponderance of probability.

Battery. The reckless or intentional application of force to another person without consent, lawful excuse or justification.

Belief. An inclination of the mind towards assenting to, rather than rejecting, a proposition based on facts that are sufficient to create that inclination of the mind to a reasonable person. Belief may be something less than knowledge, since a person can hold a belief while having a degree of doubt about the matter, but it is more than mere suspicion.

Beyond reasonable doubt. In criminal proceedings, a standard of proof that stipulates that a charge is not proved if the court is not satisfied beyond reasonable doubt that the accused committed the offence charged. Judges should not explain the term to juries because it is well understood and needs no explanation, except perhaps in cases depending on circumstantial evidence.

Birth. The act of a child being born. For a birth to take place, the whole body needs to be brought into the world; it is not sufficient that a child respires in the progress of birth. It does not include stillbirth.

Born alive. At common law, a child is born alive if it has a separate and independent existence from its mother.

Burden of proof. Under the common law adversarial system, the duty of one party (usually the party bringing the proceedings against another) to make out the case against the other party and to prove to the court that the case has been established.

Causation. The relation of cause to effect. The question of whether a plaintiff's loss is the result of the defendant's actions. The plaintiff must show a sufficient connection between the defendant's breach and the loss suffered. It is sufficient to prove that but for the defendant's breach, the loss or damage would not have been suffered. The prevailing test for causation in civil actions is the common sense test.

Cause of action. The whole set of facts that give rise to an enforceable claim.

Circumstantial evidence. Representations or information regarding a fact from which a court is asked to infer a further fact.

Citation. The year, volume, report series and page reference for a case.

Common law. The unwritten law derived from England as developed by judicial precedence, interpretation, expansion and modification. Generally a statute will not be taken to have repealed the common law unless it explicitly or implicitly shows such an intention.

Conception. The moment that an ovum is fertilized by a spermatozoon, which is the precursor to the formation of the human embryo. An embryo has no rights that a court may protect until it is born and has a separate existence from its mother.

Confinement. The state during which a pregnant woman commences labour, concluding at the birth of a child.

Consent. Affirmative acceptance, not merely a standing by and absence of objection. Actual agreement by a plaintiff to the action complained of must be genuine and obtained without fraud or duress.

Coroner. A public official statutorily appointed to inquire into the manner and cause of examinable deaths, or of fires and explosions which damage property.

Coroner's court. The primary function of the coroner's court is to inquire into the death of a person if there is reasonable cause to suspect that the person died a violent or unnatural death.

Coronial inquest. Inquiry concerning the death or suspected death of a person. The normal rules of evidence and procedure do not apply; an inquest is not adversarial and the coroner's court is not a court of blame.

Court-appointed expert. An independent person selected and directed by the judge to furnish the court with a scientific, technical, professional or specialized opinion that is likely to be outside the experience and knowledge of the judge or jury. Such an expert is appointed to inquire into and report upon a question of fact or opinion.

Damage. Loss or injury suffered by plaintiff as the foreseeable consequence of a defendant's negligent act or omission. In the case of physical injury, both the injury itself and the foreseeable consequences suffered by the plaintiff are considered to be damage for which damages are payable.

Damages. Compensation for damage suffered; a court awarded sum of money which places the plaintiff in the position he would have occupied had the legal wrong not occurred.

Death. An irreversible cessation of all functions of a person's brain, or an irreversible cessation of circulation of blood in a person's body.

Decision. A concluded opinion or determination.

Declaration. A formal, imperative statement creating or preserving a right.

Delegation. Handing down, granting, assigning or relinquishing certain powers, duties and authority to another to act on one's behalf for the implementation of a specific task.

Determine. To make an order, direction, decision or determination by a court or tribunal.

Direction to jury. Directions given to the jury by the trial judge in the summing up of the law to be applied by the jury in respect of the facts as found by it.

Discovery. A pre-trial procedure where a party to proceedings makes available for inspection all relevant documents to the other parties.

Discrimination. Any distinction, exclusion, restriction, or preference made on a particular basis, such as race, sex, religion, national origin, marital status, pregnancy, or disability, which has the purpose or effect of nullifying or impairing the recognition, enjoyment, or exercise, on an equal footing, of human rights and fundamental freedoms in the political, economic, social, cultural, or any other field of life.

Documentary evidence. Information or data, usually recorded on paper, which is produced in court to prove an occurrence. A faxed document may be admissible. In some jurisdictions, in proceedings where direct oral evidence of a fact would be admissible, computer evidence tending to establish that fact is generally admissible. Computer records have also been held to be business records and admissible under relevant provisions.

Duress. An act done by one person to another for the purpose of applying pressure or undue persuasion to do something, or refrain from doing something. Duress may take the form of constraint by injury, confinement or threats.

Duty of care. The obligation owed to anyone who it is reasonably foreseeable would be injured by the lack of care for that person. For a duty of care to arise, there must exist a relationship of proximity between plaintiff and defendant or to persons in specific categories. The duty is breached if the defendant fails to act in accordance with the required standard of care.

Duty of care and skill. The duty of an employee to perform the work agreed in the contract of employment with reasonable care and skill. An employee who accepts a job requiring a particular skill impliedly promises that they have, and will exercise, the skill required.

Employer's duty of care. The duty of care owed by an employer to their employees. The duty comprises the duty to provide safe tools and equipment, a safe place to work, and a safe system of work, including the employment of competent fellow employees.

Employer's liability. An employer is vicariously liable for the negligence of employees (but not generally independent contractors) acting in the course of their employment. Liability also arises through the employer's non-delegable duty of care towards its employees. This entails a general duty to safeguard employees from unreasonable risk of injury while at work.

Error of judgment. A mistake which does not amount to a breach of the duty of care.

Euthanasia. Generally, the bringing about of someone's death, either by the removal of or interference with, life supporting processes, or the administration of a lethal substance. Also known as 'mercy killing.'

Expert witness. A witness who is an expert in a particular field. An expert witness may express opinions upon relevant matters within the field of expertise; this is an exception to the general rule that a witness may speak only as to facts.

Eyewitness. A person who personally observes an event. An eyewitness may give evidence about what she saw where that evidence is relevant to a fact in issue.

Fact. Any act, occurrence, or other matter, other than a question of law, the existence of which is deemed legally relevant to an issue at trial. Facts are required to make out the elements of an offence or claim in a case, and are established by the parties adducing evidence. With the decline of the jury trial, the judge is required more frequently to determine both questions of fact and law.

False imprisonment. Unlawfully restraining the liberty of another person. The restraint must be a total, not merely a partial, obstruction of a person's free movement. Also known as 'detention' or 'wrongful imprisonment.'

Falsify. To state untruthfully; misrepresent. it is an offence for an employee to falsify documents of an employer.

Hearsay. Evidence which has been learnt from another person. Hearsay evidence is not admissible in court unless it falls within one of the exceptions covered by uniform evidence legislation. This can include business records, telecommunications and contemporaneous statements about a person's health, feelings, intention, knowledge or state of mind.

In need of protection. A child who has suffered or who is likely to suffer harm and does not have a parent able and willing to protect the child from harm.

Infanticide. A statutory offence by which a woman by willful act or omission causes the death of her child, being less than 12-months-old, but at the time of the act or omission, the balance of her mind was disturbed because she had not fully recovered from the effect of giving birth, or (except in Tasmania) because of the effect of lactation following the birth of the child.

Informed consent. Consent to an act after being given full or adequate disclosure.

Inference. An affirmative conclusion from circumstances proved in evidence. It is an exercise of the ordinary powers of human reason in the light of human experience; it is not affected directly by any rule of law.

Jurisdiction. The scope of a court's power to examine and determine facts, interpret and apply the law, make orders and declare judgment. Jurisdiction may be limited by geographic area, the type of parties who appear, the type of relief that can be sought and the point to be decided.

Jurisprudence. The theory of law; the study of the principles of law and legal systems and their fundamental philosophical basis.

Jury. A group of people who swear to fairly determine an issue of fact. A jury typically consists of 12 people in a criminal trial and four people in a civil trial, although this number may be increased by court order.

Law. The subject matter of the discipline of jurisprudence. Law is defined differently according to the particular jurisprudential school or methodology within which one is operating. For example, schools of legal sociology emphasise the social significance of the law and its relationship to politics; positivist schools of jurisprudence focus on the examination of the framework of rules and regulations governing society and their interrelationship; and schools of natural law jurisprudence examine more metaphysical issues about the precise essence of law and the relationship between law and morality, and positive law and natural law.

Lawyer. A barrister or solicitor; a person qualified to practice law.

Medical trespass. Medical treatment performed without the patient's informed consent. Where a patient is detained unlawfully for medical treatment, an action may lie in trespass, even if there was no medical treatment as such.

Negligence. An action in tort (civil wrong) the elements of which are: the existence of a duty of care, breach of that duty and material damage as a consequence of the breach of duty. A duty of care is a legal obligation to avoid causing harm, and arises where harm is foreseeable if due care is not taken. The type of damage, not its extent, must be foreseeable. The plaintiff (as an individual or as a member of a class of plaintiff) must also be foreseeable for a duty to arise. The defendant breaches this duty if he or she fails to avoid the risk where a reasonable person would have done so. A proximate relationship is an additional factor to foreseeability. Proximity is a situation in which persons are so closely and directly affected by the defendant's act or omission that the defendant ought reasonably to have had them in his or her contemplation as being likely to be injured by the act or omission. Proximity may be physical (the parties being close in time or space), circumstantial (due to the relationship between the parties), or causal (the injury being the direct consequence of the negligent act or omission).

Negligence calculus. The collection of factors considered in assessing whether a duty of care is owed in a certain situation and, if so, whether the requisite standard of care has been maintained. These factors include: the likelihood of injury or damage occurring, the degree of risk to others created by the defendant's activity, the practicability of taking precautions against the risk (including the cost of avoiding the risk) and the usefulness of the particular activity giving rise to the risk. These factors are balanced before the standard of response of the reasonable person placed in the defendant's position can be established as a question of fact.

Professional negligence. A breach of duty of care in tort or contract owed to a client/patient or third party arising out of the conduct of professional practice. A professional person must apply the standard of care of the ordinary skilled person exercising and professing to have that special skill. In tort law, advice or information imparted negligently in circumstances in which the actor realizes, or ought to have realized, that the plaintiff was relying on the advice or information as the basis for a course of action.

Question of fact. An issue the resolution of which requires the finding of facts or inferences arising from facts. It is to be distinguished from a question of law or a question of mixed fact and law.

Question of law. A question to be resolved by applying legal principles; an issue involving the application or interpretation of a law and reserved for a judge to decide upon.

Reasonably foreseeable. Ordinarily, properly, or fairly able to be anticipated. An event will be reasonably foreseeable if a reasonable person in the defendant's position would not brush it aside as being a far-fetched or fanciful consequence of his or her conduct.

Relevance. The ability of evidence, if accepted, to rationally affect (directly or indirectly) the assessment of the probability of a fact in issue. Generally, all relevant evidence is admissible.

Vicarious liability. The liability of an employer for the negligence of his employee while acting in the course of employment.

Ward of the court. A child who is in the care and control of the court. No important step in the life of the child may be taken without the court's consent.

Wrongful birth. The birth of a child in circumstances in which the pregnancy would have been terminated or the conception avoided but for the defendant's wrongful conduct. A wrongful birth may arise from a failure to diagnose that a fetus is deformed. Wrongful birth actions are brought by the parents.

Wrongful life. The birth of a child that would not have been born but for another's negligence. The negligence may involve an unsuccessful sterilization operation or failure to perform an abortion successfully. In Australia and England, it has been held that there is no cause of action for a wrongful life because a court cannot determine whether facing life with disabilities is worse than not being born at all.

Glossary of Medical/Midwifery Terms and Concepts

Note: Definitions based on Oxford Concise Medical Dictionary, Oxford University Press, Oxford, 2006, and the Oxford Dictionary of Nursing, Oxford, 2003.

Amniotic cavity. The fluid filled cavity between the embryo and the amnion (the membrane that forms initially over the dorsal part of the embryo but soon expands to cover it completely; it is connected to the embryo at the umbilical cord).

Amniotic fluid. The fluid contained within the amniotic cavity; it surrounds the growing fetus protecting it from external pressure.

Amniotomy. Artificial rupture of the membranes; a method of surgically inducing labour by puncturing the amnion surrounding the baby in the uterus using an amnihook or similar instrument.

Antenatal. Before birth.

Antepartum. Occurring before the onset of labour.

Antepartum haemorrhage. Bleeding from the genital tract after the 22nd week of pregnancy until the birth of the baby. Dangerous causes include abruptio plancentae and placenta praevia.

Apgar score. A method of rapidly assessing the general state of a baby immediately after birth. A maximum of 2 points is given for each of the following signs, usually measured at one minute and five minutes after delivery: type of breathing, heart rate, colour, muscle tone, and response to stimuli. An infant scoring 10 points would be in optimum condition.

When the score is low, the test is repeated at intervals as a guide to short term progress.

Aphasia. (dysphasia) A disorder of language affecting the generation and content of speech and its understanding. It is caused by damage to the language-dominated half of the brain, which is usually the left hemisphere in a right-handed person.

Asphyxia. Suffocation; a life-threatening condition in which oxygen is prevented from reaching the tissues by obstruction of or damage to any part of the respiratory system. Unless the condition is remedied by removing the obstruction (when present) and by artifical respiration if necessary, there is progressive cyanosis leading to death. Brain cells cannot live for more than about four minutes without oxygen.

Autopsy. A review of the clinical history of a deceased person followed by external examination of the body, evisceration and dissection of the internal organs, and ancilliary investigations (such as histopathology, microbiology, or toxicology) to determine the cause of death. Autopsies may be performed on the instructions of a medicolegal authority or at the request of clinicians (with consent of the family).

Bilirubin. The two most important bile pigments are bilirubin, which is orange or yellow, and its oxidized form biliverdin, which is green.

Bilirubinaemia. An excess of bilirubin in the blood. Normally, there is under 0.8 mg bilirubin per 100 ml blood; when the concentration of bilirubin is above 1-1.5 mg per 100 ml visible jaundice occurs. Jaundice is a yellowing of the skin or whites of the eyes.

Biophysical profile. A physiological assessment of fetal wellbeing based on scores for each of the following: fetal breathing, fetal movement, fetal tone, amniotic fluid volume (as observed on ultrasound) and fetal heart rate (measured by cardiotography). The maximum score is 10 (with 2 points for each component).

Breech presentation. The position of a baby in the uterus such that it will be delivered buttocks first. This type of delivery increases the risk of damage to the baby.

Brachial plexus. A network of nerves, arising from the spine at the base of the neck, from which arise the nerves supplying the arm, forearm and hand, and parts of the shoulder girdle.

Caesarean section. A surgical operation for delivering a baby through the abdominal wall. The operation most commonly performed is lower uterine segment caesarean section (LUSC), carried out through a transverse incision in the lower portion of the uterus. In addition to its use in cases of obstructed labour, malpresentation (breech, brow and shoulder), and in severe antepartum haemorrhage, caesarean section is being performed increasingly when the baby is at risk and is exhibiting signs of distress. Because of improved techniques in perinatal care, particularly of the preterm baby, the operation may be performed, if necessary, as soon as the child is viable.

Caput succedaneum. A temporary swelling of the soft parts of the head of a newly born infant that occurs during labour due to compression of the muscles of the cervix (neck) of the uterus and resolves after delivery.

Cephalic version. A procedure in which a fetus that is lying in the breech position is turned so that its head will enter the birth canal first. It may give rise to complications (e.g., abruptio placentae) and is therefore only carried out in selected cases.

Cervix. A necklike part, especially the cervix uteri (neck of the uterus), which projects at its lower end into the vagina. The cervical canal passes through it, linking the cavity of the uterus with the vagina; the cervix is capable of wide dilation during childbirth.

Cerebral palsy. A disorder of movement and/or posture as a result of non-progressive but permanent damage to the developing brain. This damage may occur before, during or immediately after delivery and has many causes, including an inadequate supply of oxygen to the brain, low levels of sugar in the blood, and infection.

Congenital. A condition that is recognized at birth or that is believed to have been present since birth. Congenital malformations include all disorders present at birth, whether they are inherited or caused by an environmental factor.

Crowning. The stage of labour when the upper part of the infant's head is encircled by, and just passing through, the vaginal opening.

CTG. Continuous cartiographic monitoring.

Delusion. A belief that is held with unshakeable conviction, cannot be altered by rational argument, and is outside the person's normal cultural or subcultural belief system. The belief is usually wrong, but can occasionally be true. The abnormal pathology lies in the irrational way in which the person comes to the belief.

Depression. A mental state characterized by excessive sadness.

Doppler ultrasound. Used to study the flow in blood vessels and the movement of blood in the heart.

Erb's palsy. Weakness or paralysis of the shoulder and arm usually caused by injury to the upper roots of the brachial plexus during traumatic childbirth. This may happen if, during a difficult delivery, excess traction applied to the head damages the fifth and sixth cervical roots of the spinal cord. The muscles of the shoulder and the flexors of the elbow are paralysed and the arm hangs at the side internally rotated at the shoulder with the forearm pronated. Recovery may be spontaneous, but in some cases nerve grafts or muscle transfers are required.

Exsanguination. Depriving the body of blood; very rarely through uncontrollable bleeding during a surgical operation.

Fetus. An unborn child from its eighth week of development.

Fetal blood sampling. Withdrawal of a sample of fetal blood either from the umbilical vein during the antenatal period or from a vein in the presenting part (usually the fetal scalp) during labour. The latter procedure is used to detect hypoxia by measuring the fetal pH and degree of acidosis. The normal pH of fetal blood is 7.35 (range 7.45 – 7.25). The lower the pH, the more likely is the fetus to be suffering from hypoxia and acidosis, indicating an urgent need to deliver the baby.

Fibrodysplasia. Abnormal development affecting connective tissue.

Forceps. Pincer-like instrument designed to grasp an object so that it can be held firm or pulled. The forceps used in childbirth are so designed as to fit firmly round the baby's head without damaging it.

Gestation. The period during which a fertilized egg cell develops into a baby that is ready to be delivered. Gestation averages 266 days in humans (or 280 days from the first day of the last menstrual period).

Gestational diabetes. Diabetes mellitus or impaired glucose tolerance that is diagnosed during pregnancy. Women at increased risk of gestational diabetes include those with a personal history of the condition or a family history of diabetes, and those who have had a previously unexplained stillbirth.

Guthrie test. A blood test performed on all newborn babies at the end of the first week of life. The blood is obtained by pricking the heel of the baby. The test can detect several inborn errors of metabolism (including phenylketonuria and hypothyroidism).

Haemoglobin. A substance contained within the red blood cells and responsible for their colour, composed of the pigment haem (an iron containing porphyrin) linked to the protein globin. Haemoglobin has the unique property of combining reversibly with oxygen and is the medium by which oxygen is transported within the body.

Haemolytic disease of the newborn. The condition resulting from destruction (haemolysis) of the red cells of the fetus by antibodies in the mother's blood passing through the placenta. This most commonly happens when the red blood cells of the fetus are Rh positive but the mother's cells are Rh negative.

Hartmann's solution. A physiological solution used for infusion into the circulation. In addition to essential ions, it also contains glucose.

Hemi. The right or left side of the body.

Hickman catheter. A fine plastic cannula usually inserted into the subclavian vein in the neck to allow administration of drugs and repeated blood samples. The catheter is tunnelled for several centimeters beneath the skin to prevent infection entering the bloodstream.

Hyaline membrane. The condition of a newborn infant in which the lungs are imperfectly expanded. Initial inflation and normal expansion of the lungs requires the presence of surfactant that reduces the surface tension of the air sacs (alveoli) and prevents collapse of the small airways. The condition is most common and serious among pre-term infants, in whom surfactant is liable to be deficient. The condition is treated by careful nursing, intravenous fluids, and oxygen, with or without positive-pressure ventilation.

Hydramnios—polyhydramnios. An increase in the amount of amniotic fluid surrounding the fetus, which occurs usually in the third trimester and may be associated with multiple diabetes, multiple pregnancy, any fetal anomaly causing impaired swallowing, or placental abnormality.

Hypertension (pregnancy-induced). Raised blood pressure (>140/90 mmHg) developing in a woman during the second half of pregnancy. It usually resolves within six weeks of delivery and is associated with a better prognosis than pre-eclampsia.

Hypoxia. A deficiency of oxygen in the tissues.

Hysterectomy. The surgical removal of the uterus, either through an incision in the abdominal wall or through the vagina. The latter is the preferred route.

Hysteroscopy. Visualization of the interior of the uterus using a hysteroscope.

Intrauterine growth restriction. Failure of a fetus to achieve its growth potential, resulting in the birth of a baby whose birth weight is abnormally low in relation to its gestational age.

Intramuscular. Within a muscle (an intramuscular injection).

Intrathecal. Within the meninges of the spinal cord (an intrathecal injection).

Intravenous. Into or within a vein (injection, infusion).

Induction. The starting of labour by artifical means. Medical induction is carried out using such drugs as prostaglandins or oxytocin, which stimulate uterine contractions. Surgical induction is performed by amniotomy (artifical rupture of membranes), usually supplemented by oxytocic drugs.

Labour. The sequence of actions by which a baby and the afterbirth (placenta) are expelled from the uterus at childbirth. The process usually starts spontaneously about 280 days after conception, but it may be started by artificial means. In the first stage, the muscular wall of the uterus begins contractions while the muscle fibres of the cervix relax so that the cervix expands. A portion of the membranous sac (amnion) surrounding the baby is pushed into the opening and ruptures under pressure, releasing amniotic fluid (liquor) to the exterior. In the second stage, the baby's head appears at the cervix and the contractions of the uterus strengthen. The passage of the infant through the vagina is assisted by contractions of the abdominal muscles and conscious pushing by the mother. When the baby's head appears at the vaginal opening, the whole infant is eased clear of the vagina, and the umbilical cord is cut. If the emergence of the head is impeded, an incision may be made in surrounding tissue (episiotomy). In the final stage, the placenta and membranes are pushed out by the continuing contraction of the uterus, which eventually returns to its unexpanded state. The average duration of labour is about 12 hours in first pregnancies and about eight hours in subsequent pregnancies.

Macrosomia. A condition in which the baby is large for its gestational age, associated with poorly controlled maternal diabetes.

Meconium. The first stools of a newborn baby, which are sticky and dark green and composed of cellular debris, mucus and bile pigments. The presence of meconium in the amniotic fluid during labour indicates fetal distress.

Microcephaly. Abnormal smallness of the head in relation to the size of the rest of the body; a congenital condition in which the brain is not fully developed.

Midwife. A midwife is a person who, having been regularly admitted to a midwifery educational programme duly recognized in the country in which it is located, has successfully completed the prescribed course of studies in midwifery and has acquired the requisite qualifications to be registered and/ or legally licensed to practise midwifery.

The midwife is recognized as a responsible and accountable professional who works in partnership with women to give the necessary support, care and advice during pregnancy, labour and the postpartum period, to conduct births on the midwife's own responsibility and to provide care for the newborn and the infant. This care includes preventative measures, the promotion of normal birth, the detecton of complications in mother and child, the accessing of medical care or other appropriate assistance and the carrying out of emergency measures.

The midwife has an important task in health counseling and education, not only for the woman, but also within the family and the community. The work should involve antenatal education and preparation for parenthood and may extend to women's health, sexual or reproductive health and child care.

A midwife may practice in any setting including the home, community, hospitals, clinics or health units. (*International Confederation of Midwives 'Definition of a Midwife': adopted July 2005 Brisbane, Australia*).

Neonate. An infant at any time during the first 28 days of life.

Nursing process. An individualized problem-solving approach to the nursing care of patients. It involves four stages: assessment (of the patient's problems), planning (how to resolve them), implementation (of the plans) and evaluation (of their success).

Nursing standard. A measure or measures by which nursing care can be judged or compared; the measures used are agreed upon by common consent.

Obstetrics. The branch of medical science concerned with the care of women during pregnancy, childbirth and the period of about six weeks following the birth, when the reproductive organs are recovering.

Occiput. The back of the head. In obstetrics, the occiput is used as a 'denominator' to describe positions when the fetus presents by the vertex. The most favourable position for delivery is occipital anterior, with the occiput of the fetus presenting towards the anterior aspect of the maternal pelvis as it enters the pelvic inlet. In the occipital transverse and occipital posterior positions, the occciput presents towards the lateral and posterior aspects respectively of the maternal pelvis; these are malpositions.

Palpation. The process of examining part of the body by careful feeling with the hands and fingertips. Palpation is used to discover the presence of a fetus in the uterus.

Panic disorder. A condition featuring recurrent brief episodes of acute distress, mental confusion, and fear of impending death.

Partogram. A graphic record of the course of labour.

Perinatal. The period starting a few weeks before birth and including the birth and a few weeks after birth.

Perineal repair. Repair of an injury to the perineum, which may be sustained during childbirth. It is vitally important that injuries are recognized and repaired by competent personnel.

Polycythemia. An abnormally high number of red blood cells which has the effect of thickening or 'sludging' the blood, thereby increasing the risk of clotting due to the hyperviscosity.

Postpartum. Relating to the period of a few days immediately after birth.

Postnatal depression. Depression that starts after childbirth. Bonding between mother and baby can be impaired, leading to attachment disorders if the illness is not diagnosed and treated (antidepressant medication, behavioural therapy, or, in rare cases, hospital admission is required).

Postpartum haemorrhage. Excessive bleeding (>500 ml) from the genital tract after delivery. Primary PPH occurs within 24 hours of delivery; secondary PPH occurs after 24 hours. Atonic PPH is due to failure of the uterus to contract after delivery; it may be caused by retained products of conception or may occur after a long labour.

Post-term pregnancy. A pregnancy that has gone beyond 42 weeks' gestation or 294 days from the first date of the last menstrual period.

Post-traumatic stress syndrome. An anxiety disorder caused by the major personal stress of a serious or frightening event. The onset is at least one month after the traumatic event. The sufferer experiences the persistent recurrence of images or memories of the event, together with nightmares, insomnia, a sense of isolation, guilt, irritability, and loss of concentration. Emotions may be deadened or depression may develop.

Pre-eclampsia. The combination of pregnancy-induced hypertension and proteinuria (0.3g in 24 hours) with or without oedema.

Proteinuria. The presence of protein in the urine.

Schizophrenia. A severe mental illness characterized by a disintegration of the process of thinking, of contact with reality and of emotional responsiveness.

Speculum. A metal instrument for inserting into a cavity of the body, such as the vagina, in order that the interior may be examined.

Stillbirth. Birth of a fetus that shows no evidence of life (heartbeat, respiration or independent movement) at any time later than 24 weeks after conception. There is a legal obligation to notify the appropriate authority of all stillbirths. In legal terms, viability is deemed to start at the 24th week of pregnancy and a fetus born dead before this time is known as a miscarriage or abortion. Some fetuses born alive before the 24th week may now survive as a result of perinatal care.

Streptococcus. A genus of Gram-positive nonmotile spherical bacteria occurring in chains.

Symphysis pubis. The joint between the pubic bones of the pelvis and the joints of the backbone, which are separated by intervertebral discs.

Septicaemia. Widespread destruction of tissues due to absorption of disease-causing bacteria or their toxins from the bloodstream; term loosely used for 'blood poisoning.'

Tachycardia. An increase in the heart rate above normal.

Traction. The application of a pulling force.

Trimester. Any one of the three successive three-month periods (the first, second and third trimesters) into which a pregnancy may be divided.

Ultrasound (ultrasonic waves). Sound waves of high frequency, inaudible to the human ear. Used to produce images of the interior of the human body as the waves reflect off structures back to the probe.

Venepuncture. The puncture of a vein for any therapeutic purpose, e.g., to extract blood for laboratory tests.

Ventouse/vacuum extractor. A device to assist delivery, consisting of a suction cup that is attached to the head of the fetus; traction is then applied slowly. Introduced in 1954, ventouse delivery has now virtually replaced delivery by rotational obstetric forceps.

Viability. When the baby is capable of living a separate existence. The legal age of viability of a fetus is 24 weeks, but some fetuses now survive birth at an even earlier age.

Notes

Notes on negligence

Most of the cases in this book are concerned with the civil action of negligence. As negligence litigation is a demanding, lengthy and uncertain process, it is not surprising that the majority of cases settle (reach agreement) out of court. In addition, legislative reforms have made negligence litigation an increasingly difficult exercise.

Legal writers Kim Forrester and Debra Griffiths also explain that:

> It is important to remember that by comparison to the actual number of medical practitioner-patient contacts, the occurrence of an adverse event is very low and the initiation of legal proceedings even lower[1]. (There is no reason why this should not apply to hospitals and maternity serves staff.)

A patient who brings a negligence action is claiming damages (compensation) for injuries and loss. A hospital itself can be negligent or it can be vicariously liable (accountable) for the negligence of its staff. Hospitals insure against this contingency. This has the effect of shifting the loss, as far as money is able to do so, from the patient who has sustained the injury or damage to the hospital or individual (for example, an obstetrician engaged by the patient) held to have caused the loss.[2]

To be successful, a patient will have to prove:

1. That a duty of care existed

At common law a hospital and its staff owes a duty of care when they can reasonably foresee that their actions may harm a patient or others. In almost all cases where care is undertaken, a court will impose a duty of care. The duty of care can be owed to both a mother and to her unborn fetus, but the right of the child to claim in negligence does not arise until it is born alive and has a separate existence from its mother.

2. That there was a breach of that duty

Whether a breach of duty occurred will be measured against what a reasonable midwife, neonatal nurse, doctor or hospital would have done in similar circumstances. A midwife, for example, is unlikely to be negligent if it can be established that she acted in a manner that was widely accepted (at the time the service was provided) by a significant number of respected midwives as competent professional practice in the circumstances. The fact that there are different peer professional opinions concerning a practice does not mean they cannot be relied upon but a court is unlikely to accept irrational or unreasonable opinions. A common practice, in itself, may be negligent.

Providing information. A different test applies to the standard of care when providing information. A medical practitioner has a duty to provide the information that a patient would require to make an informed decision about whether to undergo a procedure or diagnostic test. They have a duty to provide information on the material risks of proposed treatment.[3] The question of what is material depends not only on the doctor but also on what the patient would consider to be significant in their circumstances. Again, there is no reason why this reasoning should not apply to maternity services staff providing information that the patient/parent will rely upon. (*Sheridan* in Chapter 15.)

3. That the breach caused the damage

Legal causation is based on rules of common sense, factual causation and the scope of liability. There must be some scientific link between the breach and the injury. The law assumes factual causation if the injury would not have occurred *but for* the breach.

The judge will determine the scope of liability by considering whether and why responsibility for the harm should be imposed on the hospital or health professional. This is an important balancing exercise and one you can use when assessing risk:

What is the risk? How likely is it to occur? How serious could the damage be if the risk eventuated? What steps could be put in place to avoid or lessen the risk in terms of cost, practicality and inconvenience? What is the value of offering the service? If the service is too risky, should it be offered at all?

---

4. That the injury was reasonably foreseeable (not too remote)
The exact injury does not have to be foreseen. The law only requires that a reasonably foreseeable risk of injury was created, and that the particular injury fell within that category of risk. (Chapter 2, *McCrystal*.)

Every case is determined on its own unique circumstances.

Damages

Specific damages can be recovered for specific, actual costs that the patient has already incurred, such as medical bills, lost wages, etc., from the time of the incident to the date of the trial.

General damages are estimates of expenditure or losses flowing from the injury, including loss of future earnings, pain and suffering, loss of enjoyment/expectation of life as well as future medical, nursing, pharmaceutical costs, etc.

Thresholds and caps have been placed on the award of damages by legislation.

Damages for psychological injury can only be claimed where the patient is suffering from a recognizable psychiatric condition.

Defences. If the statutory time to bring a claim has not expired (with exceptions, usually three years from the time the injury was discovered), defences include:

- that the patient was not owed a duty of care,
- that the conduct at the time was of a reasonable standard for a skilled professional,

- that there was no damage suffered,
- that there was no causal link between the conduct and the damage;
- that the damage was not reasonably foreseeable,
- that the patient contributed to their injury (did not look after their own safety). Damages can then be reduced in proportion to the degree of responsibility or;
- that the patient was aware of the risk (when failure to disclose risk is alleged).

But on the positive side:

Medical negligence litigation is considered as one of the means by which the quality of healthcare services is improved and maintained. The threat of litigation effectively deters poor behaviour by healthcare professionals, and through the publicity of cases, educates the public and professionals about what is the appropriate standard of care.[4]

Notes on coronial investigations

The casebook also contains notes on coronial investigations. The coronial process is governed by legislation. The Legal Glossary contains information about coroners, as do web pages for the Coroners Court/Services in your state or territory.

Here is how one coroner described the process:[5]

The scope of the coroner's inquiry and findings

Coroners inquire into the cause and the circumstances of a reportable death.

(It is therefore important that hospitals and maternity services staff are clear as to what constitutes a 'reportable death': Chapter 3 *Coronial Case No: 0057/2007 [NT] 2009)* contains a warning about this)

If possible, a coroner will find:

- whether a death in fact happened;
- the identity of the deceased;
- when, where and how the death occurred; and
- what caused the person to die.

The scope of an inquest goes beyond merely establishing the medical cause of death, but it is not a trial between opposing parties. An English judge explains:

*'It is an inquisitorial process, a process of investigation quite un-
like a criminal trial where the prosecutor accuses and the accused
defends ....The function of an inquest is to seek out and record as
many of the facts concerning the death as the public interest requires.'*[6]

The focus of an inquest is on discovering what happened, not on ascrib-
ing guilt, attributing blame or apportioning liability. The purpose is to inform
the family and the public of how the death occurred with a view to reducing the likelihood of similar deaths. As a result, a coroner makes preventive
recommendations concerning public health or safety, the administration of
justice or ways to prevent deaths from happening in similar circumstances
in the future.

However, a coroner must not include in the findings or any comments or
recommendations, statements that a person is, or may be guilty of an offence
or is or may be civilly liable for something.

The admissibility of evidence and the standard of proof

Because a coronial investigation is a fact-finding exercise and not a trial,
proceedings are not bound by strict rules of evidence and the court may inform itself in any way it considers appropriate.

The civil standard of proof (balance of probabilities) is applied with a slid-
ing scale. This means that the more significant the issue to be determined,
the more serious the allegation or the more inherently unlikely an occurrence, the clearer and more persuasive the evidence needs to be.[7]

A coroner also has to comply with the rules of natural justice and to act
judicially. This means that no findings adverse to the interest of any party
may be made without that party first being given a right to be heard in op-
position to that finding. This includes the opportunity to make submissions
against findings that might be damaging to the reputation of any individual
or organization.

Findings and decision

When an inquest is held into a death, the coroner's written findings must
be given to the family and to each person/ organization who had leave to
appear at the hearing.

NOTES

1. Forrester K, Griffiths D, *Essentials of Law for Medical Practitioners,* 2011 Elsevier Ch.5 Negligence, p.85 (Chapter 5 provides a very useful overview of common law, legislation and the Ipp Reforms: Australia).
2. Ibid., Ch.5.
3. Rogers v Whittaker (1992) 175 CLR 479 at 487.
4. Forrester, Griffiths at p.85-86.
5. Christine Clements, Deputy State Coroner (Brisbane) (COR2145/05 (7).
6. *R v South London Coroner: ex parte Thompson* (1982) 126.S.J.625.
7. *Briginshaw v Briginshaw* (1938) 60 C.L.R 336 at 361 per Sir Owen Dixon J.

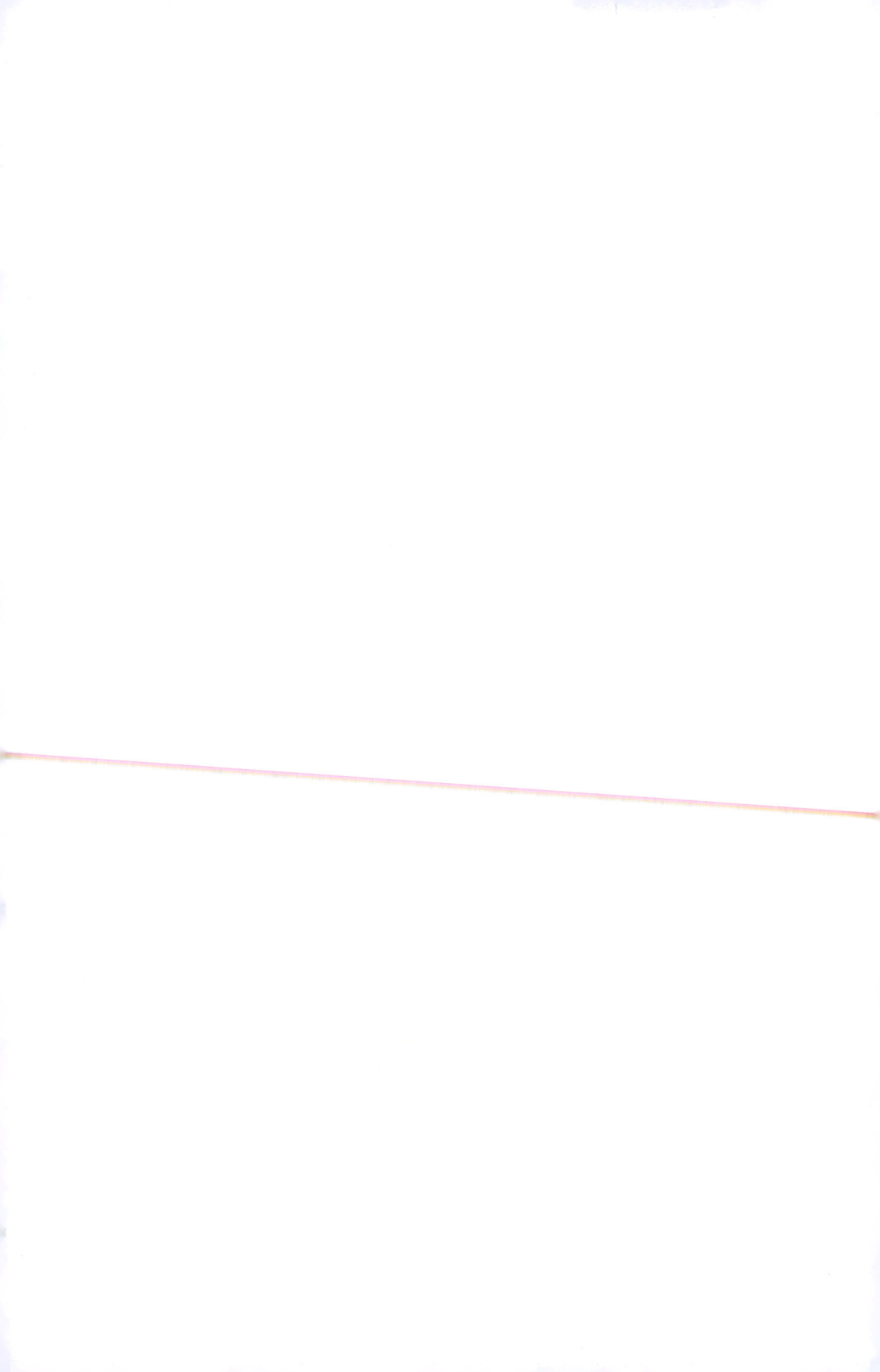

www.ingramcontent.com/pod-product-compliance
Lightning Source LLC
Chambersburg PA
CBHW041254040426
42334CB00028BA/3009